Post-Anesth

Post-Anesthesia Care

Symptoms, Diagnosis, and Management

Edited by

James W. Heitz, MD

Associate Professor of Anesthesiology and Medicine, Sidney Kimmel Medical College, Thomas Jefferson University; Medical Director, Post-Anesthesia Care Unit, Thomas Jefferson University Hospital, Philadelphia, PA, USA

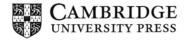

CAMBRIDGE
UNIVERSITY PRESS

CAMBRIDGE
UNIVERSITY PRESS

University Printing House, Cambridge CB2 8BS, United Kingdom

Cambridge University Press is part of the University of Cambridge.

It furthers the University's mission by disseminating knowledge in the pursuit of education, learning, and research at the highest international levels of excellence.

www.cambridge.org
Information on this title: www.cambridge.org/9781107642218

© Cambridge University Press 2016

First published 2016

Printed in the United Kingdom by Clays, St Ives plc

A catalog record for this publication is available from the British Library

Library of Congress Cataloging in Publication Data
Names: Heitz, James W., editor.
Title: Post-anesthesia care : symptoms, diagnosis, and management / edited by James W. Heitz.
Other titles: Post-anesthesia care (Heitz)
Description: Cambridge, United Kingdom : Cambridge University Press, 2016. | Includes bibliographical references and index.
Identifiers: LCCN 2015040092 | ISBN 9781107642218 (Paperback : alk. paper)
Subjects: | MESH: Postoperative Care. | Recovery Room–organization & administration. | Anesthesiology–trends.
Classification: LCC RD98.4 | NLM WO 183 | DDC 617.9/195–dc23 LC record available at http://lccn.loc.gov/2015040092

ISBN 978-1-107-64221-8 Paperback

....

To my wife, Terry, whose understanding makes it possible and whose love makes it all worthwhile.

Contents

Section III Special considerations

Contributors

Gadi Arzanipour, DO
Staff Anesthesiologist, Providence
Tarzana Medical Center, Tarzana,
CA, USA

Stephen O. Bader, MD
Staff Anesthesiologist, Northstar
Anesthesia, Heritage Valley Health
Systems, Beaver, PA, USA

Jaime Baratta, MD
Associate Professor of Anesthesiology,
Sidney Kimmel Medical College, Thomas
Jefferson University, Philadelphia,
PA, USA

Donald Baumann, DO
Assistant Professor of Anesthesiology,
Sidney Kimmel Medical College, Thomas
Jefferson University, Philadelphia,
PA, USA

Michelle Beam, DO, MBA
Assistant Professor of Anesthesiology,
Sidney Kimmel Medical College, Thomas
Jefferson University, Philadelphia, PA, USA

David Beausang, MD
Instructor of Anesthesiology, Sidney
Kimmel Medical College, Thomas Jefferson
University, Philadelphia, PA, USA

Ashley Caplan, DO
Staff Anesthesiologist, United Anesthesia
Services, P.C., Bryn Mawr, PA, USA

Min J. Chun, MD
Staff Anesthesiologist, United Anesthesia
Services, P.C., Bryn Mawr, PA, USA

Erika Davis, MD
Resident in Anesthesiology, Thomas
Jefferson University Hospital, Philadelphia,
PA, USA

Elia S. Elia, MD
Clinical Associate Professor, Department
of Anesthesiology, Thomas Jefferson
University Hospital, Philadelphia,
PA, USA

Marc Fisicaro, MD
Clinical Assistant Professor of
Anesthesiology, Sidney Kimmel Medical
College, Thomas Jefferson University,
Philadelphia, PA, USA

Peter Jonathan Gambino, DO
Staff Anesthesiologist, Tift Regional
Medical Hospital, Tifton, GA, USA

Kishor Gandhi, MD, MPH, CPE
Staff Anesthesiologist, University Medical
Center of Princeton, Plainsboro Township,
NJ, USA

Jordan E. Goldhammer, MD
Assistant Professor of Anesthesiology,
Sidney Kimmel Medical College,
Thomas Jefferson University,
Philadelphia, PA, USA

Adam W. Green, MD
Staff Anesthesiologist, Mercy Hospital
Northwest Arkansas, Rogers, AR, USA

Zvi Grunwald, MD
The James D. Wentzler Professor and
Chair, Department of Anesthesiology,
Sidney Kimmel Medical College, Thomas
Jefferson University, Philadelphia, PA,
USA

Andrea M. Hages, DO, USAF, MC
Assistant Professor in Anesthesiology,
F. Edward Hébert School of Medicine,
Uniformed Services University of the
Health Sciences, Landstuhl Regional
Medical Center, Landstuhl, Germany

Yousef Hamdeh, MD
House Officer in Anesthesiology, Thomas
Jefferson University Hospital, Philadelphia,
PA, USA

James W. Heitz, MD, FACP
Associate Professor of Anesthesiology and
Medicine Sidney Kimmel Medical College,
Thomas Jefferson University; Medical
Director, Post-Anesthesia Care Unit,
Thomas Jefferson University Hospital,
Philadelphia, PA, USA

Jeremy L. Hensley, MD
Instructor, Department of Anesthesiology
and Critical Care, Hospital of the University
of Pennsylvania, Philadelphia, PA, USA

Brian Hipszer, PhD
Distinguished Algorithm Engineer,
Critical Care, Edwards Lifesciences, Irvine,
CA, USA

George Hsu, MD
Clinical Assistant Professor of
Anesthesiology, Sidney Kimmel Medical
College, Thomas Jefferson University,
Philadelphia, PA, USA

H. Jane Huffnagle, DO, FAOCA
Clinical Professor of Anesthesiology and
Obstetrics & Gynecology, Sidney Kimmel
Medical College, Thomas Jefferson
University, Philadelphia, PA, USA

Suzanne Huffnagle, DO, FAOCA
Clinical Professor of Anesthesiology and
Obstetrics & Gynecology, Sidney Kimmel
Medical College, Thomas Jefferson
University, Philadelphia, PA, USA

Jeffrey I. Joseph, DO
Professor, Vice Chairman, and Director of
Research, Department of Anesthesiology,
Sidney Kimmel Medical College, Thomas
Jefferson University; Director, Jefferson
Artificial Pancreas Center &
Anesthesiology Program for Translational
Research, Philadelphia, PA, USA

Brian Lai, MD
Resident in Anesthesiology, Sidney Kimmel
Medical College, Thomas Jefferson
University, Philadelphia, PA, USA

Lisa Luyun, MD
Staff Anesthesiologist, United Anesthesia
Services, P.C., Bryn Mawr, PA, USA

Julie P. Ma, MD
Instructor of Anesthesiology, Sidney
Kimmel Medical College, Thomas Jefferson
University, Philadelphia, PA, USA

Emily J. MacKay, DO
Resident in Anesthesiology, Thomas
Jefferson University Hospital, Philadelphia,
PA, USA

Niels D. Martin, MD, FACS
Assistant Professor of Surgery;
Co-Medical Director, Surgical Intensive
Care Unit, University of Pennsylvania,
Perelman School of Medicine,
Philadelphia, PA, USA

Eric Massey, MD
Instructor, West Virginia University School
of Medicine, Department of
Anesthesiology, Morgantown, WV, USA

Ryan P. Maxwell, DO
Cardiac Anesthesiologist, United
Anesthesia Services, P.C., Bryn Mawr,
PA, USA

Michelle McMaster, MD
Staff Anesthesiologist, Fox Chase Cancer
Center, Philadelphia, PA, USA

Michele Mele, MD
Instructor of Anesthesiology, Sidney
Kimmel Medical College, Thomas Jefferson
University, Philadelphia, PA, USA

Zara Y. Mergan, MD
Fellow in Chronic Pain, Department
of Anesthesiology, Thomas Jefferson
University, Philadelphia, PA, USA

Boris Mraovic, MD
Associate Professor of Clinical
Anesthesiology, Department of
Anesthesiology and Perioperative Medicine,
University of Missouri, Columbia, MO, USA

Robert F. Olszewski Jr., MD
Attending Anesthesiologist, Christiana
Care Health System, Wilmington, DE, USA

Glen D. Quigley, MD, MBA
Fellow in Adult Cardiothoracic
Anesthesiology, NYU Langone Medical
Center, New York, NY, USA

Philippa Ratcliffe, RN, MA, CPAN
Nurse Manager, Post Anesthesia Care Unit,
Thomas Jefferson University Hospital,
Philadelphia, PA, USA

Nicole Renaldi, DO
Instructor of Anesthesiology, Sidney
Kimmel Medical College, Thomas Jefferson
University, Philadelphia, PA, USA

Eric S. Schwenk, MD
Assistant Professor of Anesthesiology,
Sidney Kimmel Medical College, Thomas
Jefferson University, Philadelphia, PA, USA

Megan J. Sharpe, MD
Resident in Anesthesiology, Thomas
Jefferson University Hospital, Philadelphia,
PA, USA

Allan F. Simpao, MD
Assistant Professor of Anesthesiology
and Critical Care, Department of
Anesthesiology and Critical Care Medicine,
The Children's Hospital of Philadelphia,
Philadelphia, PA, USA

Benjamin Vaghari, MD
Staff Anesthesiologist, Holy Cross
Anesthesia Associates, Wheaton, MD,
USA

John T. Wenzel, MD
Fellow, Department of Anesthesiology,
Sidney Kimmel Medical College, Thomas
Jefferson University, Philadelphia, PA,
USA

Michael Jon Williams, MD
Assistant Professor of Anesthesiology,
Sidney Kimmel Medical College, Thomas
Jefferson University, Philadelphia, PA,
USA

Elizabeth Wolo, MD
Assistant Professor of Anesthesiology,
Sidney Kimmel Medical College,
Thomas Jefferson University,
Philadelphia, PA, USA

Jon Zhou, MD
Pain Medicine Fellow, Department
of Anesthesiology and Pain Medicine,
University of California, Davis, CA, USA

Preface

James W. Heitz

"If America had contributed nothing more to the stock of human happiness than anesthetics, the world would owe her an everlasting debt of gratitude."[1]

Samuel D. Gross, MD
Professor of Surgery (1856–1882)
Jefferson Medical College

The development of the Post-Anesthesia Care Unit (PACU) is a relatively recent phenomenon, but its historical origins pre-date modern anesthesia. As early as 1801, the Newcastle Infirmary in the UK utilized two rooms adjacent to the operating room for patients after surgery or otherwise deemed to be very ill. This nascent Intensive Care Unit may have been the first recovery room, but recovery was only from the surgery, since anesthesia was not administered. William T. G. Morton's public demonstration of ether at the Massachusetts General Hospital in 1846 ushered in the era of modern anesthesia, and when this was combined with asepsis, the era of modern surgery emerged. Areas near operating rooms quickly became utilized for the induction of general anesthesia, but the benefits of specialized areas for the recovery of patients were not as rapidly recognized. In 1875, plans for the construction for The Johns Hopkins University Hospital in Baltimore included two recovery rooms adjacent to the operating rooms, but many hospitals continued to be designed up until the Second World War without dedicated recovery areas.[2]

In 1942, Dr. John Silas Lundy created the first modern PACU at the Mayo Clinic in Rochester, New York.[3] He termed this area the "post-anesthesia observation unit." At that time, the recovery room was seen as an area of the hospital where patients could be observed after surgery for untoward complications which might be more efficiently treated in an area near the operating rooms. The importance of a dedicated recovery area was soon validated, by the findings of the Anesthesia Study Commission of the Philadelphia County Medical Society in 1947 which reported that at least one-third of perioperative fatalities were potentially preventable by more vigilant monitoring.[4] Most of these were respiratory-related events requiring prompt intervention to save lives.

As surgical volume, complexity, and patient co-morbidity have increased, the PACU continues to develop, and *care* has replaced *observation*. Simply observing patients after surgery is no longer sufficient. The modern PACU now serves a multidisciplinary intensive care unit, functioning simultaneously as a recovery area for both inpatient and outpatient surgeries and more recently as a recovery area for the increasing number of procedures performed in satellite areas. It is an area to perform minor procedures such as electroconvulsive therapy, epidural blood patches, peripheral nerve blocks, and transesophageal echocardiography; a pre-procedure holding area;

and an overflow resource for the other intensive care units.[5] This has prompted the light-hearted proposal that the PACU acronym might better stand for "Put All you Can in the Unit."[6] Today, the contemporary PACU may straddle the division of past and present by simultaneously being on the forefront of modern medical care while often being the last unit in the hospital to retain an open ward design.

The early postoperative period has become a watershed, where the care of the surgical patient may be shared by surgeons, anesthesiologists, hospitalists, general internists, subspecialists, physician assistants, advanced practice nurses, and registered nurses. Each has his or her own area of expertise and interest, but none a truly comprehensive perspective of perioperative medicine.

While admittance to the PACU marks the transition from intraoperative to postoperative care for the surgical patient, it is not the "finish line" for surgery. Only about 5% of perioperative deaths occur in the operating room or the early perioperative period,[7] so much of the perioperative risk still lies ahead for the surgical patient arriving in the PACU. The anesthetic has usually ended by the time the patient arrives at the PACU, but 1 in 14 malpractice suits brought against US anesthesiologists arise from events that occur after the patient leaves the operating room.[8]

As many as one-third of patients have some sort of complication needing to be addressed in the initial hours after surgery,[9] and adequacy of treatment may profoundly affect overall outcome. A large retrospective study of the multicenter database maintained by the American College of Surgeons National Surgical Quality Improvement Program revealed a large institutional variation in mortality, but not in overall complication rate.[10] Timely diagnosis and effective management of postoperative complications is important for improving outcomes and reducing surgical mortality.

Many postoperative complications are either caused or influenced by iatrogenic factors, obscuring diagnosis and necessitating therapy specific to the perioperative period. Familiarity with the different clinical presentation of perioperative complications is just as important as dedicated recovery areas to optimal outcomes.

By taking an approach to complications based upon signs and symptoms seen in the early postoperative period among adult patients undergoing non-cardiac surgery, this book is intended to aid the practitioner in the clinical management of surgical patients during this potentially turbulent period of their care. No single reference could comprehensively review all the complications that may be encountered after surgery, and an attempt to create one would produce an unwieldy reference unlikely to be clinically useful. This volume emphasizes the most common and most serious complications, as well as complications with presentations unique to the postoperative period. Particular concerns specific to subspecialty patients, including patients requiring postoperative mechanical ventilation, pediatric patients, patients with implantable cardiac devices, morbidly obese patients, and the complex pain patient, are presented in chapters near the end. It is our hope that this reference is useful to the variety of providers caring for surgical patients after surgery.

Acknowledgements

Many thanks to Dr. Angelo Andonakakis for assistance with copy-editing and for the creation of original illustrations.

References

1. Samuel Gross, quoted in C.N. Johnson. *A Text-Book of Operative Dentistry*, third edition. Philadelphia: P. Blakiston's Son & Co, 1915, p. 323.

2. D. Zuck. Anaesthetic and postoperative recovery rooms: some notes on their early history. *Anaesthesia* 1995;50:435–438.

3. We Salute John Silas Lundy, M.D. *Anesth Analg* 1957;36:79–80.

4. H. Ruth, F. Haugen, K. Grove. Anesthesia study commission. *JAMA* 1947;135: 881–884.

5. P. Saastamoinen, M. Piispa, M.N. Niskanen. Use of postanesthesia care unit for purposes other than postanesthesia observation. *J Perianesth Nurs* 2007;22:102–107.

6. K. Litwack. *Post Anesthesia Care Nursing*. St. Louis, MO: Mosby, 1995, pp. 127–184.

7. A.J.G. Gray, R.W. Hoile, G.S. Ingram, K.M. Sherry. *The Report of the National Confidential Enquiry into Perioperative Deaths 1996/1997*. London: NCEPOD 2001. http://www.ncepod.org.uk/2001cwo .htm; accessed November 30, 2014.

8. G. Zeitlin. Recovery room mishaps in the ASA closed claims study. *ASA Newslett* 1989;53:28–30.

9. R. Hines, P.G. Barash, G. Watrous, T. O'Connor. Complications occurring in the postanesthesia care unit: a survey. *Anesth Analg* 1992;74:503–509.

10. A.A. Ghaferi, J.D. Birkmeyer, J.B. Dimick. Variation in hospital mortality associated with inpatient surgery. *N Eng J Med* 2009;361:1368–1375.

Recovery: physiological challenges

Niels D. Martin and James W. Heitz

The residual effects of anesthesia, intraoperative positioning, and surgical trespass in combination with pre-existing co-morbidity create a variety of physiological disturbances that may become evident in the Post-Anesthesia Care Unit (PACU) or the early post-operative period. While cardiac and/or respiratory problems are most frequently encountered after surgery, complications may arise from any organ system or even from the limitations within the healthcare system itself as clinicians from differing disciplines share responsibility for postoperative care. Postoperative care is by necessity multidisciplinary, and it is of critical importance that clinicians work in cooperative fashion. Errors of judgment or communication are the most commonly implicated factors contributing to PACU complications.[1] Since complications may arise from factors simultaneously within the medical, surgical, and anesthetic domains, it is important to establish and maintain effective lines of communication among healthcare providers who may view clinical problems from the differing perspectives of their respective areas of expertise.

Residual effects of anesthesia

The goals of general anesthesia including amnesia, akinesis, anxiolysis, analgesia, and autonomic stability are achieved in modern anesthetic practice by the judicious application of polypharmacy with vigilant monitoring. These medications often include volatile gases, neuromuscular blocking agents, opioids, benzodiazepines, anticholinergics, anticholinesterases, local anesthetics, and barbiturate or non-barbiturate induction agents as well as other medications administered during surgery. Each has profound physiological action, narrow therapeutic windows, and the potential to cause postoperative complications, either in isolation or in combination.

Respiratory disturbances are common after surgery and may be divided into three broad categories: disturbances in the mechanics of breathing, disturbances in ventilatory drives, and disturbances in pulmonary function.

1. **Mechanics of breathing:** Disturbances in the mechanics of breathing arise from dysfunction of either the pharyngeal muscles maintaining airway patency or the actual muscles of ventilation. Many of the drugs administered during the course of anesthesia may negatively impact pharyngeal muscle activity, leading to obstruction. Opioids and neuromuscular blocking agents are most commonly implicated, but residual effects of inhaled or intravenous agents may also contribute. Some residual

Post-Anesthesia Care: Symptoms, Diagnosis, and Management, ed. James W. Heitz. Published by Cambridge University Press. © Cambridge University Press 2016.

neuromuscular blockade is common after general anesthesia, affecting 31% of patients admitted to the PACU in one small observational study.[2] Mild weakness is usually well-tolerated by most patients, but more profound degrees of neuromuscular blockade have been associated with both upper airway obstruction and severe hypoxia after surgery.[3] The diaphragm is the major respiratory muscle and recovers relatively quickly from neuromuscular blockade, but the intercostal muscles are vulnerable to residual blockade or dysfunction after spinal or epidural anesthesia. The intercostal muscles assume a greater importance in ventilation in the supine position and in patients with lung disease including chronic obstructive pulmonary disease. Impairment of function of these muscles may place some patients at risk for postoperative hypoxic events.

2. **Ventilatory drives:** Disturbances in ventilatory drives also occur commonly after surgery. In a retrospective study of 198,103 surgical procedures, respiratory depression was the most common cause of postoperative mortality.[4] Normally, ventilation may be controlled consciously or by intrinsic ventilatory drives, of which the hypercarbic and the hypoxic drives are the most important. Consciousness may be impaired after surgery, as may the intrinsic ventilatory drives. Inhaled anesthetics have profound effects on ventilatory drives, altering both rate and tidal volume, and may exert some effect after surgery, but opioids have the most profound effect on ventilation. The magnitude of the effect of opioids is both dose-dependent and idiopathic depending upon the tolerance of the patient, and will also attenuate the hypercapnic drive. Some degree of respiratory acidosis is virtually ubiquitous after surgery owing to the use of opioids. The hypoxic drive is less reliable after the administration of opioids, so the sedated postoperative patient may become profoundly hypoxic because of the lack of ventilatory effort. The respiratory depressant effect of opioids is synergistic with other medications, especially benzodiazepines. Hypoxia therefore occurs after surgery among patients making adequate respiratory attempts but unable to maintain patent upper airways, and among patients not making adequate respiratory effort. A weaker ventilatory drive arises from pulmonary stretch receptors whose neuronal input may be lost during spinal or epidural anesthesia. This may lead to the interesting opposite phenomenon of patients who are making perfectly adequate respiratory effort and are neither hypoxic nor hypercarbic, but who may be extremely concerned that they perceive they are not breathing since they can no longer feel it.

3. **Pulmonary function:** Disturbances in pulmonary function also occur after general anesthesia. Atelectasis may occur because of effects on pulmonary surfactants, high concentrations of inspired oxygen, and mechanical ventilation. Surgical positioning in head-down position, placing the weight of abdominal organs on the diaphragm and shifting it towards the head, may further exacerbate atelectasis. Functional residual capacity is reduced under general anesthesia. The resultant small airway closure both increases the metabolic expenditure for the work of breathing, while expanding areas of poor ventilation contributing to pulmonary shunt. Ventilatory dead space is increased in the postoperative period. Volatile agents inhibit hypoxic pulmonary vasoconstriction, which may additionally contribute to postoperative hypoxia. In susceptible individuals, volume resuscitation may contribute to pulmonary edema, or airway manipulation may cause bronchospasm, further compromising pulmonary function.

Cardiac disturbances are also common after surgery and are observed with approximately the same frequency as respiratory complications. Electrocardiogram (ECG) changes in axis, intraventricular conduction delays, T-wave changes, and QT prolongation may be observed. Pharmacological alterations in both sympathetic and parasympathetic nervous system activity may also alter cardiac rate and activity. Reductions in cardiac preload occur during general anesthesia because of the venous dilatation coupled with intravascular volume depletion due to hemorrhage and insensible fluid loss from evaporative loss through surgical incisions. As these effects dissipate after surgery, fluctuations in cardiac preload may occur from changes in venous tone, intraoperative volume resuscitation, and third-spacing. Pharmacological depression of cardiac contractility may also occur from medications administered during surgery.

Hepatic blood flow is decreased during general anesthesia, but a greater demand is placed upon the liver to metabolize and detoxify the myriad of medications administered. Inadequacies in hepatic function may be revealed after surgery. Volume shifts and fluid administration may stress renal function, but urine concentrating ability may be impaired from the metabolism of fluorinated hydrocarbons used in anesthesia into renal toxic fluoride ions.

Residual effects of intraoperative positioning

Positioning of the patient for surgery is primarily determined by the need for surgical exposure. All patients are at increased risk for compression neuropathy or skin breakdown from prolonged immobility during the procedure. If surgical positioning places the incision above the level of the heart, there is also the risk of venous air embolism. However, apart from the discrete complications that may be seen after surgical positioning, there are transient physiological effects that may manifest in the postoperative period.

Many of the effects of intraoperative positioning are caused by the exertion of gravity on the body and circulation. For example, "head-down tilt" position (Trendelenburg position) is associated with visceral force against the diaphragm (see Figure 1.1). In this position, functional residual capacity is reduced, atelectasis is promoted, and intrathoracic pressure during mechanical ventilation is increased. These factors increase the risk of pulmonary

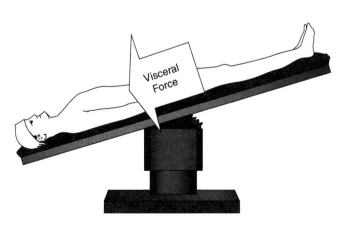

Figure 1.1 Trendelenburg position

barotrauma. Atelectasis may persist after return to supine positioning, and central obesity and longer duration in this position may exacerbate this problem.

Gravity also exerts hemodynamic effects related to positioning. Some of these effects may be clinically beneficial. For example, the sitting position may be used for posterior fossa craniotomy or high cervical spine surgery, providing good surgical access while promoting gravity-dependent venous and cerebral spinal fluid drainage and lowering of intracranial pressure. Position in lateral decubitus positioning for thoracotomy promotes pulmonary blood flow to the dependent (non-operative) lung, minimizing shunt fraction and improving oxygenation during one lung ventilation. However, some of the gravitational effects on hemodynamics may produce untoward effects. These include edema formation in body parts positioned below the level of the heart and arterial ischemia in body parts above the level of the heart.

Procedures performed in extreme head-down tilt position, such as robot-assisted prostatectomy, may be associated with edema accumulation in the head and torso. Sclera edema may be seen after prolonged duration in this position. Although usually benign and self-limited, when this position has been prolonged and large amounts of crystalloid have been infused, delayed extubation of the trachea may be prudent to allow for edema resolution to avoid potential airway compromise. Increases in periocular venous pressure from face-down (prone) positioning have been implicated in postoperative visual loss from posterior ischemic optic neuropathy, although the etiology of this complication is not fully understood and causality has not been proven.

Systemic arterial pressure is much higher than normal pulmonary artery or venous pressures and therefore less affected by gravity. However, intraoperative positioning may still contribute to tissue ischemia. Mean arterial pressure falls by 2 mmHg for each inch above the level of the heart.[5] When portions of the body are placed high above the level of the heart, the risk for arterial ischemia increases. In high lithotomy position, the feet may be 36 inches or more above the level of the heart, greatly reducing pedal perfusion pressure. Limb ischemia and lower extremity compartment syndromes have been observed post-operatively, if higher mean arterial pressures are not maintained during surgery. Similarly, "beach chair" position, which places the head above the level of the heart, may predispose to cerebral ischemia by a similar mechanism. It is important to note that great care is taken to mitigate this risk and cerebral ischemia in the beach chair position is no more common than in other surgical positions.[6] However, anatomical variations may place some patients at unrecognized increased risk.[7]

Physiological effects of surgical trespass

The "stress" of surgery is a systemic physiological load above and beyond basal metabolic activities. This global burden has a multifactorial etiology including previously discussed pharmacological effects of the anesthetic drugs, as well as the systemic release of inflammation modulating hormones from the site of surgery, and the macroscopic, mechanical alterations in function from regional structures affected by surgical manipulation.

Local inflammatory responses with global, systemic effects: Varying body tissues respond differently to physical surgical manipulation. In a similar fashion to a surgeon's hand causing release of vaso active substances from a pheochromocytoma, surgical manipulation in any of the body's tissues can cause local release of inflammatory cytokines that may gain access to the systemic circulation. This systemic inflammatory response syndrome (SIRS) can be initiated anywhere in the body and can be accentuated by pre-existing conditions, especially infection.

1. **Postoperative fever**: Fever in the first 24 hours following surgery is not uncommon. Clinically, early postoperative fever is often attributed to atelectasis, but there is little evidence to support the role of atelectasis in the etiology of postoperative fever.[8] Atelectasis resolves rapidly and spontaneously with innate mechanisms such as coughing and sighing, which were suppressed during general anesthesia, but occur once emergence from anesthesia is complete. This process occurs in 1 to 2 days, and fever that persists beyond 24 to 48 hours should not be attributed to atelectasis.

   The astute clinician must be aware of the less common but much more pathological causes of fever in the postoperative period. An acute necrotizing skin and soft tissue infection at the surgical site must always be considered, and direct examination of the surgical wound should be performed in all febrile patients. If this requires removal of the surgical dressing, then that should be done. Erythema, acute edema, and crepitus should all prompt immediate surgical consultation and evaluation.

   Fever may also represent transient bacteremia, especially in a clean-contaminated, contaminated, or dirty surgical field. As long as no major source of infection remains present in the patient, this is generally spontaneously cleared in the immune-competent patient. In the face of immunosuppression or altered immunity, antibiotics should be considered more strongly, and close observation for subsequent development of SIRS or frank sepsis should be performed. This may include subsequent monitoring in a higher level of care post the PACU stay.

2. **Postoperative hypotension**: There are many causes of postoperative hypotension, most of which will be addressed in other sections. These include acute coronary syndrome, SIRS, sepsis, and basic hypovolemia. However, hypovolemia from acute hemorrhagic shock must be considered in all post-surgical patients. Prompt evaluation for surgical hemorrhage should involve interrogation of the surgical site dressing for saturation, and measurement and character evaluation of any surgical drain output. Additionally, the surgical site should be examined for hematoma formation. If direct examination of the surgical space is not possible (deeper cavity not palpable transdermally), then other means of imaging or reexploration should be considered. Site-specific signs and symptoms of hemorrhage will be further addressed in the following section on the systems-based evaluation of surgical trespass.

3. **Secondary (direct-inflammatory) end-organ injury**: Surgical manipulation can cause direct inflammation and injury to structures physically handled by the surgical team. These same structures, on a cellular level, have the potential to release cytokines systemically and drive a global response to local stimulation.[9] This secondary inflammatory process can take place throughout the body, but those organs most susceptible include the lungs, kidneys, liver, heart, and brain.

   An acute lung injury can manifest as interstitial edema causing pulmonary edema and hypoxia; acute kidney injury causes acute tubular necrosis with or without oliguria; acute liver injury can manifest as cholestasis; cardiac injury via cardiomyopathy of critical illness; and injury in the brain as delirium. All of these secondary injuries are treated with supportive care and alleviation, if possible, of the inflammatory cytokine source. Of note, these SIRS reactions can occur in 7% to 44% of operative cases, and occur with greater frequency in longer procedures.[10]

Macroscopic, mechanical alterations caused by surgical manipulation: It is important to be familiar with surgical disease processes and how surgical intervention functions to resolve the condition. Knowledge of this pathophysiology allows for the intuitive comprehension of potential complications, not only intraoperative, but those that present in the post-anesthesia period.

1. **Neurological and spine surgery:** The brain and spinal cord are within an enclosed space. Any fluid build-up, including blood, can cause an acute deterioration in central nervous system (CNS) function.[11] Further, vascular manipulation leading to or within the CNS can be complicated by thrombosis or an acute embolic event. Therefore, any change in neurological exam postoperatively needs to be evaluated urgently. This includes lethargy or a depressed mental state and any lateralizing signs such as an unequal pupillary exam, facial asymmetry, or discrepancy in extremity motor/sensory exam. In this setting, an acute intervention is needed to prevent permanent injury; therefore, prompt recognition is imperative.

2. **Maxillofacial and neck surgery:** Maxillofacial and neck surgery either involves or is closely related to the airway. Airway obstruction is therefore the most dreaded complication and can occur secondary to infection, edema, or hematoma. The first step of treatment involves rapidly establishing a patent airway, usually via reintubation. This intubation can be complicated by abnormal anatomy from the inciting factor. Opening the surgical wound can often decompress the airway obstruction and allow for intubation, but should only be done when major bleeding and exsanguination are less likely. This is based on the type of surgery; thyroid surgery or mass excisions are much less likely to cause exsanguination than a carotid endarterectomy with a fresh major vascular anastomosis. The presence of the surgeon is of paramount importance when deciding to open an incision.

   Creation of a myocutaneous free tissue flap in the head and neck area has become very prevalent in the past several years to allow for coverage after major tumor resections. Along with hematoma formation, these procedures are also complicated by flap ischemia. A PACU practitioner must be able to evaluate the blood flow to and from the flap. Often, a site for Doppler scanning is marked by the surgeon, but flap color, capillary refill, and temperature should be a part of ongoing flap assessments in the PACU.[12]

3. **Thoracic surgery:** An acute hemothorax in the postoperative period can cause several problems. The hemothorax can occupy thoracic cavity volume that would otherwise allow for lung expansion and gas exchange. With a large enough hemothorax, tension physiology may occur if the blood not only affects the unilateral lung but places pressure on the mediastinal structures. Tension on the mediastinum can affect venous blood return to the heart and cause hypotension as well. Finally, global hemorrhagic shock can occur from the blood loss, and it must be treated with intravascular volume resuscitation.

   Most thoracic surgery procedures result in the placement of a chest tube, which can drain some of the accumulating hemothorax and clue the practitioner to an ongoing bleed. It should be noted that the chest tubes themselves can become non-functional from clot and therefore should never used as a reason to rule out a hemothorax. Other signs include hypoxia, tachycardia, shortness of breath, and anxiety. The diagnosis can usually be confirmed via chest X-ray. After thoracic surgery, a low threshold for an interval chest X-ray should be considered if any issues arise in the PACU.

In a similar fashion to hemothorax, an acute pneumothorax can obstruct lung function and similarly place tension on the mediastinum. Tension pneumothorax can occur quite acutely. Classic signs include decreased breath sounds, tracheal deviation away from the side of the pneumothorax, hypoxia, and hypotension. The diagnosis here can be made either by recognizing the clinical presentation or confirmed by chest X-ray, if the diagnosis is in doubt. Treatment involves placing an additional chest tube with or without needle decompression first. If an indwelling chest tube is already present, it is prudent to search for the cause for its malfunction. Loss of the tidal movement of the fluid in the tubing may be an indicator of a non-functional tube. Kinking and occlusion of the tubing, as well as malfunction of the chest tube drain itself should be sought out.

Intrathoracic manipulation, even exterior to the pericardium, can cause cardiac irritability and result in dysrhythmias. These dysrhythmias may start as tachycardia and degenerate to more malignant rhythms. Atrial fibrillation is the most common dysrhythmia after thoracic surgery. First-line treatment involves the use of β-blockers, both in a prophylactic and therapeutic manner.[13] Second-line therapies include calcium channel blockers, amiodarone, or digoxin. Cardioversion should be reserved for hemodynamically unstable patients.

Treatment of additional underlying contributing factors of the dysrhythmia should be investigated. This differential should include endotracheal tube obstruction, electrolyte abnormalities, intravascular volume abnormalities, and myocardial ischemia/infarction.

Lung and pleural cavity manipulation can also result in direct trauma and subsequent atelectasis. Segmental hypoventilation during surgery can also result in pooling of bronchial secretions causing subsequent mucous plugging that can become clinically significant in the postoperative setting. Finally, pulmonary mobilization, even to small degrees, can allow lobar torsion and result in acute decompensation. Diagnosis is made on chest X-ray and treatment is emergent operative de-torsion.

4. **Intra-abdominal surgery:** Intra-abdominal hypertension (IAH) is caused by increased pressure in the abdominal cavity. If left untreated, abdominal compartment syndrome can result. The patients at most risk for IAH are those who required large amounts of volume in the operating room or postoperatively and patients who underwent a hernia repair with a loss of domain for the abdominal viscera. This loss of domain comes from returning the viscera back into the formal peritoneal cavity from the hernia sac or actual contraction of the peritoneal cavity via the hernia repair process itself. Besides abdominal pain, IAH also places increased pressure on the diaphragm, causing respiratory difficulty, and occlusive pressure on the renal veins, causing an acute kidney injury.

The bedside clinician should maintain a high index of suspicion for IAH based on abdominal exam along with respiratory status and kidney function. The diagnosis is usually confirmed indirectly by measuring the pressure in the bladder via a commercial bladder pressure kit that gets connected to the Foley catheter. If close observation of IAH is warranted, the patient should transition to an intensive care setting for monitoring. If abdominal compartment syndrome is imminent or present, immediate surgical decompression of the abdominal wall should be performed.

Postoperative intra-abdominal hemorrhage can be difficult to recognize as the abdomen can accommodate a fair volume of blood before distension ensues. Abdominal pain is generally the earliest sign, although not specific. Any abdominal drains such as Jackson–Pratt drains should be interrogated. Ultimately, physiology suspicious for bleeding (tachycardia and hypotension) is usually the determining factor in persuading the surgeon to re-explore the abdomen.

5. **Vascular surgery:** Vascular surgery can be complicated by surgical site bleeding, which is generally quite obvious. More conspicuously, vascular anastomoses can thrombose and place down stream organs and/or extremities at risk of ischemia. Neurovascular evaluation at least hourly is warranted in the postoperative period following vascular surgery, whether open or endovascular. Any change in examination should prompt evaluation by the vascular surgeon; this includes pulse, pallor, paresthesias, pain, or paralysis.[14]

6. **Orthopedic surgery:** Acute hardware failure following orthopedic surgery is generally visible as a deformity at the surgical site. If this site is wrapped, pain out of proportion to postoperative recovery is usually the first sign. Diagnosis is made on radiological imaging.

   Surgical manipulation can also result in an extremity compartment syndrome. Pain is again the first sign. A thorough neurovascular exam should be performed and if there is any question, compartment pressures should be measured by the orthopedic surgeon.[15] Vascular compromise can also be direct following orthopedic surgery if the vessels were injured or kinked during the surgery. A change or abnormal vascular exam should prompt early evaluation by a vascular surgeon.

7. **General issues:** Hypovolemia will be addressed in several locations throughout this book. For the purposes of surgical trespass, it should be noted that generally, during an exploratory laparotomy, the patient does have evaporative losses that equate to approximately one liter per hour. This certainly changes based on patient demographics, and other physiological measures should be used to maintain euvolemia.

   Despite optimal resuscitation, acute kidney injury may still present in the PACU. Those at greatest risk are those with pre-existing dysfunction, those undergoing surgery involving the aorta, and those with predisposing conditions such as sepsis or shock.[16] Evaluation of oliguria should be algorithm-based and treated based on underlying cause. This will be addressed in further detail elsewhere in this book.

   Hypothermia can result from any surgery but abdominal surgery is specifically prone to heat losses due to the exposed surface area. Both active and passive rewarming postoperatively should be initiated in hypothermic patients as hypothermia can result in increased blood loss and increased transfusion requirements.[17]

References

1. M. Kluger, M. Bullock. A review of Anesthetic Incident Monitoring Study. *Anesthesia* 2002; 57:1060–1066.

2. P.C. Yip, J.A. Hannam, A.J. Cameron, D. Campbell. Incidence of residual neuromuscular blockade in a post-anesthesia care unit. *Anaesth Intensive Care* 2010; 38:91–95.

3. G.S. Murphy, J.W. Szokol, J.H. Marymont, *et al.* Residual neuromuscular blockade and critical respiratory events in the postanesthesia care unit. *Anesth Analg* 2008; 107:130–137.

4.   L. Tiret, J.M. Desmonts, F. Hatton, G. Vourc'h. Complications associated with anaesthesia–a prospective survey in France. *Can Anaesth Soc J* 1986; 33:336–344.

5.   G.E.H. Enderb. Postural ischaemia and blood pressure. *Lancet* 1954; 266:185–187.

6.   D.J. Friedman, N.Z. Parnes, Z. Zimmer, L.D. Higgins, J.J. Warner. Prevalence of cerebrovascular events during shoulder surgery and association with patient position. *Orthopedics* 2009; 32:256–261.

7.   J.C. Drummond, R.R. Lee, J.P. Howell. Focal cerebral ischemia after surgery in the "beach chair" position: the role of a congenital variation of circle of Willis anatomy. *Anesth Analg* 2012; 114:1301–1303.

8.   M.N. Mavros, G.C. Velmahos, M.W. Falagas. Atelectasis as a cause of postoperative fever: where is the clinical evidence? *Chest* 2011; 140:418–424.

9.   D.E. Fry. Sepsis, systemic inflammatory response, and multiple organ dysfunction: the mystery continues. *Am Surg* 2012; 78:1–8.

10. R.D. Becher, J.J. Hoth, P.R. Miller, J.W. Meredith, M.C. Chang. Systemic inflammation worsens outcomes in emergency surgical patients. *J Trauma* 2012; 72:1140–1149.

11. S.I. Stiver. Complications of decompressive craniectomy for traumatic brain injury. *Neurosurg Focus* 2009; 26:E7.

12. A.D. Kruse, H.T. Luebbers, K.W. Gratz, J.A. Obwegeser. Factors influencing survival of free-flap in reconstruction for cancer of the head and neck: a literature review. *Microsurgery* 2012; 31:572–579.

13. J.J. Baltimore. Perianesthesia care of cardiac surgery patients: a CPAN review. *J Perianesth Nurs* 2001; 16:246–254.

14. C. Bryant, C. Ray, T.L. Wren. Abdominal aortic aneurysm repair: a look at the first 24 hours. *J Perianesth Nurs* 2002; 17:164–169.

15. B. Shadgan, M. Menon, D. Sanders, *et al.* Current thinking about acute compartment syndrome of the lower extremity. *Can J Surg* 2010; 53:329–334.

16. L. Agodo. Acute renal failure in the PACU. *J Perianesth Nurs* 2002; 17:377–383.

17. M. Bock, J. Muller, A. Back, *et al.* Effects of preinduction and intraoperative warming during major laparotomy. *Brit J Anaesth* 1998; 80:159–163.

Recovery: goals and standards

Philippa Ratcliffe

- Standards for recovery from anesthesia have been proposed by numerous organizations.
- These guidelines have both commonality and areas of dissimilarity.
- Institutional policies should be individually established.
- Discharge scales employing objective scoring systems offer the most clinical utility.

The function of the Post-Anesthesia Care Unit (PACU) is to monitor and care for patients of all ages that are admitted following procedures where general anesthesia, sedation, or regional anesthesia has been administered. These patients may be discharged home on the day of surgery or admitted for continuing care and treatment depending upon need. The PACU performs a vital role in promoting patient health and recovery after the surgical procedure. The primary goals are patient safety, recovery from anesthesia, and treatment of postoperative complications.

Each institution should develop policies and standards for recovery from anesthesia. In the United States, the guidelines from the American Society of Anesthesiologists (ASA)[1] and the American Association of PeriAnesthesia Nurses (ASPAN)[2] serve as the foundation of institutional policies. Oversight and maintenance of policies should be established jointly with the anesthesia medical director and the nurse manager and educator of PACU. All policies and procedures should be reviewed annually to ensure that clinical or institutional changes are reflected in accurate and up-to-date information and guidelines for staff.

Recovery after anesthesia may be divided into three phases, which require different levels of care which may or may not be delivered in geographically distinct locations within the institution. Phase One is for patients who require intense respiratory and hemodynamic monitoring as well as management of pain and nausea, and fluid management. Phase Two occurs when the patient no longer requires intensive monitoring and the attention shifts towards planning for discharge from the unit or home readiness. Phase Three, or Extended Care, may occur for patients who otherwise complete Phase Two, but are awaiting discharge to another area of the hospital.

Post-Anesthesia Care: Symptoms, Diagnosis, and Management, ed. James W. Heitz. Published by Cambridge University Press. © Cambridge University Press 2016.

The PACU should be staffed by qualified registered nurses (RNs) experienced in Phase One care, although the specific level of certification required of the PACU RN will be dependent on the patient population. Basic Life Support is obligatory for all RNs and ancillary staff such as nursing assistants, nurse externs, and any unlicensed personnel. Although guided by individual institutional policy, certification in Advanced Cardiac Life Support and Pediatric Advanced Life Support is best practice for RNs caring for the adult and pediatric population in tertiary care facilities. The RN should have a strong critical care background, owing to increasing numbers of acutely ill patients and intensive care patients cared for in the PACU. Although this may be less essential in outpatient surgery locations, it is still desirable. Many RNs in the United States and abroad have multiple qualifications in peri-anesthesia nursing and/or critical care nursing, and pain and regional anesthesia. These skill sets create an experienced and broadly educated workforce that provides for a professional learning environment and considerable managerial flexibility. Beyond the United States, there are many nursing organizations that support and educate the peri-anesthesia nursing population, including the British Anaesthetic and Recovery Nurses Association, and organizations in Denmark, Belgium, Ireland, New Zealand, Australia, and Canada.

ASPAN standards

To provide guidance to the large cohort of registered nurses in the United States, ASPAN standards have been developed which offer a framework for peri-anesthesia nursing practice. These authoritative statements describe the responsibilities and specific competencies necessary including Scope of Practice, Standards, Practice Guidelines, and Resources and Position Statements. Utilization of these recommendations elevates practice, ensures patient safety, and is mandatory in a best practice environment.

American and European guidelines

In 2001 the ASA formed a task force of 10 members to evaluate the current literature and get expert opinion from a large representative body of anesthesiologists throughout the country. They systematically evaluated research, interviewed leading experts, surveyed a random sample of active members, held open forums, and collaborated on the feasibility of implementing these guidelines.[1] Their study formed the foundation for the ASA guidelines and standards for post-anesthesia care. The European Society of Anaesthesiology (ESA) also evaluated current literature giving recommendations on "relevant aspects of organization, responsibilities, methods, safety and quality control of postanaesthesia care."[3]

The many physiological needs and challenges for post-anesthesia patients are addressed in the three guidelines discussed. These guidelines share many elements of commonality as each outlines a framework for delivering safe patient care (see Table 2.1). Where the European and American medical societies differ is that the ESA focuses more on structure while the ASA focuses more on specifics of monitoring. There are some variances between these guidelines. An electrocardiogram (ECG) is required by the ASA and recommended but not required by the ESA; however, the ESA places a stronger emphasis on capnography for mechanically ventilated patients.

Table 2.1 Comparison between practice guidelines for care and discharge from the European Society of Anaesthesiology, the American Society of Anesthesiologists, and the American Society of PeriAnesthesia Nurses

Function	ESA	ASA	ASPAN
Transfer from OR to PACU with monitoring and supplemental oxygen	Yes, recommended	Yes, recommended	Yes
Capacity of beds per OR	1.5–2 per room	Not specified	Not specified
Length of stay	Surgery type dependent No min or max	No mandatory minimum stay	Surgery type dependent No min or max
Bedside monitoring equipment: ECG, SpO_2, temperature regulation	Yes	Yes	Yes
Staffing	Minimum of two RNs	Not specified	Minimum of two registered nurses, one of whom is experienced in peri-anesthesia care
Postoperative assessment and monitoring			
Respiratory status	SpO_2 and capnography	Airway patency, SpO_2, and RR	Yes, capnography if indicated and available
Cardiovascular	BP and ECG	HR, BP, and ECG monitors	Yes
Neuromuscular	Physical exam or neuromuscular blockade monitoring	Physical exam or neuromuscular blockade monitoring	Yes. Equipment available as needed to assess
Mental status	Assess periodically	Assess periodically	Yes
Temperature	Yes	Yes	Yes
Nausea and vomiting	Yes	Yes	Yes
Hydration status and fluid management	Yes	Yes	Yes

Table 2.1 (cont.)

Function	ESA	ASA	ASPAN
Urine output and voiding	Yes – voiding on a case by case basis	Yes – voiding on select patients only	Yes, bladder scanning
Drainage and bleeding	Yes	Yes	Yes
Treatment			
Oxygen	Yes, recommended	Yes, recommended	Yes
Shivering & hypothermia	Active rewarming and meperidine IV	Active rewarming and meperidine IV	Forced air warming
PONV prophylaxis	Yes	Selective prophylaxis	Yes
Benzodiazepine antagonists	Flumazenil not used routinely, but used in select patients. Note: no observation time specified	Flumazenil not used routinely, but used in select patients. Note: no observation time specified	No position
Opioid antagonist	Used in select patients for reversal. Note: no observation time specified	Used in select patients for reversal. Note: no observation time specified	No position
Neuromuscular blockade reversal	Train of Four recommended on case by case basis	Specific antagonists may be used for reversal	No position
Postoperative pain management	Yes – ensure trained staff administering	Periodic assessment	Yes, by a registered nurse

OR = operating room, SpO$_2$ = hemoglobin saturation by pulse oximetry, HR = heart rate, RR = respiratory rate, BP = blood pressure, ECG = electrocardiogram, PONV = postoperative nausea and vomiting

Discharge criteria

A variety of scoring systems have been proposed to define recovery from anesthesia. One of the earliest was the Notre Dame Hospital Post-Anesthetic Scoring System, but this cumbersome tool required observation over a period of days and was not appropriate to serve as Phase One discharge criteria.[4] In 1970, Drs. Aldrete and Kroulik introduced a simple scoring system[5] which is still in widespread use, being only slightly modified after the clinical introduction of pulse oximetry. The Modified Aldrete scoring values include respiration, blood, oxygen saturation, consciousness, and activity (see Table 2.2).[6] The Modified Aldrete scoring system has received widespread international support.

Table 2.2 The Modified Aldrete scoring system

Criteria	Score
Respiration	
Able to take a deep breath and cough	2
Dyspnea or shallow breathing	1
Apnea	0
Oxygen saturation	
Maintains >92% on room air	2
Supplemental O_2 to maintain saturation greater than 90%	1
<90% with supplemental O_2	0
Consciousness	
Fully awake	2
Arousable on calling	1
Not responsive	0
Circulation	
Blood pressure +/− 20 mmHg of preoperative value	2
Blood pressure +/− 20–50 mmHg of preoperative value	1
Blood pressure +/− 50 mmHg of preoperative value	0
Activity	
Able to move all extremities	2
Able to move two extremities	1
Unable to move any extremities	0
Sum of 9 or greater needed for discharge	

Also notable is the Post-Anesthetic Discharge Scoring System Scale (PADSS). Similar in use to the Modified Aldrete Score, the PADSS derives its score by evaluating slightly different criteria, specifically vital signs, activity level, nausea, pain, and bleeding (see Table 2.3).[7] The PADSS is used to determine transition from Phase Two to Extended Care.

It is important to emphasize that standardized discharge criteria are helpful clinical tools to assess readiness for transitioning to the next phase of recovery, but cannot entirely replace the need for individualized physician evaluation. Specific co-morbidities (e.g. malignant hyperthermia susceptibility) cannot be accounted for by these simple systems and may necessitate longer periods of monitoring or therapy.

Table 2.3 The Post-Anesthetic Discharge Scoring System

Criteria	Score
Vital signs	
Blood pressure and pulse within 20% of preoperative values	2
Blood pressure and pulse within 20–40% of preoperative values	1
Blood pressure and pulse <40% or >40% of preoperative values	0
Activity	
Steady gait, no dizziness, or return to preoperative baseline	2
Requires assistance	1
Unable to ambulate	0
Nausea and vomiting	
Minimal, treated with oral medication	2
Moderate, treated with parenteral or rectal medication	1
Severe, refractory to treatment	0
Pain	
Controlled with oral medication and acceptable to patient	2
Not controlled with oral medication or not acceptable to patient	1
Surgical bleeding	
Minimal – no dressing changes	2
Moderate – up to two dressing changes	1
Severe – three or more dressing changes	0
Sum of 9 or greater needed for discharge	

Fast-tracking and the Modified Aldrete Score

Fast-tracking refers to the practice of bypassing Phase One and taking the patient to Phase Two care directly from the operating room. In institutions where Phases One and Two are geographically separate, this may have cost savings. The landmark legal case of Laidlaw v. Lions Gate Hospital referred to the Phase One PACU as "the most important room in the hospital"[8] and it is paramount that patient safety not be compromised when this step is omitted. Additionally, poor patient selection may delay care and use resources inefficiently, ultimately increasing financial costs.[9] Proper patient selection for fast-tracking is critical.

Drs. White and Song evaluated the Modified Aldrete Score and concluded that, although it was appropriate for determining patient readiness for discharge from Phase One, it was less suited to determining appropriateness for fast-tracking. They proposed a six-criteria scoring system including level of consciousness, activity, hemodynamic

Table 2.4 Fast-tracking criteria of White and Song

Criteria	Score
Level of consciousness	
Awake	2
Arousable with minimal stimulation	1
Responsive only to tactile stimulation	0
Physical activity	
Able to move all extremities to command	2
Some weakness in movement of extremities	1
Unable to voluntarily move extremities	0
Hemodynamic stability	
Blood pressure +/− 15% of baseline	2
Blood pressure +/− 30% of baseline	1
Blood pressure +/− 50% of baseline	0
Oxygen saturation	
$SpO_2 > 90\%$ on room air	2
Requires supplemental O_2 to maintain $SpO_2 > 90\%$	1
$SpO_2 < 90\%$ on supplemental O_2	0
Pain	
None or mild	2
Moderate or severe controlled with IV analgesia	1
Persistent to severe	0
Emetic symptoms	
None or mild without emesis	2
Transient emesis controlled with IV anti-emetics	1
Persistent moderate to severe nausea and emesis	0

Sum of 12 or greater needed to fast-track with no individual score <1

stability, oxygen saturation, pain, and emetic systems to determine fast-tracking eligibility (see Table 2.4).[10]

The safe recovery of patients from anesthesia requires a coordinated practice between physicians and specialized perioperative nurses. The adoption of formal guidelines and scoring systems aids in this process, but institutional guidelines are also essential because of the significant variations in care that may exist between institutions.

References

1. J.L. Apfelbaum, J.H. Silverstein, F.F. Chung, *et al.*; American Society of Anesthesiologists Task Force on Postanesthetic Care. Practice guidelines for postanesthetic care: an updated report by the American Society of Anesthesiologists Task Force on Postanesthetic Care. *Anesthesiology* 2013; 118:291–307.

2. Perianesthesia Nursing. Standards, Practice Recommendations and Interpretive Statements. 2015–2017. New Jersey: America Society of PeriAnesthesia Nurses.

3. L. Vimlati, F. Gilsanz, Z. Goldik. Quality and safety guidelines of postanaesthesia care. Working Party on Post Anaesthesia Care. European Society of Anaesthesiology. *Eur J Anaesthesiol* 2009; 26:715–721.

4. G. Carighan, M. Kerri-Szanto, J. Lavelle. Post-anesthetic scoring system. *Anesthesiology* 1964; 25:396–397.

5. J.A. Aldrete, D. Kroulik. The postanesthetic recovery. *Anesth Analg* 1970; 49:924–933.

6. J.A. Aldrete. The post anesthesia recovery score revisited. *J Clin Anesth* 1995; 7:89–91.

7. F. Chung, V.W.S. Chan, D. Ong. A post-anesthetic discharge scoring system for home readiness after ambulatory surgery. *J Clin Anesth* 1995; 7:500–506.

8. *Laidlaw v. Lions Gate Hospital* (1969), 70 WWR 727 (BC SC).

9. D. Song, F. Chung, M. Roranye, *et al.* Fast-tracking (bypassing the PACU) does not reduce nursing workload after ambulatory surgery. *Br J Anaesth* 2004; 93:768–777.

10. P. White, D. Song. New criteria for fast tracking after outpatient anesthesia: a comparison with the modified Aldrete's scoring system. *Anesth Analg* 1999; 88:1069–1072.

Chapter

3

Hypertension

James W. Heitz

- Secondary causes of hypertension are common after surgery.
- Pain is the most common cause of secondary hypertension in the surgical patient.
- Management of postoperative hypertension should be directed at the underlying cause.
- Severe or potentially dangerous elevation of blood pressure should be treated with easily titrated intravenous antihypertensive agents.

Hypertension is a global problem affecting approximately 40% of adults over the age of 25 years.[1] In the United States, approximately 78 million adults have hypertension.[2] This represents 33% of all adults over the age of 20 years. By age 55 years, a majority of American men and women have developed chronic hypertension. While most Americans with hypertension have been diagnosed by their physician, only 53% of known hypertensive patients are controlled at or below their target blood pressure. In the United Kingdom, 2 of every 3 adults with hypertension are either undiagnosed or inadequately treated.[3] Hypertension is therefore a very common morbidity among surgical patients and frequently observed after surgery.

There is no consensus on the hemodynamic parameters to define postoperative hypertension. Generally, a systolic blood pressure greater than 160 mmHg, a diastolic blood pressure greater than 90 mmHg, or an elevation of 20%–30% above the baseline is significant. In a prospective study of 1,844 general surgery patients in the Post-Anesthesia Care Unit (PACU) after general anesthesia, the incidence of hypertension was 3.25%.[4] For 50% of the affected patients in this study, there was no preoperative history of hypertension. The incidence of postoperative hypertension after certain types of surgical procedures may be higher. The incidence of postoperative hypertension has been reported to be between 9% and 64% after carotid endarterectomy, 22% to 54% after cardiac surgery, 10% to 20% after neck dissection, and 57% to 91% after intracranial procedures.[5]

The 2014 Guidelines of the Eighth Joint National Committee recommend a blood pressure goal of below 150/90 mmHg in adults over the age of 60 years and a diastolic goal of below 90 mmHg in adults aged 30 to 59 years.[6] These goals are for medical patients and cannot be extrapolated to surgical patient populations. Postoperative hypertension is distinct from hypertension observed in medical patient populations.[7]

Post-Anesthesia Care: Symptoms, Diagnosis, and Management, ed. James W. Heitz. Published by Cambridge University Press. © Cambridge University Press 2016.

Hypertension in the medical setting is typically essential hypertension. Management involves titrating oral medications to control blood pressure to prevent long-term sequelae. Only about 5% of hypertension in medical populations is due to secondary causes, where management is directed at correction of the underlying cause, rather than merely reducing the blood pressure. Postoperative hypertension commonly occurs in patients without pre-existing hypertension. These patients typically have a secondary cause for their hypertension. Even patients with a history of essential hypertension often have a secondary cause exacerbating their hypertension. Management of postoperative hypertension is often directed at a correction of a secondary cause rather than direct reduction of blood pressure. Non-pharmacological treatment and administration of pharmacological agents are instituted in the management of post-operative hypertension with the goal of reducing short-term sequelae. Target blood pressure is dependent on both the clinical situation and the preoperative baseline blood pressure.

Secondary causes of hypertension

Secondary causes of hypertension in medical patient populations are uncommon, but have been described by the mnemonic ABCDE (see Table 3.1).[8] Since many of the causes of hypertension observed in the postoperative setting are unique, the ABCDE mnemonic requires substantial modification for application to that setting.

Pathophysiology: The pathophysiology of postoperative hypertension may be variable because of its individual etiology, with sympathetic nervous system activation with elevation of serum catecholamines appearing to be the final common pathway.[16–21] Activation of the renin–angiotensin–aldosterone system seems to be less important in acute postoperative hypertension than it is in chronic essential hypertension, except perhaps when hypertension is due to bladder over-distension. Plasma renin, angiotensin II, and aldosterone levels are not elevated in acute postoperative hypertension.[17,21]

Prognosis: Acute postoperative hypertension typically occurs within 20 to 30 minutes after emergence from general anesthesia and resolves within 6 to 8 hours.[22] The impact of hypertension, either acute postoperative or chronic essential, upon perioperative outcome is controversial. A retrospective review of surgical outcome published in 1929 revealed a 32% increase in cardiovascular mortality among patients with hypertension.[23] However, this study was conducted in an era when the therapeutic options for blood pressure management were severely limited and anesthetic management was less advanced. Significant clinical attention has been focused upon controlling hypertension prior to elective surgery with the aim of improving cardiovascular outcome. The evidence of benefit to this practice on clinical outcome is equivocal. A more recent retrospective review of 30-day cardiac mortality after general anesthesia revealed an odds ratio of 1.9 for having hypertension compared with matched controls without hypertension.[24] A prospective observational study of patients having non-cardiac surgery established a similar odds ratio of 1.9 for perioperative myocardial ischemia in patients with hypertension.[25] This contrasts with a prospective observational study that was unable to detect an outcome difference for surgical patients with mild hypertension.[26] More recently, several large (17,000 and 183,039 patients) retrospective studies have been unable to detect a difference in outcome for patients with hypertension after surgery.[27,28] The most recent American Heart Association guidelines recommend postponement of elective surgery when systolic blood pressure exceeds 180 mmHg

Table 3.1 Common etiologies of secondary hypertension

	Medical patients	Surgical patients
A	Accuracy, Apnea (obstructive sleep apnea), Aldosteronism	Accuracy, Anxiety, Analgesic deficiency (pain), Autonomic dysreflexia
B	Bruits (renovascular), Bad kidney (renal parenchymal disease)	Breathing (hypoxia, hypercapnia), Bladder distension
C	Catecholamines, Coarctation of the aorta, Cushing's syndrome	Catecholamines, Cold (hypothermia)
D	Drugs, Diet	Drugs, Drug withdrawal, Diabetes (hypoglycemia)
E	Erythropoietin (endogenous or exogenous), Endocrine disorders	Elevated ICP, Emergence excitation, Excessive hydration, Endocrine disorders

A: Pain (analgesic deficit) is the most common cause of hypertension in the postoperative setting in both patients with and without prior history of hypertension. Pain is implicated in as many as 35% of hypertension observed in the PACU.[4] Pain increases serum catecholamines, with greater severity causing greater elevations and pain relief lowering of serum catecholamine levels.[9] Anxiety may also contribute to postoperative hypertension. Autonomic dysreflexia may be observed in paraplegics with spinal levels above the dermatome. Distension of a hollow viscus, such as may occur with a full bladder, can cause profound hypertension with reflex bradycardia in susceptible individuals. Similar to medical hypertension, accuracy of the measurement needs to be considered in order to avoid treating erroneous blood pressure values. In the medical setting the most common cause of spuriously elevated blood pressure is improper size or application of the cuff upon the arm. In the postoperative setting, problems with patient movement including shivering may interfere with proper measurement[10] as well as improper zeroing or transducer placement of arterial lines.

B: Disorders of breathing including hypoxia and hypercapnia may contribute to hypertension after surgery. Pulse oximetry may detect hypoxia, but unless end-tidal carbon dioxide monitoring is employed a high degree of clinical suspicion is needed to recognize hypercapnia. The evaluation of hypertension in the PACU setting should begin with a clinical assessment of ventilation. Bladder distension causes increases in systolic and diastolic blood pressure by increasing sympathetic outflow.[11] Bladder distension can be a potent cause of postoperative hypertension which may be resistant to treatment with antihypertensive medications. Difficult-to-treat postoperative hypertension should raise suspicion for overlooked postoperative urinary retention.

C: Hypothermia (cold) raises blood pressure primarily through increases in serum norepinephrine levels.[12] The catecholamine surge that patients may experience during surgical procedures can also elevate blood pressure.

D: Postoperative hypertension may be caused by the administration of a new medication or the withdrawal from a chronic medication or other drug. Interruption of an antihypertensive medication, because of fasting or inability to tolerate pills, may unmask previously treated essential hypertension. The acute cessation of α-agonists or β-blockers may cause rebound hypertension. Alcohol or opioid withdrawal is also associated with hypertension. Systemic absorption of topical cocaine or oxymetazoline,[13] or subcutaneous epinephrine administered with local anesthetic for analgesia, may cause postoperative hypertension. Elevation in blood pressure, sometimes profound, may be caused by the administration of vasopressors (ephedrine, phenylephrine, isoproterenol, dopamine, dobutamine, vasopressin), bronchodilators (terburtaline, albuterol, aminophylline), anticholinergics (atropine, glycopyrrolate), or dissociative anesthetics (ketamine). Hypoglycemia may cause hypertension by sympathetic stimulation.[14]

E: Elevated intracranial pressure (ICP) may be associated with both hypertension and bradycardia in the surgical patient. Emergence excitation results in a catecholamine surge upon emergence from general anesthesia and may be responsible for as many as 1 in 6 cases of postoperative hypertension in the PACU.[4] Intravascular volume overload (excessive hydration) may also contribute to elevated blood pressure. Hypertension is an expected finding of transfusion-associated circulatory overload.[15] Endocrinological causes including pheochromocytoma, thyroid storm, or pregnancy-induced hypertension may rarely be observed after surgery.

or diastolic blood pressure exceeds 110 mmHg, but recognizes that this is at most a weak risk factor for adverse outcome.[2]

If equivocal evidence supports the need for blood pressure control prior to elective surgery, is it a clinical necessity to treat hypertension that is observed after surgery? There are theoretical reasons to suspect that postoperative hypertension may affect outcome and be more clinically significant than preoperative hypertension. Elevations in postoperative blood pressure may contribute to more postoperative hemorrhage, stress fresh suture lines, and increase strain upon an already over-taxed heart. There is insufficient literature to validate these hypotheses, but one large retrospective study (n = 18,380 patients) of admissions to the PACU found either tachycardia or hypertension to be associated with adverse postoperative events and perioperative mortality.[29] It is unclear whether treating this hypertension would reduce adverse events, but effective treatment of postoperative hypertension (Figure 3.1) is clinically prudent.

Management: A treatable cause of secondary hypertension should be remedied. Treatment of blood pressure directly is rarely indicated for secondary causes. Hypoxia or hypercapnia should be corrected if present. A full bladder should be drained and analgesics administered for pain. The hypothermic surgical patient should be rewarmed with forced air warming. Pain is more appropriately treated with analgesics than with antihypertensive medication. However, for hypertension causing end-organ damage (encephalopathy, myocardial ischemia) and for patients in whom elevated blood pressure is potentially acutely dangerous (carotid endarterectomy with a fresh patch, aneurysms,

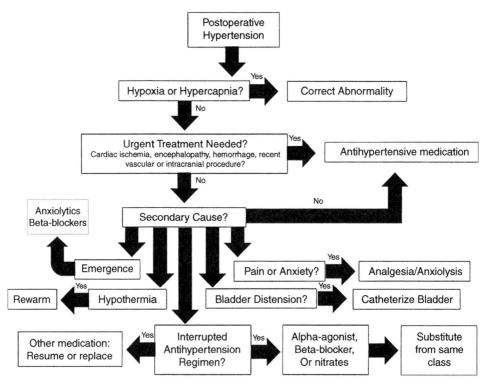

Figure 3.1 Initial evaluation of postoperative hypertension.

Table 3.2 Antihypertensive medications administered by continuous infusion

Medication	Typical dose	Time to onset	Duration of action	Mechanism	Comments
Clevidipine	1–2 mg/hr Max 21 mg/hr	1–2 min	5–15 min	Calcium entry blocker	Ultrafast titration, increase infusion every 90 seconds to target blood pressure, causes fever
Esmolol	Bolus 500 mcg/kg, 25–200 mcg/kg/min	6–10 min	<20 min	Cardioselective β-antagonist	Metabolism by plasma esterases
Fenoldopam	0.1 mcg/kg/min, increase by 0.05–0.1 mcg / kg/min q 20 min, max 1.6 mcg/kg/min	20–40 min	15–30 min	Dopamine type 1-receptor antagonist	Increased renal blood flow, ↑ ICP, no coronary steal
Nicardipine	5 mg/hr Max 15 mg/hr Increase 1–2.5 mg q 5–15 min	10–15 min	15–20 min	Calcium entry blocker	Beneficial in cerebral vasospasm and subarachnoid hemorrhage
Nitroglycerin	5–300 mcg/min	<1 min	5–10 min	Primarily venodilator, ↓ preload	Coronary vasodilatation, tolerance
Sodium nitroprusside	0.5–5 mcg/kg/min	<1 min	1–3 min	Direct venous and arterial vasodilator	Cyanide toxicity, coronary steal

intracranial procedures, cardiac ischemia), antihypertensive therapy should immediately be directed at blood pressure management. Rapid-onset and quick-offset medications are preferred in the perioperative setting. There are no established guidelines for target blood pressure in the treatment of postoperative hypertension, and attention must be given to co-morbidities and baseline blood pressure. In cases of interruption of the antihypertensive regimen owing to an inability to take oral medications, choice of a substitute intravenous medication with the same mechanism of action is practical, but little evidence validates this common clinical practice. Replacement of an α-agonist or β-blocker with a similar medication is advantageous to prevent rebound hypertension. Clonidine is available as a transdermal preparation, but this is not appropriate as sole agent for postoperative hypertension since therapeutic blood levels may take 2 to 3 days to be established after initial application of the patch.[30]

Table 3.3 Antihypertensive medications administered by intermittent bolus

Medication	Typical dose	Time to onset	Duration of action	Mechanism	Comments
Hydralazine	5–20 mg	15–30 min	4–6 hr	Direct arterial smooth muscle relaxation	Reflex tachycardia limits effect, safe in pregnancy
Labetalol	10–20 mg	5–10 min	3–5 hr	α_1 non-selective β-antagonist	Use with caution if heart block, cardiac conduction abnormalities, reactive airway disease
Enalaprilat	1.25–5 mg IV over 15–20 min q 6 hr Max dose 20 mg/day	15 min	Up to 12 hr	Angiotensin-converting enzyme (ACE) inhibitor	Caution in renal dysfunction, contraindicated in pregnancy, IV to oral conversion is 1:1
Metoprolol	0.1 mcg/kg/min, increase by 0.05–0.1 mcg/kg/min q 20 min, max 1.6 mcg/kg/min	20–40 min	15–30 min	β_1 selective blocker	Increased renal blood flow, ↑ renal blood flow, ↑ ICP, no coronary steal
Nitroglycerin paste	1–2 inches	<30 min	12–18 hr	Primarily venodilator, ↓ preload	Coronary vasodilatation, tolerance, headache, poorly titratable

Medications

The pharmacological options for treating acute postoperative hypertension are vast. Clinical consideration should be paid to severity of hypertension and associated symptoms, underlying co-morbidities, cost, and where the patient is to be cared for after the PACU. Continuous infusions (see Table 3.2) generally offer the most rapid and easily titrated control of blood pressure, but will necessitate intra-arterial blood pressure monitoring and more intensive nursing care. Intermittent bolus medications (see Table 3.3) may be more appropriate for less severe cases.

Postoperative hypertension after the PACU

Secondary causes of hypertension remain important considerations throughout the postoperative setting. The etiology and frequency are slightly different after the PACU period.

Hypothermia and bladder distension are less common causes of hypertension later in the recovery phase. Hypoxia and hypercapnia need to be considered in the etiology of post-operative hypertension throughout the hospitalization, particularly for patients receiving parenteral opioids with a history of sleep apnea. Insufficiently controlled pain remains an important cause of secondary hypertension, but becomes less clinically significant later in the postoperative course as pain scores naturally wane. The effects of drug withdrawal, especially interruption of chronic antihypertensive therapy, rebound hypertension from α-agonist or β-blocker withdrawal, or alcohol withdrawal syndrome, all become more clinically likely after the PACU period as the time of abstinence increases. Secondary causes of hypertension should not be overlooked in surgical patients with or without previous histories of hypertension while recovering from procedures on the surgical wards.

References

1. World Health Organization. A global brief on hypertension: silent killer, global public health crisis. WHO/DCO/WHD/2013.2 http://www.who.int/cardiovascular_ diseases/publications/global_brief_ hypertension/en/. Accessed Dec 26, 2014.

2. A.S. Go, D. Mozaffarian, V.L. Roger *et al.* on behalf of the American Heart Association Statistics Committee and Stroke Statistics Subcommittee. Heart Disease and Stroke Statistics – 2014 update. A report from the American Heart Association. *Circulation* 2013; 129:e28–e292.

3. T. McCormack, C. Arden, A. Begg *et al.* Optimising hypertension treatment: NICE/BHS guideline implementation and audit for best practice. *Br J Cardiol* 2013; 20 (Suppl 1): S1–S16.

4. T.J. Gal, L.H. Cooperman. Hypertension in the immediate postoperative period. *Br J Anaesth* 1975; 47:70–74.

5. C.E. Hass, J.M. LeBlanc. Acute postoperative hypertension: a review of therapeutic options. *Am J Health-Sys Pharm* 2004; 61:1661–1675.

6. P.A. James, S. Oparil, B.L. Carter *et al.* 2014 evidence-based guideline for the management of high blood pressure in adults: report from the panel members appointed to the eighth joint national committee. *JAMA* 2014; 311:507–520.

7. J.H. Levy. The ideal agent for perioperative hypertension and potential cytoprotective effects. *Acta Anaesthesiol Scand* 1993; 37:20–25.

8. E. Onusko. Diagnosing secondary hypertension. *Am Fam Physician* 2003; 67:67–74.

9. E.C. Huskisson. Catecholamine excretion and pain. *Br J Clin Pharmacol* 1974; 1:80–82.

10. J.G. De Courcy. Artefactual "hypotension" from shivering. *Anaesthesia* 1989; 44:787–788.

11. J. Fagius, S. Karhuvaara. Sympathetic activity and blood pressure increases with bladder distension in humans. *Hypertension* 1989; 14:511–517.

12. S.R. Hart, B. Bordes, J. Hart, D. Corsino, D. Harmon. Unintended perioperative hypothermia. *Ochsner J* 2011; 11:259–270.

13. A.S. Ramesh, R. Cartabuke, G. Essig, J.D. Tobias. Oxymetazoline-induced postoperative hypotension. *Pediatr Anesth Crit Care J* 2013; 1:72–77.

14. S. Feldman-Billard, P. Massin, T. Meas, P.-J. Guillausseau, E. Héron. Hypoglycemia-induced blood pressure elevation in patients with diabetes. *Arch Intern Med* 2010; 170:829–831.

15. R.C. Skeate, T. Eastlund. Distinguishing between transfusion related acute lung injury and transfusion associated circulatory overload. *Curr Opin Hematol* 2007; 14:682–687.

16. R. Wallach, R.B. Karp, J.G. Reves *et al.* Pathogenesis of paroxysmal hypertension developing during and after coronary artery bypass surgery: a study of hemodynamics and humoral factors. *Am J Cardiol* 1980; 46:559–560.

17. M. Breslow, D.A. Jordan, R. Christopherson *et al.* Epidural morphine decreases postoperative hypertension by attenuating sympathetic nervous system hyperactivity. *JAMA* 1989; 261;3577–3581.

18. G.S. Weinstein, P.M. Zabetakis, A. Clavel *et al.* The renin-angiotensin system is not responsible for hypertension following coronary bypass grafting. *Ann Thorac Surg* 1987; 43:74–77.

19. A.J. Roberts, A.P. Niarchos, V.A. Subramanian *et al.* Systemic hypertension association with coronary bypass surgery. *J Thorac Cardiovasc Surg* 1977; 74:846–859.

20. J.H. Kataja, S. Kaukinen, O.V. Viianamaki *et al.* Hemodynamic and hormonal changes in patients pretreated with captopril for surgery of the abdominal aorta. *J Cardiothorac Anesth* 1989; 3:425–432.

21. K.S. Olsen, C.B. Pedersen, J.B. Madsen *et al.* Vasoactive modulators during and after craniotomy: relation to postoperative hypertension. *J Neurosurg Anesthesiol* 2002; 14:171–199.

22. C. Pyrs-Roberts. Anaesthesia and hypertension. *Br J Anaesth* 1984; 50:711–724.

23. H.B. Sprague. The heart in surgery. An analysis of the results of surgery on cardiac patients during the past ten years at the Massachusetts General Hospital. *Surg Gynecol Obstet* 1929; 49:54–58.

24. S.J. Howell, Y.M. Sear, D. Yeates *et al.* Risk factors for cardiovascular death after elective surgery under general anesthesia. *Br J Anaesth* 1998; 80:14–19.

25. M. Hollenberg, D.T. Mangano, W.S. Browner *et al.* Predictors of postoperative myocardial ischemia in patients undergoing noncardiac surgery. The Study of Perioperative Ischemia Research Group. *JAMA* 1992; 268:205–209.

26. L. Goldman, D.L. Caldera. Risks of general anesthesia and elective operation in the hypertensive patient. *Anesthesiology* 1979; 50:285–292.

27. J.B Forrest, K. Rehder, M.K. Cahalan, C.H. Goldsmith. Multicenter study of general anesthesia. III: Predictors of severe perioperative adverse outcomes. *Anesthesiology* 1992; 76:3–15.

28. D.L. Davenport, V.A. Ferraris, P. Hosokawa *et al.* Multivariable predictors of postoperative cardiac adverse events after general and vascular surgery: results from the Patient Safety in Surgery study. *J Am Coll Surg* 2007; 204:1199–1210.

29. D.K. Rose, M.M. Cohen, D.P. DeBoer. Cardiovascular events in the postanesthesia care unit: contribution of risk factors. *Anesthesiology* 1996; 84:772–781.

30. D.T. Lowenthal, S. Saris, E. Paran *et al.* Efficacy of clonidine as transdermal therapeutic system: the international clinical trial experience. *Am Heart J* 1986; 112:893–900.

Chapter

4

Hypotension

James W. Heitz

- Most postoperative hypotension is responsive to fluid administration.
- A pulse pressure variation greater than 15% during mechanical ventilation predicts fluid responsiveness.
- A high degree of suspicion may be necessary to recognize occult hemorrhage or myocardial ischemia which may initially present as postoperative hypotension.

Hypotension is common after general surgery. Although there is no single definition, postoperative hypotension may be defined as a systolic blood pressure (SBP) below 90 mmHg or mean arterial pressure (MAP) below 60 mmHg. Significant postoperative hypotension has been observed to occur in 1 in 31 patients admitted to the Post-Anesthesia Care Unit (PACU).[1] Evaluation of postoperative hypotension should consider the baseline blood pressure of the patient. Hypotension typically becomes clinically significant when blood pressure falls 20% to 30% below baseline. Often, baseline blood pressure may not be known precisely and the immediate pre-procedure blood pressure may overestimate true baseline blood pressure because of the hypertensive effects of anxiety or pain. If available, blood pressure readings taken days or weeks prior to the procedure are often more helpful in establishing a baseline than are measurements immediately prior to surgery. When blood pressure falls 30% below baseline or is associated with signs of organ hypoperfusion, including change in mental status, chest pain, electrocardiogram (ECG) changes, or oliguria, it requires treatment. Therapy is directed at correction of the underlying cause for the hypotension.

Hypotension may be caused by disturbances in preload, cardiac output, or systemic vascular resistance (see Table 4.1). Clinically, it is important to identify the cause and severity of hypotension. Therapy will differ according to the etiology, and more severe hypotension will require more aggressive resuscitation.

Preload

Decreased venous return to the heart causes decreased cardiac preload and decreased blood pressure. Decreased intravascular volume or increased venous capacitance will decrease preload. Effective intravascular volume may be decreased by operative blood loss, insensible losses, and the loss of intravascular volume into the third space. Preoperative restrictions regarding oral fluid intake and fluid loss from bowel cleansing preparations may exacerbate

Post-Anesthesia Care: Symptoms, Diagnosis, and Management, ed. James W. Heitz. Published by Cambridge University Press. © Cambridge University Press 2016.

Table 4.1 Differential diagnosis of postoperative hypotension

↓Preload	• Hypovolemia (blood loss, insensible fluid loss, third spacing) • ↑Venous capacitance (venodilatation/neuraxial anesthetics) • ↑Intrathoracic pressure (mechanical ventilation)
↓Cardiac output	• ↓Chronotropy • ↓Inotropy
↓SVR	• SIRS (sepsis, burns, trauma, pancreatitis) • Anaphylaxis • Transfusion reaction • Endocrine (myxedema, secondary hypoadrenalism)

SIRS = systemic inflammatory response syndrome, SVR = systemic vascular resistance

hypovolemia. Venous capacitance may be increased from the venodilatory effects of spinal or general anesthetic agents or from epidural infusion for postoperative analgesia, effectively decreasing preload. A fluid challenge with crystalloid or colloid solution is appropriate for most postoperative patients with hypotension in the absence of signs of intravascular volume overload. However, a fluid challenge in the surgical patient is not necessarily benign, and excessive volume administration is to be avoided since it may contribute to adverse outcomes.[2]

Predicting response to fluid challenge: The responsiveness of hypotension to volume administration may be predicted by beat-to-beat respiratory variations in blood pressure during positive pressure ventilation. The magnitude of the effect of positive intrathoracic pressure on stroke volume across different portions of the cardiac cycle is reflected in the pulse pressure (PP). PP may be defined as systolic blood pressure (SBP) minus the diastolic blood pressure (DBP). This is typically 30 to 40 mmHg in adults. PP varies with stroke volume during the respiratory cycle and is known as pulse pressure variation (PPV). PPV may be defined as the difference between the highest and lowest PP divided by the average PP.

$$PP = SBP - DBP$$

$$PPavg = \frac{PPmax + PPmin}{2}$$

$$PPV = \frac{PPmax - PPmin}{PPavg} \times 100\%$$

Some modern monitors have the ability to calculate the PPV automatically from an arterial line tracing. A PPV >15% strongly predicts fluid responsiveness, a PPV <10% strongly predicts fluid-unresponsive hypotension.[3] To be able to interpret the PPV to guide fluid therapy, the patient should be receiving mechanical ventilation with tidal volumes of 8 to 10 ml/kg.[4] The cardiac rhythm must be regular, since the variations in stroke volume associated with irregular rhythms make the PPV unreliable in predicting fluid responsiveness. Additionally, decreased chest wall compliance (obesity, circumferential third degree burns) will cause the PPV to rise and may inappropriately suggest fluid responsiveness. PPV must also be interpreted cautiously in patients with chronic obstructive pulmonary disease. It is important to note that PPV predicts the responsiveness of hypotension to fluid administration, since it reflects the dependence of cardiac output upon preload. PPV is not validated as an assessment tool for volume status and has no clear clinical implications in the absence of hypotension. Respiratory variation in pulse oximeter plethysmographic waveform may be used to predict fluid responsiveness if an arterial waveform is not available.[5]

While PPV is a very useful tool for intraoperative fluid management, it has less application to the postoperative setting where only a minority of patients receive mechanical ventilation. PPV is not reliable in predicting fluid responsiveness of hypotension patients during spontaneous ventilation.[6] In contrast to positive pressure ventilation in which inspiration is associated with increased intrathoracic pressure and decreased right ventricular preload, spontaneous ventilation is associated with negative intrathoracic pressures and increased right ventricular preload. PPV performs poorly in predicting fluid responsiveness of spontaneously breathing patients. Approximately 1 in 2 patients predicted to have fluid-responsive hypotension fail to respond appropriately to fluid challenge.[7,8] In animal models, spontaneous ventilation through an expiratory threshold resistor may be used to amplify PPV and better discriminate between fluid-responsive and fluid-unresponsive hypotension,[9] but this technique has no current clinical application. Having patients take a maximal deep breath rather than normal tidal volume may improve the discrimination of PPV to predict fluid responsiveness of blood pressure, but this technique has yet to be validated in the postoperative setting.[10]

Ultrasound may be utilized to accurately assess volume status and predict fluid responsiveness in the spontaneously ventilating hypotensive postoperative patient. An inferior vena cava of normal diameter with <50% respirophasic variation suggests euvolemia. Progressively diminishing vessel diameter and greater respirophasic variation are correlated with lesser central venous pressures.[11] Although this technique is well validated, its applicability is limited by the need for both specialized equipment and skills to adequately assess volume status. More recently, respirophasic variation in carotid artery flow during mechanical ventilation has been identified as a measure of volume responsiveness of hypotension to fluid challenge.[12] This technique may allow for easier imaging with ultrasound, but its utility in the postoperative setting is not yet validated.

Fluid challenge is appropriate for mechanically ventilated patients with PPV >15% in absence of signs of fluid overload. Increasing peak airway pressures during mechanical ventilation or increasing oxygen requirements may be early diagnostic clues to the development of pulmonary edema. For surgical patients without arterial lines or mechanical ventilation, other parameters must be examined. If a central line is present, a central venous pressure of <5 mmHg also suggests hypovolemia, but central venous pressures may be clinically misleading in some situations. For the majority of postoperative patients, assessment of skin turgor, urine output, and clinical judgment needs to direct fluid management.

Hemorrhage: Although hypotension is infrequently due to hemorrhage after surgery, ongoing blood loss should be considered in the differential diagnosis of postoperative hypotension. Hemorrhage may be occult and may not be reflected in surgical drains or chest tube output. Additionally, "minor" parts of the procedure may be overlooked when evaluating for hemorrhage. For example, hemodynamically significant hemothorax may occur after central venous catheter placement even though the main procedure occurred outside of the thorax. The absence of a central line postoperatively does not guarantee that there was not an unsuccessful attempt to place one. Acute hemorrhage without volume resuscitation does not reliably produce anemia, so laboratory testing may not initially detect ongoing blood loss. A high degree of clinical suspicion and a pertinent physical examination are required. The treatment of postoperative hemorrhage may require return to the surgery, so preparation should begin early to facilitate this process. Intravenous access may need to be upgraded; the access sufficient for the initial surgery may not be adequate in the presence of ongoing hemorrhage. Blood should be made available, and coagulation studies and platelet count should be measured as consumptive coagulopathy may occur.

Increased intrathoracic pressure: Special attention must be paid to patients requiring positive pressure mechanical ventilation. Auto-PEEP (positive end-expiratory pressure) occurs when there is insufficient time for expiration, as may occur with patients with asthma or chronic obstructive pulmonary disease during bronchospasm or during hyperventilation. If an expiratory flow waveform is available, it may demonstrate a failure to return to baseline prior to inspiration. Often, an expiratory flow waveform may not be available, and auto-PEEP may be difficult to diagnosis. Auto-PEEP causes hypotension which may progress to pulseless electrical activity if not corrected. Peak airway pressures may increase and neck veins may be distended. Disconnection from mechanical ventilation for 30 seconds may be life-saving. Although auto-PEEP may first be recognized by hypotension, therapy is directed at correction of bronchospasm and increasing the expiratory time. Auto-PEEP has been implicated as a possible etiology for auto-resuscitation after cessation of cardiopulmonary resuscitation. This rare phenomenon is poorly understood.[13]

Other causes of excessively high peak inspiratory pressures during mechanical ventilation may also cause hypotension. When hypotension is precipitated by high peak pressures on mechanical ventilation, hypotension is merely a symptom of a more serious problem and therapy should be directed at correction of the ventilator problem. Bronchospasm, pneumothorax, endobronchial intubation, auto-PEEP, increased chest wall rigidity, or bucking on the ventilator may each cause increased intrathoracic pressures and systemic hypotension.

Cardiac output

Cardiac output is defined as the product of heart rate and stroke volume, and reduction in either will decrease cardiac output. A variety of problems related to chronotropy or inotropy are encountered after surgery and may cause hypotension by impairing cardiac output.

$$CO = SV \times HR$$
$$CO = \text{cardiac output}, \quad SV = \text{stroke volume}, \quad HR = \text{heart rate}$$

Chronotropy-mediated hypotension: When hypotension occurs with bradycardia, initial therapy is directed at increasing heart rate. Bradycardic rhythms are common in the perioperative period and may be related to increased parasympathetic tone or sympathetic exhaustion.

Bezold–Jarisch reflex: The Bezold–Jarisch reflex is mediated by chemoreceptors in the heart.[14] Parasympathetic outflow via the vagal nerve can cause bradycardia, hypotension, and hypopnea. Hypotension may be disproportionate to the degree of bradycardia. The Bezold–Jarisch reflex may often be observed during myocardial infarction and responds to treatment with atropine. Bezold–Jarisch reflex may occasionally be elicited by severe hemorrhage. Reduced circulatory volume may cause increased parasympathetic activity with decreased blood pressure and heart rate.[14] Serotonin released from activated platelets may exacerbate this response.[15] In one retrospective review of 750 trauma patients, 28.9% presented with a heart rate inappropriately low for the severity of hemorrhage.[16] This lack of tachycardia may result in delay of diagnosis of hemorrhage and in some instances may be due to the Bezold–Jarisch reflex. Vasopressors or atropine may paradoxically worsen the hypotension by exacerbating the reflex. In animal models, propranolol administration increased stroke volume and blood pressure, but not heart rate, during severe hemorrhage with Bezold–Jarisch reflex physiology.[17]

Vaso-vagal presyncope: Vaso-vagal phenomenon including hypotension and bradycardia may occur after surgery, especially in conjunction with nausea or pain. Management is directed at increasing the heart rate to increase blood pressure and at treating the underlying precipitator. Although the administration of opioid may be clinically counterintuitive during hypotension, it is sometimes necessary.

"High spinal" anesthesia may be associated with neuraxial anesthesia and may present as hypotension when the sensory level rises above the fourth thoracic dermatome. Cardiac accelerator fibers originate from T1 to T4, and once blocked, bradycardia may ensue. High spinal would be uncommon after surgery, but may occur in the Holding Area when spinal anesthesia is delivered. The same effect may occur with epidural infusion, and this may occur if the epidural catheter is bolused after surgery for postoperative analgesia, particularly if the catheter has migrated into the subarachnoid space.

Bradycardia may be triggered by perioperative medications, including β-blockers which may be initiated preoperatively. Bradycardia and hypotension may be associated with local anesthetic overdose, which is an emergency and requires immediate treatment with 20% intralipid infusion to bind the local anesthetic. Neurological toxicity, including seizures, usually precedes cardiac toxicity, but may not when the local anesthetic is bupivacaine. Local anesthetic overdose presenting postoperatively as hypotension would be unusual, but may occur with delayed absorption of local anesthesia, such as when absorbed through mucosal surfaces during bronchoscopy.

Inotropy-mediated hypotension: When hypotension occurs because of decreased cardiac contractility, therapy needs to be tailored to the clinical situation. This is the uncommon situation where volume expansion is not indicated for postoperative hypotension. Inadequacy of ventilation producing either hypoxia or hypercapnia may initially increase contractility via increased catecholamine release, but as these conditions become more severe, contractility is impaired.[18] Acidosis from any etiology may impair contractility.

Atrial fibrillation is a common postoperative dysrhythmia. Atrial contraction accounts for 15 to 25% of stroke volume, and the loss of the atrial kick can precipitate hypotension. Severe hypotension requires synchronized cardioversion. Stable atrial fibrillation usually requires rate control to reduce the risk of cardiac ischemia. Chemical cardioversion is seldom necessary for postoperative atrial fibrillation. Perioperative volume shifts and intraoperative fluid administration can cause atrial stretching, precipitating atrial fibrillation. Unless this was a preoperative dysrhythmia, spontaneous conversion to sinus rhythm is common.

Myocardial ischemia may present as hypotension. Dyspnea and chest pain may not be present, as postoperative myocardial ischemia is often silent after cardiac[19] and non-cardiac[20] procedures. Myocardial ischemia is 2–2.5 times more likely to be silent in surgical (50–70%) than in medical (20–40%) patients.[21–24] Residual anesthetic effects, analgesic administration, and competing somatic stimulation (e.g. incisional pain) may mask angina pain. Myocardial ischemia may occur in as many as 40% of patients after non-cardiac surgery.[25] While it is most often transient and silent, new-onset hypotension or arrhythmia in the postoperative setting should raise suspicion for a possible cardiac ischemic event.

Afterload

Reduction in systemic vascular resistance may cause postoperative hypotension. Arterial vasodilation will reduce systemic vascular resistance and, if severe, cause hypotension.

$$SVR = 80 \times \frac{MAP - CVP}{CO}$$

SVR = systemic vascular resistance; MAP = mean arterial pressure; CVP = central venous pressure; CO = cardiac output

Systemic inflammatory response syndrome (SIRS): SIRS is an inflammatory state due to an infectious or non-infectious insult (see Table 4.2). SIRS was first defined by the American College of Chest Physicians in 1992.[26] It may be caused by the release of pro- and anti-inflammatory mediators by trauma or surgery. SIRS may also be caused by third degree burns or pancreatitis. Extensive research into targeting specific inflammatory mediators has yielded little benefit. Management is directed at treating the underlying cause and at supportive care including volume resuscitation and vasopressors to maintain organ perfusion.

Sepsis: Sepsis may be defined as a SIRS in the presence of infection. Severe sepsis is accompanied by lactic acidosis, an absolute SBP less than 90 mmHg or a fall of SBP of 40 mmHg from baseline. Severe sepsis with hypotension despite volume resuscitation is septic shock. Severe sepsis needs to be considered in the hypotensive surgical patient. Management includes treatment of the precipitating infection and supportive care including vasopressors as needed.

Anaphylaxis: Perioperative anaphylaxis is a rare phenomenon reported to occur in the range of 1:6,000[27] to 1:34,000[28] surgical procedures. Neuromuscular blocking agents, latex, and antibiotics are the most frequently implicated agents in causing perioperative anaphylaxis.[29] More recent data suggest that several neuromuscular blocking agents may carry a particularly elevated risk of allergic reaction. In a retrospective observation study of anaphylaxis to neuromuscular blocking agents, succinylcholine was associated with allergic reaction in 1 in 2,080 administrations, rocuronium was associated with allergic reaction in 1 in 2,499 administrations.[30] Allergic reaction needs to be considered in the differential diagnosis of hypotension during the polypharmacy of the perioperative period. Hypotension due to allergic reaction may be accompanied by bronchospasm, hives,

Table 4.2 Systemic inflammatory response syndrome[26]

Body temperature >38 °C or <36 °C
Heart rate >90 beats/min
Respiratory rate >20/min or $PaCO_2$ <32 mmHg
Leukocyte count >12,000/µl, <4,000/µl, or >10% immature (band) forms
Two or more necessary for diagnosis

or urticaria. Although perioperative anaphylaxis most often occurs in the operating room, in one large retrospective study, 7.9% of cases were first identified in the PACU.[28] Anaphylactoid reactions may also occur perioperatively and are commonly associated with morphine or intravenous (IV) contrast dye. Management includes epinephrine, H_1 and H_2 antagonists, and intravenous steroids.

Transfusion reaction: If blood products are administered during or after surgery, hypotension may be due to a transfusion reaction. The incidence of reported transfusion reaction is 0.24%.[31] A number of complications related to transfusion may cause hypotension. Acute hemolytic transfusion reaction is typically due to ABO incompatibility because of clerical error and the transfusion of mislabeled blood product. Hypotension may be severe and is typically accompanied by other signs including tachycardia, fever, chills, flank pain, hematuria, and, possibly, bleeding from incision sites. This fulminant reaction typically occurs while the blood is transfusing. Management includes immediate discontinuation of the blood product, notification of the Blood Bank, and laboratory testing of recipient and donor blood. Volume resuscitation, vasopressor support, and mannitol administration may be necessary, with the clinical aim of protecting the patient from acute kidney injury caused by myoglobinuria. Acute allergic reactions to blood are rare, but may occur when the recipient has IgA deficiency or allergens are present in the donor blood. Discontinuation of the transfusion and treatment of anaphylaxis, as necessary, is the treatment of choice. Patients on chronic angiotersin-converting enzyme (ACE) inhibitor therapy may experience profound hypotension from blood transfusion which is believed to be mediated by bradykinin accumulation in the transfused product.[32] Discontinuation of the transfusion and supportive care of the blood pressure is indicated.

A particularly insidious transfusion reaction which may occur in the postoperative setting is bacterial contaminated blood product. Diagnosis may be difficult since this may present after the unit has been transfused. This may first be recognized in the

Table 4.3 Effect of commonly used pressors on hemodynamic parameters

Medication	Bolus dose	Infusion dose	CO	HR	SVR	Inotropy
Ephedrine	5–25 mg IV		↑	↑	↑	↑
Phenylephrine	40–200 mcg IV	40–180 mcg/min IV	↔	↓	↑	↔
Epinephrine		0.1–1 mcg/kg/min	↑	↑	↑	↑
Norepinephrine		0.05–3 mcg/kg/min IV	↑	↑	↑	↑
Vasopressin	2–10 units IV	0.01–0.04 units/min IV	↔	↔	↑	↔
Dopamine (low dose)		1–5 mcg/kg/min IV	↔	↔	↔	↔
Dopamine (medium dose)		5–15 mcg/kg/min IV	↑	↑	↔	↑
Dopamine (high dose)		20–50 mcg/kg/min IV	↑	↑	↑	↑
Dobutamine			↑	↑	↓	↑
Milrinone		0.375–0.75 mcg/kg/min	↔	↔	↓	↑
Isoproterenol		2–10 mg/min	↑	↑	↓	↑

CO = cardiac output, HR = heart rate, SVR = systemic vascular resistance

PACU setting.[33] A high degree of clinical suspicion is therefore necessary to make the diagnosis. Platelets are the most commonly contaminated blood product since they are typically stored at warmer temperatures.

Hypoadrenalism: Hypotension may be observed in the postoperative period among surgical patients on chronic preoperative steroid therapy. The incidence of symptomatic hypoadrenalism in this cohort is about 1–2%.[34,35] Intraoperative administration of etomidate suppresses the enzyme β-11-hydroxylase[36] and may contribute to hypoadrenalism for 24 to 72 hours after administration.[37]

Miscellaneous: Hypotension is a very non-specific sign with many etiologies. This chapter addressed causes that may occur in broad populations of surgical patients, but numerous unusual causes still exist for individual patient populations: spinal shock after acute spinal cord injury, hypotension after carotid endarterectomy, hemodynamic instability after cardiac surgery to name a few. The evaluation of hypotension requires assessment of the entire clinical situation.

References

1. C.M. Barbour, D.M. Little. Postoperative hypotension. *JAMA* 1957; 163:1529–1532.

2. S. Brandt, T. Regueira, H. Bracht, *et al.* Effect of fluid resuscitation on mortality and organ function in experimental sepsis models. *Crit Care* 2009; 13:R186. doi:10.1186/cc8179.

3. F. Michard. Changes in arterial pressure during mechanical ventilation. *Anesthesiology* 2005; 103:419–428.

4. D. De Backer, S. Heenen, M. Piagnerelli, M. Koch, J.L. Vincent. Pulse pressure variations to predict fluid responsiveness: influence of tidal volume. *Intensive Care Med* 2005; 31:517–523.

5. M. Cannesson, O. Desebbe, P. Rosamel, *et al.* Pleth variability index to monitor the respiratory variations in the pulse oximeter plethysmographic waveform amplitude and predict fluid responsiveness in the operating theatre. *Br J Anaesth* 2008; 101:200–206.

6. S. Heenen, D. De Backer, J.-L. Vincent. How can the response to volume expansion in patients with spontaneous respiratory movements be predicted? *Crit Care* 2006; 10:R102. doi:10.1186/cc4970.

7. S.A. Magner, D.G. Georgiadis, T. Cheong. Respiratory variations in right atrial pressure predict response to fluid challenge. *J Crit Care* 1992; 7:76–85.

8. S. Magder, D. Lagonidis, F. Erice. The use of respiratory variations in right atrial pressure to predict the cardiac output response to PEEP. *J Crit Care* 2002; 18:108–114.

9. M.K. Dahl, S.T. Vistisen, J. Koefoed-Nielsen, A. Larsson. Using an expiratory resistor, arterial pulse pressure variations predict fluid responsiveness during spontaneous breathing: an experimental porcine study. *Crit Care* 2009; 13:R39. doi: 10.1186/cc7760.

10. D.M. Hong, J.M. Lee, J.H. Seo, *et al.* Pulse pressure variation to predict fluid responsiveness in spontaneously breathing patients: tidal vs forced inspiratory breathing. *Anaesthesia* 2014; 69:717–722.

11. D.J. Blehar, D. Resop, B. Chin, M. Dayno, R. Gaspari. Inferior vena cava displacement during respirophasic ultrasound imaging. *Crit Ultrasound J* 2012; 4:18. doi:10.1186/ 2036-7902-4-18.

12. Y. Song, Y.L. Kwak, J.W. Song, Y.J. Kim, J.K. Shim. Respirophasic carotid artery peak velocity variation as a predictor of fluid responsiveness in mechanically ventilated patients with coronary artery disease. *Br J Anaesth* 2014;113:61–66.

13. K. Hornby, L. Hornby, S.D. Shemie. A systematic review of autoresuscitation after cardiac arrest. *Crit Care Med* 2010; 38:1246–1253.

14. D.M. Aviado, D.G. Aviado. The Bezold–Jarisch reflex: a historical perspective of cardiopulmonary reflexes. *Ann NY Acad Sci* 2001; 940:48–58.

15. A.J.M. Verbene, M. Saita, D.M. Sartor. Chemical stimulation of vagal afferent neurons and sympathetic vasomotor tone. *Brain Res Rev* 2003; 41:288–305.

16. D. Demetriades, L.S. Chan, P. Bhasin, *et al.* Relative bradycardia in patients with traumatic hypotension. *J Trauma* 1998; 45: 534–539.

17. G. Wisbach, S. Tobias, R. Woodman, A. Spalding, W. Lockette. Preserving cardiac output with beta-adrenergic receptor blockade and inhibiting the Bezold–Jarisch reflex during resuscitation from hemorrhage. *J Trauma* 2007; 63:26–32.

18. T.V. Serebrovskaya. Comparison of respiratory and circulatory human responses to progressive hypoxia and hypercapnia. *Respiration* 1992; 59:34–41.

19. J.E. Adams, G.A. Sicard, B.T. Allen, *et al.* Diagnosis of perioperative myocardial infarction with measurement of cardiac troponin I. *N Engl J Med* 1994; 330:670–674.

20. R.C. Smith, J.M. Leung, D.T. Mangano. Postoperative myocardial ischemia in patients undergoing coronary artery bypass graft surgery. S.P.I. Research Group. *Anesthesiology* 1991; 74:464–473.

21. D.T. Mangano. Perioperative cardiac morbidity. *Anesthesiology* 1990; 72:153–184.

22. P.F. Cohn. Silent myocardial ischemia. *Ann Intern Med* 1988; 109:312–317.

23. W.B. Kannel, R.D. Abbott. Incidence and prognosis of unrecognized myocardial infarction: an update on the Framingham Study. *N Engl J Med* 1984; 311:1144–1147.

24. A.A. Knight, M. Hollenberg, M.J. London, *et al.* Perioperative myocardial ischemia: importance of the preoperative ischemic pattern. *Anesthesiology* 1988; 68:681–688.

25. D.T. Mangano, W.S. Browner, M. Hollenberg, *et al.* and the Study of Perioperative Ischemia Research Group. Association of perioperative myocardial ischemia with cardiac morbidity and mortality in men undergoing noncardiac surgery. *N Engl J Med* 1990; 323:1781–1788.

26. R.C. Bone, R.A. Balk, F.B. Cerra, *et al.* Definitions for sepsis and organ failure and guidelines for the use of innovative therapies in sepsis. The ACCP/SCCM Consensus Conference Committee. American College of Chest Physicians/ Society of Critical Care Medicine. *Chest* 1992; 101:1644–1655.

27. S. Fasting, S.E. Gisvold. Serious intraoperative problems – a five year review of 83,844 anesthetics. *Can J Anaesth* 2002; 49:545–553.

28. C. Gurrieri, T.N. Weingarten, D.P. Martin, *et al.* Allergic reactions during anesthesia at a large United States referral center. *Anesth Analg* 2011; 113:1202–1212.

29. D.L. Hepner, M.C. Castells. Anaphylaxis during the perioperative period. *Anesth Analg* 2003; 97;1381–1395.

30. J.I. Reddy, P.J. Cooke, J.M. van Schalkwyk, *et al.* Anaphylaxis is more common with rocuronium and succinylcholine than with atracurium. *Anesthesiology* 2015; 122:39–45.

31. The 2011 National Blood Collection and Utilization Survey Report. Report of the US Department of Health and Human Services. Available at http://www.hhs.gov/ ash/bloodsafety/2011-nbcus.pdf. Accessed November 30, 2014.

32. C. Doria, E. Elia, Y. Kang, *et al.* Acute hypotensive transfusion reaction during liver transplantation in a patient on angiotensin converting enzyme inhibitors from low aminopeptidase P activity. *Liver Transpl* 2008; 14:684–687.

33. M.D. Rollins, A.B. Molofsky, A. Nambia, *et al.* Two septic transfusion reactions presenting as TRALI from a split plateletpheresis unit. *Crit Care Med* 2012; 40:2488–2491.

34. H. Kehlet, C. Binder. Adrenocortical function and clinical course during and after surgery in unsupplemented

glucocorticoid-treated patients. *Br J Anaesth* 1973; 45:1043–1048.

35. L. Knudsen, L.A Christiansen, J.E. Lorentzen. Hypotension during and after operation in glucocorticoid-treated patients. *Br J Anaesth* 1981; 51:295–301.

36. F.H. de Jong, C. Mallios, C. Jansen, P.A. Scheck, S.W. Lamberts. Etomidate suppresses adrenocortical function by inhibition of 11 beta-hydroxylation. *J Clin Endocrinol Metab* 1984; 59:1143–1147.

37. A. Majesko, J.M. Darby. Etomidate and adrenal insufficiency: the controversy continues. *Crit Care* 2010; 14:338. doi:10.1186/cc9338.

Chapter

5

Dysrhythmia

Eric Massey and Stephen O. Bader

- New perioperative dysrhythmia requires assessment of adequacy of ventilation, hemodynamics, electrolytes, and possible cardiac ischemia.
- Atrial fibrillation is a common dysrhythmia in the adult surgical patient and after non-thoracic surgery is often attributable to atrial stretch from intravascular volume expansion.
- Many dysrhythmias are transient and require only supportive care.

Dysrhythmias in the perioperative period can pose unique challenges to a physician in the Post-Anesthesia Care Unit (PACU). Diagnosing a dysrhythmia, finding an underlying etiology, and providing an appropriate treatment must all be accomplished quickly. Many perioperative arrhythmias are transient, while others can be sustained and symptomatic. The cause for dysrhythmias may be secondary to a patient's pathology, but can result from the many physiological disruptions caused by surgery and anesthesia.

Dysrhythmia classification and diagnosis requires an understanding of normal cardiac electrophysiology. Normally, the heart beats in an ordered electrical pathway. The sino-atrial (SA) node is the "pacemaker" of the heart and determines the heart rate. The SA node discharges an electrical signal to initiate atrial contraction. These impulses travel to the atrioventricular (AV) node via internodal atrial conduction pathways. The AV node serves to delay this signal on its way to the bundle of His conduction system of the ventricles. This delay allows for full atrial contraction prior to ventricular contraction, which optimizes stroke volume and cardiac output. The signal then passes from the bundle of His conduction system to divide into a left and right bundle branch. Finally the impulse travels down the ventricles via the Purkinje system to initiate ventricular contraction.[1] Abnormalities in signal initiation due to physiological disruption can cause ectopic beats, tachycardia, or bradycardia depending on the cause of disruption or location of the abnormal pacemaker.[2]

PACU standards dictate electrocardiogram (ECG) monitoring throughout recovery, and a systematic analysis of the ECG is helpful in diagnosis of dysrhythmia. The decision tree in Figure 5.1 shows one approach.

The initial assessment of the dysrhythmia patient should include pulse, blood pressure, peripheral perfusion demonstrated by capillary refill, and any indication of impaired organ perfusion, such as acute change in mental status. Acute cardiovascular collapse, indicated by

Post-Anesthesia Care: Symptoms, Diagnosis, and Management, ed. James W. Heitz. Published by Cambridge University Press. © Cambridge University Press 2016.

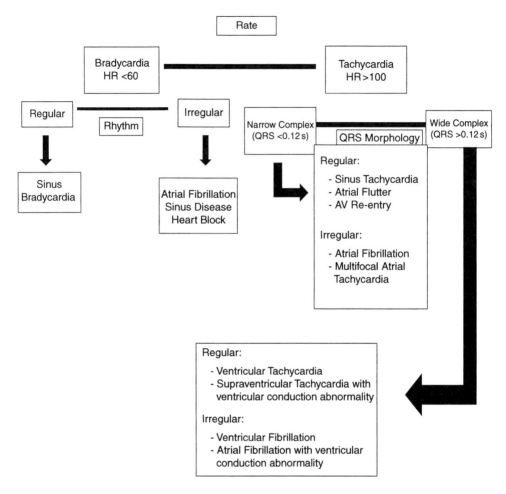

Figure 5.1 Decision tree.

loss of consciousness, pulselessness, or severe hypotension, necessitates immediate therapy. In a hemodynamically stable patient, establishing an etiology and treatment plan can be accomplished with less urgency.

Predisposing factors in the perioperative patient

Many predisposing factors result directly from recent surgery or anesthesia. Medical history and co-morbidities are important components in the initial work-up of patients with arrhythmia. Patients with diabetes, chronic obstructive pulmonary disease (COPD), and coronary artery disease (CAD) are more likely to have negative outcomes than those without.[3] Cardiac surgeries, craniotomies, and dental and ocular procedures have been correlated with increased incidences of arrhythmias. A recent medication history can be helpful in the differential diagnosis, as many chronic prescriptions are withheld prior to surgery, and many drugs new to the patient may be given on the day of surgery. Increased sympathetic outflow is common postoperatively and increases the risk of many dysrhythmias. Factors that contribute to the postoperative predisposition toward dysrhythmia can include:

- Hypercarbia or hypoxia
  - Obstructive sleep apnea (OSA) is a particularly dangerous cause of hypercarbia and hypoxia. Postoperatively, OSA frequently leads to hypercapnic respiratory acidosis and failure.
- Hyper/hypothermia
- Anemia
- Intravascular hypo/hypervolemia
- Pre-existing disease
  - Coronary disease: CAD is an important predisposing factor toward arrhythmias in the perioperative period.[4]
  - Pre-existing congenital arrhythmia disorders such as Wolff Parkinson White (WPW) are exacerbated postoperatively.
  - Intracranial disease, especially subarachnoid hemorrhage, can commonly lead to ST-T-wave changes and may easily mimic myocardial ischemia and infarction.[5]
- Myocardial infarction
  - Catecholamine levels (endogenous or iatrogenic) – catecholamine release increases cellular potassium uptake, leading to lower serum levels.
- Electrolyte, acid–base, and metabolic derangements
  - Intraoperative fluid therapy may lead to derangements in electrolytes vital for appropriate cardiac depolarization and contraction. Hypomagnesemia, hypo or hyperkalemia, and hypocalcemia are common in the PACU.
  - Hyperventilation due to inadequately treated pain or mechanical ventilation can lead to alkalosis and decrease levels of serum potassium. This phenomenon may precipitate severe cardiac arrhythmias.[6]
- Drug effects
  - Perioperative drugs that increase or potentiate endogenous catecholamines, such as ephedrine, cocaine, and ketamine, can facilitate the development of tachyarrhythmias.
  - Neuraxial anesthesia causes vasodilation and hypotension, leading to a compensatory tachycardia or to a bradycardia if the level of sympathectomy involves high thoracic cardiac accelerator nerves.
  - Intravascular injection or high total doses of infiltrated local anesthetics, particularly bupivacaine, may lead to asystole and cardiac arrest. This form of cardiac arrest can be very difficult to treat and requires prolonged CPR in many cases.[7]
    - 20% intralipid is the treatment option of choice in this situation; however, the exact mechanism of action is unclear.[8]
- Mechanical factors
  - Intravascular catheter or device placement
- Surgical factors
  - Cardiac surgery: Cannulation of the major vessels of the heart, cross clamping of the aorta, and direct manipulation of the myocardium lead to higher incidences of arrhythmias following cardiac surgery.

- Dental surgery leads to sympathetic and parasympathetic excitation and can be associated with generation of arrhythmias.[9] Junctional rhythms can be directly correlated to trigeminal nerve (CN V) irritation.
- Eye surgery can induce the oculocardiac reflex, leading to severe bradycardia in response to traction on the rectus muscles of the orbit. The reflex arc comprises CN V stimulation and subsequent stimulation of the vagus nerve (CN X). Children and neonates following strabismus surgery may demonstrate an exaggerated response.

Increased vagal tone in any fashion can be pro-arrhythmic. Profound sinus bradycardias, ventricular escape beats, heart block, and asystole have been observed following actions that increase vagal tone. Traction of peritoneum and abdominal mesentery, direct pressure on the vagus nerve during carotid surgery, jugular vein cannulation, and carotid sinus palpation are all possible causes of increased vagal tone.[1] It seems appropriate that an initial goal in postoperative dysrhythmia therapy should be to identify and remove causative and correctable predisposing factors in the recovery room. The stress response and derangements in normal physiology resulting from surgery continue past the recovery phase, and therefore, appropriate post-recovery therapy, consultation, level of care, and monitoring should be considered prior to discharge from the PACU.

Bradyarrhythmias

Bradycardia is defined as a heart rate <60 bpm. Bradycardia can occur frequently in healthy patients and is often of little clinical consequence. However, heart rates <40 bpm are poorly tolerated in most individuals and can lead to hemodynamic compromise. Transient bradycardias are frequent in the PACU, but therapy is not indicated unless bradycardia recurs or is symptomatic. As described previously, increased vagal tone can be an etiology for bradyarrhythmias. Sustained symptomatic bradycardias should be treated initially with intravenous (IV) atropine 0.5 to 1 mg, while an external pacing system is retrieved.[10] The total dose of atropine should not exceed 3 mg.[11] Beta-agonists such as epinephrine or dopamine may be useful if the bradycardia is refractory to anticholinergic therapy. Percutaneous or transvenous pacing should follow if pharmacological intervention is not successful.

Tachycardias

A QRS segment is either described as narrow complex (<0.12 seconds) or wide complex (>0.12 seconds). Narrow complex arrhythmias usually demonstrate supraventricular tachycardia (SVT), and wide complex arrhythmias originate in the ventricle or represent SVT with a pre-existing bundle branch block (BBB) or other intraventricular conduction delay.

Supraventricular tachycardias

Supraventricular tachycardias usually are narrow QRS complex, unless the patient has a concurrent BBB, have a heart rate >100 bpm, and they may or may not contain P waves. Supraventricular indicates an atrial or nodal origin for the tachycardia. Estimated incidence following non-cardiac surgery is about 3–4% and even as high as 37% following total pneumonectomy.[12]

Sinus tachycardia

Sinus tachycardia is common postoperatively. Causes can include anxiety, pain, fever, hypovolemia, anemia, hypoxemia, hypercarbia, and perioperative medications. There is no conduction abnormality in sinus tachycardia, and treatment consists of improving the underlying cause. Rate control with β-blockers or calcium channel blockers is reasonable, especially in patients with coronary or stenotic valvular heart disease.

Atrial tachycardia

Atrial tachycardias often originate from a separate ectopic pacer focus than the SA node, or they are caused by reentrant pathways. Atrial tachycardias are more common in children than in adults, but they comprise about 8% of paroxysmal SVTs in adults. These tachycardias can be identified by P-wave morphologies that are different than that of sinus rhythm.

Multifocal atrial tachycardia (MFAT)

This atrial tachycardia is usually seen in acutely ill, elderly patients. It is also seen in patients with significant pulmonary disease.[13] In MFAT, there are three or more different P-wave morphologies, and the rhythm is irregularly irregular. Predisposing factors include hypoxia, hypercapnia, myocardial infarction, congestive heart failure, and electrolyte disturbances. Beta-blockers, calcium channel blockers, and amiodarone are mainstays in therapy.[14]

AV nodal reentry tachycardia

AV nodal reentry is the most common SVT, accounting for 60% of SVTs.[15] Accessory pathways from the atria to ventricle lead to multiple depolarizations of the ventricle. P waves are usually absent, or unusually shaped. Simultaneous forward and reverse signal conduction across the AV node and accessory pathway cause the aberrant P-wave morphology. Management can consist of maneuvers designed to increase vagal tone and obliterate the reentrant signal propagation. These include Valsalva maneuvers and carotid massage among others. Adenosine (6–12 mg IV) can also break the reentry process, and owing to its short half-life, it has few side effects. Adenosine has some diagnostic usefulness as well. If significant cardiovascular compromise exists, electrical cardioversion may be indicated. Calcium channel blockers and digoxin can inhibit AV nodal conduction and allow for unopposed accessory pathway conduction and rapid atrial fibrillation (AF) in susceptible patients, such as those with WPW.[10]

Atrial fibrillation

AF is an irregularly irregular rhythm, usually with a narrow QRS. Rate control is the acute goal in AF, because the shortened filling time during diastole due to tachycardia can lead to decreased stroke volume and cardiac output.

AF is the most common postoperative arrhythmia. AF has been reported in up to 15% to 40% of patients[16] following coronary artery bypass graft (CBAG) surgery, as high as 85%[17] following CABG and valve surgeries, and is less frequent at around 3%[18] in non-cardiac surgery. Postoperative factors that contribute to AF include pericardial inflammation, hypovolemia or volume overload, cardiac ischemia, electrolyte imbalances, and increased sympathetic tone. AF is associated with significant morbidity and mortality even when it occurs briefly and can increase the risk of stroke 3–4 fold.[19]

Preoperative and early postoperative β blockade has been recommended to prevent AF.[20] Unless contraindicated, IV β blockade with metoprolol 1–5 mg IV can be repeated until rate control is achieved. Diltiazem infusion is commonly used in patients that may not tolerate β blockade.

Amiodarone is effective at acutely controlling rate and converting AF to a sinus rhythm. Digoxin can also be used for acute rate control and is especially useful in heart failure patients. Conversion to sinus rhythm in patients with undiagnosed chronic AF without first ruling out atrial thrombus may lead to embolic events.

Ventricular tachycardia

Ventricular arrhythmias are traditionally wide complex. They can contain ectopic ventricular beats, non-sustained ventricular tachycardia (VT), and sustained VT and fibrillation (VF). Sustained VT is defined as three or more consecutive beats or >30 seconds in duration.

Identifying dangerous ventricular arrhythmias should primarily consist of determining whether the rhythm is benign or malignant, paroxysmal or sustained, and whether hemodynamic compromise exists. Pre-existing structural heart disease is a key feature in determining outcome and progression to dangerous VTs. When caring for patients with significant heart disease and concurrent ventricular ectopy or limited runs of ventricular arrhythmias, one should have a high level of caution.[10] These ECG anomalies can be predictors for more dangerous sustained ventricular arrhythmias and sudden cardiac death. These patients should receive prompt evaluation and reversal of possible predisposing factors.

The treatment of VT, if stable with a pulse, is amiodarone 150 mg IV over 10–30 minutes followed by an infusion of 1 mg/min for 6 hours, which is then followed by 0.5 mg/min for 18 hours or more. Repeat loading doses of amiodarone, synchronized cardioversion, lidocaine, and procainamide are secondary treatments that may be useful if the rhythm persists.

Sustained ventricular arrhythmia can cause cardiovascular collapse (pulseless VT), and immediate intervention must be instituted to treat the patient using American Heart Association Advanced Cardiac Life Support (ACLS) algorithms, which now support a CAB (circulation, airway, and breathing) model instead of the traditional ABCs of American Heart Association Basic Life Support (BLS). The provider should start immediate chest compressions, secure effective ventilation with patent airway or with ETT, and synchronized electrical cardioversion or defibrillation with 200–360 J for monophasic devices or 120–200 J for a biphasic device. Epinephrine is given 1 mg at 3-minute intervals, vasopressin 40 U at 10-minute intervals. If pulseless VT persists give 300 mg amiodarone IV bolus, and if unsuccessful after 10 minutes, follow with another bolus of amiodarone 150 mg IV. This should be followed with amiodarone 1 mg/min IV infusion for 6 hours. Lidocaine 1–1.5 mg/kg IV loading dose and a 0.5–0.75 mg/kg repeat dose at 3-minute intervals may also be helpful.[21]

Ventricular fibrillation

VF is an irregular rhythm that results from one or multiple rapidly firing foci of electrical activity. Ventricular contractions resulting from this erratic electrical activity are uncoordinated and provide little or no cardiac output. A patient in VF needs CPR or other artificial means to maintain perfusion. Heart rate is indeterminable, and there is no discernible rhythm. There are no P waves or QRS complexes seen. VF accounts for 80% to 85% of sudden cardiac deaths.[22] It is usually preceded by VT, but also may occur as a primary arrhythmia. The most common cause of VF is acute myocardial infarction. It also is observed in patients with chronic ischemic heart disease, hypoxia, acidosis, hypokalemia, and massive hemorrhage.

The management of VF is identical to treatment of pulseless VT as above: immediate initiation of chest compressions and electrical defibrillation according to ACLS algorithms. Epinephrine 1 mg at 3-minute intervals, vasopressin 40 U at 10-minute intervals, and magnesium 1 g are all used in addition to antiarrhythmics.[22]

Torsades de pointes

VT is differentiated by the morphology of the complexes. If all complexes are alike the arrhythmia is termed monomorphic, and if they are constantly changing in appearance the arrhythmia is termed polymorphic. Torsades de pointes is a polymorphic VT that results from a prolonged QT interval and is often secondary to medications. Torsades can be caused by "R on T" phenomena, when pacing or unsynchronized cardioversion electrical energy is delivered during repolarization of the myocardium.[23] Torsades de pointes can quickly degenerate into VF. Premature ventricular contractions that occur during a prolonged repolarization period can initiate torsades, and the chance of converting to a torsades rhythm is higher if a patient has bradycardia. This concept supports the use of agents that increase heart rate, e.g. isoproterenol, or external pacing as immediate treatment in patients with related torsades.[21] Magnesium therapy is a mainstay in treatment for torsades that is refractory to cardioversion.[24]

References

1. S.A. Irefin. Anesthesia for correction of cardiac arrhythmias in *Miller's Anesthesia*, 7th edition (ed. R.D. Miller) Philadelphia: Churchill Livingstone, 2010, Chapter 61, pp. 1977–1986.

2. R.D. Gajulapalli, F. Rader. *Postoperative Arrhythmias*, Case Western Reserve University; http://www.intechopen.com/.

3. U. Wolters, T. Wolf, H. Stutzer, T. Schrode. ASA classification and perioperative variables as predictors of postoperative outcome. *Br J Anaesth* 1996; 77:217–222.

4. L. Angelini, M.I. Feldman, R. Lufschonowski, R.D. Leachman. Cardiac arrhythmias during and after heart surgery: diagnosis and management. *Prog Cardiovasc Dis* 1974; 16:469–495.

5. M.A. Samuel. The brain–heart connection. *Circulation* 2007; 116:77–84.

6. R. Edwards, A.P. Winnie, S. Ramamurthy. Acute hypocapneic hypokalemia: an iatrogenic anesthetic complication. *Anesth Analg* 1977; 56:786–792.

7. S. Reiz, S. Nath. Cardiotoxicity of local anesthetic agents. *Br J Anaesth* 1986; 58:736–746.

8. G. Weinberg. Lipid infusion resuscitation for local anesthetic toxicity: proof of clinical efficacy. *Anesthesiology* 2006; 105:7–8.

9. J.P. Alexander. Dysrhythmia and oral surgery. *Br J Anaesth* 1971; 43:773–778.

10. S.M. Hollenberg, R.P. Dellinger. Noncardiac surgery: postoperative arrhythmias; *Crit Care Med* 2000; 28(10 Suppl):N145–N150.

11. D. Dublin. *Rapid Interpretation of EKGs*, 6th edition. New York: Cover Publishing Company, 2000.

12. T. Saran, G.D. Perkins, M.A. Javed, et al. Does the prophylactic administration of magnesium sulphate to patients undergoing thoracotomy prevent postoperative supraventricular arrhythmias? A randomized controlled trial. *Br J Anaesth* 2011; 106:785–791.

13. J. McCord, S. Borzak. Multifocal atrial tachycardia. *Chest* 1998; 113:203–209.

14. J.H. Levine, J.R. Michael, T. Guarneri. Treatment of multifocal atrial tachycardia with verapamil. *N Engl J Med* 1985; 312:21–25.

15. J.A. Kastor. *Arrhythmias*. Philadelphia: WB Saunders, 1994.

16. J.P. Mathew, M.L. Fontes, I.C. Tudor, et al.; Investigators of the Ischemia Research and Education Foundation. Multicenter study of perioperative ischemia research group: a multicenter risk index for atrial fibrillation after cardiac surgery. *JAMA* 2004; 291:1720–1729.

17. S.B. Sloan, H.H. Weitz. Postoperative arrhythmias and conduction disorders. *Med Clin North Am* 2001; 85:1171–1189.

18. L. Goldman. Supraventricular tachyarrhythmias in hospitalized adults after surgery. Clinical correlates in patients over 40 years of age after major noncardiac surgery. *Chest* 1978; 73:450–454.

19. P.P. McKeown. American College of Chest Physicians guidelines for the management of postoperative atrial fibrillation after cardiac surgery. *Chest* 2005; 128(Suppl):6S–8S.

20. K.A. Eagle, R.A. Guyton, R. Davidoff, et al. ACC/AHA 2004 guideline update for coronary artery bypass graft surgery: Summary article. A report of the American College of Cardiology/American Heart Association Task Force on practice guidelines (Committee to Update the 1999 Guidelines for Coronary Artery Bypass Graft Surgery). *J Am Coll Cardiol* 2004; 44:e213–e310.

21. J.M Field. *Advanced Cardiovascular Life Support Provider Manual* Part 4 p. 42.

22. J.P. DiMarco. Work-up and management of sudden cardiac death survivors. *Cardiol Clin* 1993; 11:11–19.

23. C. Napolitano, S.G. Priori, P.J. Schwartz. Torsade de pointes: mechanisms and management. *Drugs* 1994; 47:51–65.

24. D. Tzivoni, S. Banai, C. Schuger, et al. Magnesium therapy for torsades de pointes. *Circulation* 1988; 77:392–397.

Chest pain

Jeremy L. Hensley and Stephen O. Bader

- Myocardial ischemia after non-cardiac surgery may peak during the early postoperative period, as opposed to postoperative day 2 as previously thought.
- Postoperative cardiac ischemia may not present with chest pain, so hemodynamic instability should alert the care giver to possible ischemia.
- A high degree of suspicion for pulmonary embolism or pneuomothorax should be held for the surgical patient in the early postoperative period.
- Referred pain to the left shoulder or arm from diaphragmatic irritation of retained insufflation gas may mimic angina after laparoscopic procedures.

Healthcare providers in the Post-Anesthesia Care Unit (PACU) may infrequently encounter patients experiencing chest pain in the immediate postoperative period. Because of the life-threatening nature of many causes of chest pain, a thorough evaluation should begin in the PACU. Some of these patients may require immediate intervention before any diagnostic work-up can be initiated. This may include application of supplemental oxygen, intubation and mechanical ventilation, intravenous fluid administration, and treatment with vasopressors. At a minimum, diagnostic tests including routine laboratory evaluation with cardiac biomarkers, a 12-lead electrocardiogram (ECG), and a chest film should be obtained. As with all patients experiencing chest pain, the patient in the immediate postoperative period must be evaluated in the context of individual medical history, hospital diagnoses, and the procedures performed.

Myocardial ischemia and infarction

Myocardial ischemia occurs when there is an imbalance between myocardial oxygen supply and demand. This imbalance may occur in the perioperative period by several mechanisms. Perioperative catecholamine elevations may contribute to increases in both heart rate and blood pressure (increased cardiac demand) while simultaneous increases in coronary artery sheer forces may contribute to coronary plaque rupture (decreasing blood supply). Additionally, surgically induced release of cytokines and other proinflammatory mediators may contribute to a hypercoagulable state, precipitating coronary thrombosis. Most patients experiencing perioperative myocardial infarction (MI) have pre-existing coronary atherosclerosis. The chest discomfort of myocardial ischemia, or angina pectoris, is frequently

Post-Anesthesia Care: Symptoms, Diagnosis, and Management, ed. James W. Heitz. Published by Cambridge University Press. © Cambridge University Press 2016.

described as heaviness, pressure, or squeezing. The location of the pain is usually retrosternal but may radiate to the neck, jaw, teeth, arms, or shoulders. The pain experienced with acute coronary syndromes such as unstable angina and MI is usually similar in quality but more prolonged and severe. Some patients with myocardial ischemia may experience atypical chest pain syndromes without traditional retrosternal pain or heaviness. Atypical chest pain is more common in the elderly, females, diabetics, and those with gastroesophageal reflux disease. Perioperative MI is often silent after both non-cardiac[1] and cardiac procedures,[2] so a high degree of suspicion for ischemia must be held for patients with hemodynamic instability after surgery even in the absence of classic chest pain or anginal symptoms.

Ischemia is an infrequent event in the PACU. One study demonstrated an incidence of 0.3% of PACU patients being admitted to the Intensive Care Unit (ICU) to rule out MI.[3] Of these, only 7.5% actually sustained an MI. However, the outcomes can be devastating, as 50% died during their hospital stay as a result of complications associated with their acute MI. In addition, another study noted that the incidence of perioperative MI was higher (5.6%) in patients with documented ischemic heart disease diagnosed by cardiac biomarkers and ECG monitoring.[4] Another major finding of this study was that peak incidence of perioperative MI occurred during the first postoperative night, in contrast to previous studies which showed a peak around postoperative day 2. Only 17% of these patients presented with chest pain, an unexpectedly low number which may have been reduced by concomitant opioid use.

Evaluation: As with any patient experiencing acute chest discomfort, the patient with suspected ischemia should be assessed for hemodynamic and respiratory compromise. Once initially stabilized, the patient should be evaluated for potentially life-threatening conditions. Currently the American Society of Anesthesiologists (ASA) acknowledges that routine ECG monitoring may not be necessary for all patients and all procedures.[5] However, consultants for the ASA Task Force on Postanesthetic Care and surveyed ASA members agreed that routine pulse rate, blood pressure, and ECG monitoring detect cardiovascular complications and reduce adverse outcomes during emergence and recovery. Commonly, at least one lead is monitored. Lead I is best for detecting ischemia of the anterior wall, Lead II is best for inferior wall ischemia and often shows the P wave well, allowing for proper rhythm determination. There are institutional and practitioner preferences for choosing which lead to monitor; however, monitoring of additional leads, especially precordial V3–6, should be considered if left ventricular ischemia is likely.

If ischemia is suspected based on the presence of chest pain or cardiopulmonary instability, diagnosis should begin with a 12-lead ECG as well as cardiac biomarker levels. It should be noted that many postoperative ECGs are non-diagnostic, and pre-test probability must be taken into account. Non-specific ECG changes, new-onset dysrhythmias, and non-cardiac hemodynamic instability can obscure the diagnosis. In addition, false positive elevations in CK-MB are more common than true positives.[1] This finding is thought to be the result of tissue injury during surgery. The measurement of troponin-I levels avoids this problem and appears to be the ideal marker of myocardial injury in the perioperative period.[6] In addition, transthoracic echocardiography (Figure 6.1) may be a useful tool in evaluating global cardiac function and regional wall motion abnormalities, although this has not been studied in the PACU setting.

Management: Patients should be admitted to the ICU for at least 24 hours of observation. An ECG should be obtained in most patients. Invasive hemodynamic

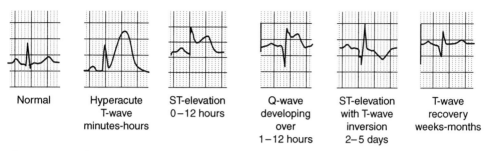

| Normal | Hyperacute T-wave minutes-hours | ST-elevation 0–12 hours | Q-wave developing over 1–12 hours | ST-elevation with T-wave inversion 2–5 days | T-wave recovery weeks-months |

Figure 6.1 Transthoracic echocardiography

monitoring, including an arterial line, central venous, or possibly pulmonary artery catheter, may be needed. All causes of tachycardia, hypertension, hypotension, anemia, and pain should be treated aggressively. Heart rate control is of paramount importance in acute ischemia. Six-month mortality and troponin levels are reduced by administration of β-blockers and optimization of the oxygen supply–demand ratio.[7] Reduced heart rate improves myocardial perfusion time during diastole. However, care must be taken to maintain adequate blood pressure with intravenous fluids while optimizing the heart rate. Nitroglycerin can be administered in the absence of hypotension. Nitroglycerin reduces ventricular wall tension by decreasing preload via venodilation, and may vasodilate coronary arteries. Morphine can be used to treat chest pain unresponsive to nitroglycerin. Morphine relieves anxiety and decreases heart rate, thereby reducing myocardial oxygen demand. Among medical patients experiencing MI, orally administered aspirin contributes substantial reduction (23%) to mortality.[8] With aspirin administration for the surgical patient one must weigh the risk of postoperative bleeding against the potential survival benefits. For most surgical patients, the benefits of aspirin will outweigh the risks when the clinical suspicion for MI is high. Patients for whom small quantities of bleeding may be devastating, including patients with recent intracranial, spinal, or ocular procedures, require special attention before a decision to administer aspirin is made. For patients who may benefit from aspirin but are not yet able to take oral medications, aspirin may be administered per rectum. Emergent coronary intervention, anticoagulants, or glycoprotein IIb/IIIa antagonists are rarely indicated owing to the risk of bleeding unless ST-segment elevation or intractable cardiogenic shock ensues.[9] In the perioperative setting, the use of these agents must be individualized based upon risk–benefit analysis, taking into account the risk of bleeding posed by the recent surgery.

Pulmonary embolism

Although surgical patients are a diverse group, there are characteristics that put this population at high risk of deep venous thrombosis (DVT) and thus pulmonary embolism (PE). These factors include total hip and knee replacement, surgery for hip fracture, surgery for cancer, trauma patients, following spinal cord injury, and immobilization.[10] Pleuritic chest pain is seen in 44% of patients experiencing acute pulmonary embolism.[11] Other symptoms include dyspnea, cough, orthopnea, lower extremity pain or swelling, and wheezing. Signs include tachypnea, tachycardia, rales, decreased breath sounds, an accentuated pulmonic component of the second heart sound, and jugular venous

Table 6.1 Wells criteria and modified Wells criteria: clinical assessment for pulmonary embolism

Clinical symptoms of DVT (leg swelling, pain with palpation)	3.0
Other diagnosis less likely than (PE)	3.0
Heart rate >100 bpm	1.5
Immobilization (>3 days) or surgery in the previous 4 weeks	1.5
Previous DVT/PE	1.5
Hemoptysis	1.5
Malignancy	1.0
Probability	**Score**
Traditional clinical probability assessment (Wells criteria)	
High	>6.0
Moderate	2.0 to 6.0
Low	<2.0
Simplified clinical probability assessment (modified Wells criteria)	
PE likely	>4.0
PE unlikely	≤4.0

Data from van Belle, A. *et al.* JAMA 2006; 295:172–179. [12]

distension. Circulatory collapse is uncommon, but massive PE may be accompanied by acute right heart failure. It is important to keep in mind that many of these symptoms, including chest pain, may be masked in the acute postoperative period.

Evaluation: Many tests can be used to contribute to the diagnosis of PE. However, in 2006, The Christopher Study proposed a simplified algorithm for evaluating the patient suspected of having a PE.[12] Here, patients were first evaluated by the modified Wells criteria and categorized as PE unlikely (score ≤4) or PE likely (score >4). Scoring for the modified Wells criteria can be found in Table 6.1. If PE was unlikely by these criteria, the diagnosis was excluded if the D-dimer level was normal. All other patients underwent CT-pulmonary angiography (CT-PA). The application of these criteria in immediately postoperative patients can be difficult, and many postoperative patients will have a positive D-dimer due to surgical trauma. Therefore, most patients clinically suspected of having PE in the PACU should be evaluated by CT-PA as soon as possible. If CT-PA is inconclusive, pulmonary angiography is recommended.

Management: The initial management of suspected PE should focus on respiratory and hemodynamic support. Severe hypoxemia and respiratory failure should be treated with intubation and mechanical ventilation, keeping in mind that patients with right heart failure are prone to hypotension. Hypotension should be managed initially with intravenous fluid administration. One study found that administration of 500 ml of dextran significantly improves cardiac index in patients with PE.[13] If hemodynamic status does not improve, vasopressors may be required; however, an optimal agent has yet to be determined. Beyond supportive therapy, anticoagulation with unfractionated heparin is the next step of therapy for acute PE. Patients in the immediate postoperative period are likely to be at high risk for excessive bleeding; thus anticoagulation and thrombolytic therapy may not be possible after many procedures. In these cases, placement of an inferior vena cava filter is an acceptable alternative to prevent further embolism. Percutaneous or open surgical embolectomy may be considered in cases with severe hypotension or hypoxemia despite supportive therapy.

Pneumothorax

Pneumothorax (PTX) may occur in the perioperative patient because of complications of central venous access placement, barotrauma from positive pressure ventilation, or direct surgical trauma. PTX usually presents in the mechanically ventilated patient shortly after the inciting event. In the intubated patient, PTX may be suspected following the onset of high peak inspiratory pressures and possibly hypotension. However, the presentation may be delayed until PACU admission. Signs and symptoms of PTX include chest pain, dyspnea, tachypnea, unequal or unilaterally absent breath sounds, and hyperresonance to percussion on the affected side. Suspicion of PTX should be increased in the setting of recent subclavian central line placement, intercostal nerve blocks, chest trauma, or surgery at or near the diaphragm (liver resection, nephrectomy, splenectomy, hiatal hernia repair, gastric or esophageal resection).

Evaluation: Tension PTX can lead to rapid hemodynamic collapse and therefore requires rapid diagnosis and treatment. Signs include hypotension, tachycardia, tracheal deviation, completely absent breath sounds on the affected side, and jugular venous distension. PTX is often evaluated initially by chest X-ray. This evaluation can be performed in upright, supine, or lateral decubitus positions. Frequently, portable anteroposterior chest X-ray in the semi-upright position is the most quickly obtained exam in the PACU. However, the lateral decubitus position is most sensitive and is able to detect as little as 5 ml of pleural gas.[14] CT scanning is the most accurate diagnostic modality. Bedside ultrasound has also been used to screen for evidence of PTX in emergent situations. A systematic review has demonstrated that this modality is more sensitive and specific than the supine chest X-ray.[15] Although bedside ultrasound may be useful to the anesthesiologist in diagnosing PTX in the PACU, its use has not been well-documented in this setting.

Management: Small pneumothoraces (<15% of the hemithorax) may be observed for spontaneous reabsorption by serial chest radiographs. Suspected tension PTX should be treated with immediate tube thoracostomy or needle decompression. For the latter, a 14-gauge angiocatheter can be used. A length of up to 7 cm may be needed. Acceptable puncture sites include the second or third intercostal space in the midclavicular line or the fifth intercostal space in the midaxillary line. Needle decompression should produce an audible rush of air, and be followed by chest tube placement as soon as possible.

Chest pain following laparoscopic surgery

Following laparoscopic surgery, the majority of patients report pain in the upper abdomen, but many may report pain radiating to the chest or right shoulder. This pain is thought to result from the presence of residual pneumoperitoneum following surgery. In fact, one study demonstrated decreased opioid requirement in patients in whom residual pneumoperitoneum was actively aspirated following laparoscopic cholecystectomy.[16]

Evaluation: Residual pneumoperitoneum as a cause of postoperative chest pain should be considered a diagnosis of exclusion. The anesthesiologist should first evaluate the patient for potentially life-threatening causes of chest pain. If the pain persists or is accompanied by abdominal pain, a CT scan may be ordered to rule out a perforated viscus.

Management: A review of literature has found that non-steroidal anti-inflammatory drugs (NSAIDs), intraperitoneal bupivacaine, saline, and wound infiltration of local anesthetic can decrease postoperative pain following laparoscopic cholecystectomy.[17] Interestingly, one study demonstrated that blockade of the right phrenic nerve following intubation, and before abdominal insufflation, decreased the incidence of shoulder pain. Since the pain related to laparoscopy is likely multifactorial, a multimodal approach to analgesia in the PACU is warranted.

Chest wall pain

Chest pain occurring in the PACU may be the result of direct injury to the chest wall. This may be due to positioning, for example improper placement of an axillary roll for procedures in the lateral decubitus position. Blunt chest trauma and rib fractures are also common causes. In addition, chest wall pain may be the result of surgical trauma, i.e. post-thoracotomy pain. The latter is particularly important to the practice of anesthesiology because it is considered to be one of the most severe postoperative pain experiences known. Post-thoracotomy pain contributes to morbidity as postoperative pulmonary dysfunction. In addition, chronic post-thoracotomy pain is a common problem that may be seen in up to 50% of patients evaluated 2 years after surgery.[18]

Evaluation: Chest wall pain should be considered only after potentially life-threatening causes of chest pain have been ruled out. These may include MI or chest tube complications such as malfunction or improper placement.

Management: The management of post-thoracotomy pain in the acute postoperative period has been studied extensively. Recommendations have been made for the management of acute post-thoracotomy pain based on the few studies that are well-designed and controlled.[19] Systemic opioids are considered the cornerstone of therapy to which all other modalities are compared. The following techniques are associated with decreased opioid requirement and pain scores: indwelling intercostal catheters with bupivacaine, indwelling intrapleural catheters with bupivacaine, epidural morphine (with an infusion via the thoracic route or bolus administration via the lumbar route), combined thoracic epidural infusion of bupivacaine with either thoracic epidural or intravenous sufentanil, thoracic epidural fentanyl, and systemic NSAIDs as adjuncts to systemic opioids. Low-dose intramuscular ketamine is another promising adjunct. Regardless of the approach used, adequate control of pain in the acute postoperative period may decrease the likelihood of developing chronic post-thoracotomy pain.[16] In the PACU, the treatment options should be based on the pain management plan that was chosen preoperatively. For example, if the patient has an epidural catheter in place, the anesthesiologist may choose bolus administration of either opioid or local anesthetic via this route. Systemic opioids and NSAIDs should also be considered.

Patients with multiple rib fractures are likely to come to the operating room for other injuries. Patients with fewer than three rib fractures may have intercostal nerve blocks in place. For patients requiring immediate operative management, postoperative pain control is usually instituted with systemic opioids. Epidural analgesia is often considered once the patient's condition is stabilized.[20] Thus, treatment of chest wall pain from rib fractures in the PACU depends on the patient's condition as well as the presence or absence of an epidural catheter.

References

1. J.E. Adams, G.A. Sicard, B.T. Allen, et al. Diagnosis of perioperative myocardial infarction with measurement of cardiac troponin I. *N Engl J Med* 1994; 330:670–674.

2. R.C. Smith, J.M. Leung, D.T. Mangano. Postoperative myocardial ischemia in patients undergoing coronary artery bypass graft surgery. S.P.I. Research Group. *Anesthesiology* 1991; 74:464–473.

3. R. Hines, P.G. Barash, G. Watrous, et al. Complications occurring in the postanesthesia care unit: a survey. *Anesth Analg* 1992; 74:503–509.

4. N.H. Badner, R.L. Knill, J.E. Brown, et al. Myocardial infarction after noncardiac surgery. *Anesthesiology* 1998; 88:572–578.

5. J.L. Apfelbaum, Silverstein JH, Chung FF, et al.; American Society of Anesthesiologists Task Force on Postanesthetic Care. Practice guidelines for postanesthetic care: an updated report by the American Society of Anesthesiologists Task Force on Postanesthetic Care. *Anesthesiology* 2013; 118:291–307.

6. J.E. Adams, G.S. Bodor, V.G. Davila-Roman, et al. Cardiac troponin I: a marker with high specificity for cardiac injury. *Circulation* 1993; 88:101–106.

7. E. Martinez, L. Kim, B. Rosenfeld, et al. Early detection and real-time intervention of postoperative myocardial ischemia: the STOPMI study. *Abstract presented at: Association of University Anesthesiologists*; May 16–18, 2008; Durham, NC.

8. ISIS-2 (Second International Study of Infarct Survival) Collaborative Group. Randomized trial of intravenous streptokinase, oral aspirin, both, or neither among 17,187 cases of suspected acute myocardial infarction: ISIS-2. *Lancet* 1988; 332:349–360.

9. P.B. Berger, V.R. Bellot, M.R. Bell, et al. An immediate invasive strategy for the treatment of acute myocardial infarction early after noncardiac surgery. *Am J Cardiol* 2001; 87:1100–1102.

10. V.F. Tapson. Acute pulmonary embolism. *N Engl J Med* 2008; 358:1037–1052.

11. P.D. Stein, A. Beemath, F. Matta, et al. Clinical characteristics of patients with acute pulmonary embolism: data from PIOPED II. *Am J Med* 2007; 120:871–879.

12. A. van Belle, H.R. Buller, M.V. Huisman, et al. Effectiveness of managing suspected pulmonary embolism using an algorithm combining clinical probability, D-dimer testing and computed tomography. *JAMA* 2006; 295:172–179.

13. A. Mercat, J.L. Diehl, G. Meyer, et al. Hemodynamic effects of fluid loading in acute massive pulmonary embolism. *Crit Care Med* 1999; 27:540–544.

14. J.J. Carr, J.C. Reed, R.H. Choplin, et al. Plain and computed radiography for detecting experimentally induced pneumothorax in cadavers: implications for detection in patients. *Radiology* 1992; 183:193–199.

15. R.G. Wilkerson, M.B. Stone. Sensitivity of bedside ultrasound and supine anteroposterior chest radiographs for the identification of pneumothorax after blunt trauma. *Acad Emerg Med* 2010; 17:11–17.

16. B. Fredman, R. Jedeikin, D. Olsfanger, et al. Residual pneumoperitoneum: a cause of postoperative pain after laparoscopic cholecystectomy. *Anesth Analg* 1994; 79:152–154.

17. V.L. Wills, D.R. Hunt. Pain after laparoscopic cholecystectomy. *Br J Surg* 2000; 87:273–284.

18. W.A. Pluijms, M.A.H. Steegers, A.F.T.M. Verhagen, et al. Chronic post-thoracotomy pain: a retrospective study. *Acta Anaesthesiol Scand* 2006; 50:804–808.

19. B.P. Kavanagh, J. Katz, A.N. Sandler, et al. Pain control after thoracic surgery: a review of current techniques. *Anesthesiology* 1994; 81:737–759.

20. M.K. Karmakar, A.M. Ho. Acute pain management of patients with multiple fractured ribs. *J Trauma* 2003; 54:615–625.

ECG changes

Adam W. Green and Stephen O. Bader

- Non-specific ECG changes are common after surgery and anesthesia.
- Mild QT-interval prolongation is commonly observed after surgery and anesthesia.
- ST-segment depression or elevation should raise suspicion for possible cardiac ischemia.

Just as general anesthesia is considered the greatest medical discovery of the nineteenth century, electrocardiography (ECG) may be considered one of the greatest discoveries of the twentieth century.[1] First invented in 1901 by William Einthoven, the ECG still aids today in clinical cardiac diagnosis and therapy.[2] The consultants and American Society of Anesthesiology (ASA) members surveyed for the ASA practice advisory on post-anesthetic care recommend using pulse rate, blood pressure, and ECG (in selected patients) for monitoring circulation along with attention to oxygenation, ventilation, level of consciousness and temperature in the Post-Anesthesia Care Unit (PACU).[3] There are many ECG changes that occur commonly in the PACU. Some ECG changes could represent a normal variant within the population requiring no intervention, while others can signal life-threatening conditions that require immediate intervention. ECG interpretation consists of specific findings such as the heart rate, the rhythm, the axis, evidence of hypertrophy, and any evidence of ischemia or infarction. Combining these specific findings with the patient's presenting signs and symptoms can lead to a final diagnosis and management plan.

Tachycardia

The normal QRS complex lasts from 0.06 to 0.12 seconds. Tachycardia can be classified as either narrow or widened QRS complex tachycardia. Narrow QRS complex tachycardia reflects rapid activation of the ventricles. Widened QRS complex tachycardia reflects abnormally slow ventricular activation. One of the most common ECG changes found in the PACU is sinus tachycardia.[4] A normal heart rate ranges from 60 to 100 beats per minute (bpm). Tachycardia increases myocardial oxygen consumption, decreases myocardial oxygen supply, and decreases cardiac output by shortening ventricular filling time, which could be detrimental to a patient with an already

Post-Anesthesia Care: Symptoms, Diagnosis, and Management, ed. James W. Heitz. Published by Cambridge University Press. © Cambridge University Press 2016.

compromised myocardium. Patients with underlying coronary disease are at an increased risk for myocardial infarction (MI), when tachycardic.

Symptoms: The symptoms of tachycardia are broad. Patients could complain of acute chest pain, shortness of breath, a feeling of impending doom, or palpitations could be the lone symptom. Tachycardia is frequently the result of incisional pain, hypotension secondary to hypovolemia, hemorrhage, or fever.

Diagnosis: Narrow QRS complex tachycardia is characterized by QRS complex <120 ms. Sinus tachycardia, atrial fibrillation, and paroxysmal supraventricular tachycardias (PSVTs) are examples of frequently encountered narrow complex tachycardias in the PACU. Sinus tachycardia can be easily diagnosed with an ECG tracing showing a heart rate >100 bpm and sinus rhythm. Sinus tachycardia has a broad differential diagnosis. It is important to rule out the life-threatening causes initially. Widened QRS complex tachycardias are characterized by QRS complex >120 ms, such as ventricular tachycardia.

Management: Management of most tachycardias involves treating the inciting disorder. If the patient is unstable, with hypotension, impaired vital organ function, or imminent cardiac arrest: immediate intervention is required.[5] Unstable wide complex tachycardia should be treated by the ACLS algorithm immediately. Synchronized cardioversion should be performed with sedation if the patient is still stable and conscious. For stable PSVT, vagal maneuvers such as bearing down to increase abdominal pressure will terminate up to 25% of cases.[6] Intravenous adenosine can be used when vagal maneuvers fail, as an alternative to electrical cardioversion. For all tachycardic patients, the preload should be optimized with intravenous fluids or blood transfusion when anemic, pain should be controlled, patient body temperature should be corrected with antipyretics or warming blankets, and acidosis, electrolyte abnormalities, or respiratory disorders should be corrected. Reduction of the heart rate while correcting the underlying cause can be initially accomplished with β-blockers or calcium channel blockers in most patients with narrow complex tachycardia, including atrial fibrillation.

Bradycardia and AV block

Bradycardia may be seen as a normal variant in the absence of heart disease in well-conditioned athletes, some elderly, and in otherwise healthy patients. In the postoperative period, bradycardias are common secondary to anesthetics and analgesics given in the operating room and PACU. Increased vagal tone due to heightened central parasympathetic activity and sympathetic withdrawal on the sinoatrial node can be associated with profound bradycardia. The normal PR interval is 0.12 to 0.20 seconds. This represents the amount of time an impulse travels from the beginning of atrial depolarization to the beginning of ventricular depolarization. These impulses become delayed or interrupted in atrioventricular (AV) block. AV blocks are classified as first, second, or third degree. These blocks may be caused by medications, electrolyte disturbances, and anatomical or structural problems.

Symptoms: Patients can have asymptomatic bradycardia with or without AV block. Bradycardia may be an incidental finding on ECG or present with symptoms such as fatigue, syncope, decreased mental status, or nausea and vomiting.

Diagnosis: Sinus bradycardia is classified as sinus rhythm with a rate below 60. *First degree AV block* is characterized on ECG by a prolonged PR interval >0.20 seconds, infrequently causes symptoms, and may be a side effect of β-blockers and many other medications. *Second degree AV block: Mobitz type I (Wenckebach)* consists of a progressive prolongation of the PR interval with successive beats followed by a dropped QRS complex. *Second degree AV block: Mobitz type II* is characterized on ECG by a non-conducted P wave, or "dropped QRS" not preceded by PR prolongation. *Third degree AV block* is characterized on ECG by complete dissociation between the atria and ventricles, with P waves and QRS complexes showing complete independence from one another. Along with ECG interpretation, the patient should be evaluated for signs and symptoms. Some causes of bradycardia could be exaggerated vagal activity from vomiting, coughing, or even from a tight collar with pressure on the carotid sinus, increased intracranial pressure, MI, obstructive sleep apnea, and medications. The Trendelenburg position following spinal anesthesia has been associated with severe bradycardia.[5]

Management: Asymptomatic or minimally symptomatic bradycardia requires no intervention. First degree AV block is generally benign and found incidentally on ECG. Second degree AV block: Mobitz type I (Wenckebach) is a block at the AV node and is usually transient, asymptomatic, and generally does not require immediate intervention, but may be the only sign of an underlying disorder. Second degree AV block: Mobitz type II is usually caused by pathology below the AV node, usually symptomatic, and may progress to third degree AV block. Management of symptomatic bradycardia depends on the severity. If the patient is unstable – hypotensive, showing signs of impaired vital organ function or imminent cardiac arrest – then ACLS should be initiated.[6] The initial treatment for symptomatic bradycardia is atropine. Atropine is an anticholinergic drug that increases the heart rate by blocking the effects of acetylcholine on the SA node.[7] The recommended dose is 0.5 mg IV every 3 to 5 minutes with a maximum dose of 3 mg.[6] Medication may be a temporary measure and transcutaneous pacing should be considered. Immediate pacing should be considered with third degree AV block and unstable patients unresponsive to atropine. Alternative medications to consider are catecholamines such as dopamine, epinephrine, isoproterenol, and dobutamine. Dopamine and epinephrine have α- and β-adrenergic actions, and infusions of either can be started at 2 to 10 mcg/kg/min. Isoproterenol is a β-adrenergic agent with a recommended dose of 2 to 10 mcg/min by infusion titrated to effect.[6] Dobutamine is another commonly used β-adrenergic agent, started at 2 to 10 mcg/kg/min. While both of these β-agonists are effective at increasing the heart rate, they can be associated with hypotension secondary to vasodilation.

Ventricular premature contractions/atrial premature contractions

The normal QRS interval is 0.06 to 0.12 seconds. This time reflects depolarization of the ventricles. The P wave represents atrial depolarization and is normally <0.12 seconds and amplitude <0.25 mV. APC is a common and insignificant finding both in the young and in the elderly. Atrial premature contractions (APCs) are commonly associated with medical conditions such as acute or chronic pulmonary disease, chronic renal failure, and neurological disorders. Ventricular premature contraction (VPC) is common during anesthetic recovery and most of the time is insignificant. However, new-onset VPC could progress to a more serious arrhythmia such as ventricular tachycardia or ventricular fibrillation.[2] VPCs are more likely to precede ventricular fibrillation when they are multiple, multifocal, or bigeminal.[2]

Symptoms: Most patients with APCs or VPCs are asymptomatic. Some may present with symptoms such as palpitations, chest pain, fatigue, or syncope. VPCs are common in patients with pre-existing cardiac disease.

Diagnosis: APC is characterized on ECG by an irregular rhythm, variable heart rate, and a premature P wave with aberrant morphology. APC may or may not create an abnormal QRS complex, making it difficult to distinguish from a VPC. One distinguishing feature is that there is no compensatory pause interval from the APC to the next sinus beat. The VPC often blocks the next depolarization of the SA node leading to a compensatory pause between the interval from VPC to the expected normal QRS complex.[2] VPC is characterized on ECG by an irregular rhythm, variable heart rate, no P wave, QRS complex >0.12 seconds. Consider underlying causes with VPC such as electrolyte abnormalities, trauma, and brainstem stimulation.

Management: No intervention is required for asymptomatic patients. Treat the underlying disorder such as electrolyte abnormalities, or acidosis. If VPCs are believed to be a herald to a more serious arrhythmia or are of any hemodynamic significance initial therapy with lidocaine 1.5 mg/kg intravenous may be appropriate.[2] Other medications to consider are β-blockers and calcium channel blockers. If progression to a more serious arrhythmia such as ventricular tachycardia or ventricular fibrillation develops, ACLS protocol should be initiated.

ST-segment and T-wave changes

The normal ST segment is isoelectric and represents the interval from the end of ventricular depolarization to the beginning of ventricular repolarization. The T wave represents repolarization of the ventricles. There are many types of abnormalities involving the ST segment and T wave, ranging from non-specific changes to an acute MI. One of the most important aspects of ECG is the ability to identify areas of ischemic or injured myocardium.

Symptoms: Signs and symptoms of acute myocardial ischemia can range from chest pain, nausea, jaw pain, shock, and arrhythmias, to being asymptomatic.

Diagnosis: Patients who are suspected of developing an acute MI should be diagnosed based on clinical presentation along with 12-lead ECG, and laboratory tests including creatine kinase, troponin, and myoglobin. ECG can show an ST-elevation MI or a non-ST-elevation MI. An acute ST-elevation MI evolves on ECG beginning with peaked T waves reflecting an increase in serum potassium concentration in the area of infarction, followed by elevation of the ST segment which appears concave then convex, and then merges with the T wave in different leads depending on the area of injury. These finding are also symmetric in at least two contiguous leads. This is followed by the development of Q waves and T-wave inversions as the ST segments return to baseline.[8,9] Patients who have a non-ST-elevation MI have T-wave flattening or inversion preceding ST segment depression. Q waves are typically absent but may occur[8,9] Non-specific changes can range from subtle straightening to flattening/depression of the ST segment, flattening or T-wave inversion. Differential diagnosis such as fever, electrolyte abnormalities, acidosis or alkalosis, and medications should be included.

Management: Acute ST-elevation MI is a medical emergency and therefore multiple therapies should be instituted simultaneously. The patient should receive supplemental oxygen and morphine for chest pain or anxiety relief. Nitrates should be considered if the patient is hypertensive, but avoided in cases where hypotension is more likely to occur, such as the hypovolemic postoperative patient, or patients with severe aortic stenosis. Beta-blockers should be given to reduce the heart rate if not contraindicated, and statin therapy should be initiated as early as possible. Cardiology should be consulted for possible percutaneous coronary intervention. Anticoagulation, as with aspirin therapy, must be carefully considered in the postoperative setting to assess whether the benefit outweighs the risk of bleeding.[10]

QT interval

The normal QT interval is between 0.33 and 0.44 seconds. This interval represents the total time for ventricular depolarization and repolarization. Prolongation of the QT interval can lead to a life-threatening arrhythmia known as torsades de pointes. QT prolongation can be congenital or acquired. QT prolongation is a common finding in stroke patients.[11] Many commonly used medications in the operating room and PACU can cause QT prolongation. QT prolongation is a common postoperative finding in patients undergoing non-cardiac surgery under general anesthesia, with an incidence of 4%.[12]

Symptoms: The vast majority of patients are asymptomatic, but they may present with palpitations, dizziness, chest pain, nausea, or shortness of breath.

Diagnosis: The QT interval varies inversely with the heart rate, and a QT interval corrected for the heart rate is known as the QTc. The QTc = QT interval ÷ square root of the RR interval.[13] The QT interval is considered prolonged when QTc >0.44 seconds in men and is extended to >0.46 seconds in women.[13] Causes of prolongation of the QT interval include hypokalemia, hypomagnesemia, and hypocalcemia. Many different drug classes prolong the QTc, such as anti-emetics (ondansetron, droperidol), antiarrhythmic drugs (quinidine, sotalol, and amiodarone), macrolide antibiotics (e.g. erythromycin), methadone, and many others.

Management: Most cases of simple QT prolongation require no treatment other than discontinuing the inciting medication and correcting the electrolytes. If hemodynamically unstable torsades de pointes develops, then prompt non-synchronized defibrillation is indicated. In conscious, stable patients with torsades, first-line therapy is IV magnesium. If no response to IV magnesium, temporary pacing should be considered.

References

1. N.J. Mehta, I.A. Khan. Cardiology's 10 greatest discoveries of the 20th century. *Tex Heart Inst J* 2002; 29:164–171.

2. Z. Hillel, G. Landesberg. Electrocardiography. In Miller R., editor. *Miller's Anesthesia.* 7th edition, vol. 1. Philadelphia, PA: Churchill Livingstone; 2010 pp. 1357–1386.

3. J.L. Apfelbaum, J.H Silverstein, F.F. Chun, et al. Practice guidelines for postanesthetic care: an updated report by the American Society of Anesthesiologists Task Force on Postanesthetic Care. *Anesthesiology* 2013; 118:291–307.

4. R. Hines, P. Barash, G. Watrous, T. O'Connor. Complications occurring in the postanesthesia care unit: a survey. *Anesth Analg* 1992; 74:503–509.

5. H. Ponhold, M.N. Vicenzi. Incidence of bradycardia during recovery from spinal anaesthesia: influence of patient position. *Br J Anaesth* 1998; 81:723–726.

6. R.W. Neumar, C.W. Otto, M.S. Link, et al. Adult advanced cardiovascular life support:

2010 American Heart Association guidelines for cardiopulmonary resuscitation and emergency cardiovascular care. *Circulation* 2010; 122: S729–S767.

7.   R.K. Stoelting, S.C. Hillier. *Pharmacology & Physiology in Anesthetic Practice*. 4th edition. Philadelphia, PA: Lippincott Williams & Wilkins; 2006.

8.   K. Thygesen, J.S. Alpert, A.S. Jaffe, et al. Third universal definition of myocardial infarction. *Circulation* 2012; 126:2020–2035.

9.   R.E. Casas, H.J. Marriot, D.L. Glancy. Value of leads V7–V9 in diagnosing posterior wall acute myocardial infarction and other causes of tall R waves in V1–V2. *Am J Cardiol* 1997; 80:508–509.

10. Writing Committee Members, E.M. Antman, D.T. Anbe, P.W. Armstrong, et al. ACC/AHA guidelines for the management of patients with ST-elevation myocardial infarction. Executive Summary: A Report of the American College of Cardiology/American Heart Association Task Force on Practice Guidelines (Writing Committee to revise the 1999 guidelines for the management of patients with acute myocardial infarction). *Circulation* 2004; 110:588–636.

11. D.S. Goldstein. The electrocardiogram in stroke: relationship to pathophysiological type and comparison with prior tracings. *Stroke* 1979; 10:253–259.

12. P. Nagele, S. Pal, F. Brown, et al. Postoperative QT interval prolongation in patients undergoing noncardiac surgery under general anesthesia. *Anesthesiology* 2012; 117:321–328.

13. A.J. Moss. Measurement of the QT interval and the risk associated with QTc interval prolongation: a review. *Am J Cardiol* 1993; 72:23B–25B.

Chapter

Heart failure

Glen D. Quigley and Elia S. Elia

- The risk of postoperative heart failure (HF) ranges from 1% to 6% after major surgery in patients with no cardiac history, and from 6% to 25% in patients with a history of cardiac disease.
- The most likely symptoms and signs are shortness of breath, hypoxia, hypotension, and/or peripheral edema.
- Diagnostic work-up should immediately assess the adequacy of circulation and rule out myocardial ischemia; after this, investigate possible precipitating factors.
- Management depends on severity of symptoms. Acute decompensated HF (cardiogenic shock) should be managed in a systematic fashion by first improving the "metabolic milieu" (hypoxia, hypercarbia, acid–base status, hypocalcemia, anemia, and hyper/hypokalemia), then optimizing heart rate and rhythm, and finally adjusting preload, contractility, and afterload.

Heart failure (HF) can present significant challenges in both diagnosis and management during the postoperative period. Studies have shown that 6% to 7% of patients undergoing non-cardiac surgery have either current HF or a history of HF; this number is even higher for the cardiac surgical population.[1] This fact is significant, as several studies have noted that patients with HF undergoing surgery have longer hospital stays, increased likelihood for hospital readmission, and elevated long-term mortality rates.[2] Postoperative HF is not limited to patients with a prior history of HF and is seen with surprising frequency in patients with no prior history of cardiac disease. Studies have reported a risk of postoperative HF ranging from 1% to 6% after major surgery in patients with no cardiac history and from 6% to 25% in patients with a history of cardiac disease (coronary disease, valvular disease, history of HF).[3–5] This chapter will discuss the common symptoms and signs of postoperative HF and a pragmatic approach to the diagnostic work-up. Afterwards, a stepwise, algorithmic approach will be presented regarding the selection of appropriate pharmacological and invasive treatment modalities.

Classification

Heart failure is a condition in which the heart has lost the ability to pump enough blood to the body's tissues. With too little blood being delivered, the organs and other tissues do not

Post-Anesthesia Care: Symptoms, Diagnosis, and Management, ed. James W. Heitz. Published by Cambridge University Press. © Cambridge University Press 2016.

receive enough oxygen and nutrients to function properly. Heart failure can be due to either systolic or diastolic dysfunction. Systolic HF occurs when the pumping ability of the heart is reduced, which is diagnostically defined as a reduced left ventricular (LV) ejection fraction and/or global or regional wall motion abnormalities. Diastolic dysfunction occurs when impaired relaxation of the ventricle leads to decreased ventricular filling; ejection fraction is preserved, but stroke volume and cardiac output are reduced. Diastolic function can be evaluated with echocardiography by measuring transmitral inflow velocities, pulmonary venous flow patterns, and tissue Doppler imaging (TDI). Another important determination is whether HF involves the left ventricle, the right ventricle (RV), or both ventricles (biventricular). Determination of RV dysfunction is an important part of choosing an appropriate pharmacological therapy. Also, determining whether the HF is reversible or irreversible may assist in deciding between management options. Examples of reversible causes include myocardial stunning following an ischemic event, stress- or tachycardia-induced cardiomyopathy, hypertensive crisis, drug- and alcohol-induced myocardial depression, electrolyte abnormalities, peripartum cardiomyopathy, and high-output HF states (e.g. sepsis, thyrotoxicosis).

Symptoms and signs

The most likely symptoms and signs are shortness of breath, hypoxia, hypotension, and/or peripheral edema.[6] A thorough review of the patient's medical history should be performed. Key information includes the procedure performed, any surgical difficulties, any anesthetic or airway issues, and intraoperative fluid and medication administration.

Physical examination should confirm findings from the history and help to determine the severity of HF present. A complete set of vitals should be taken and rechecked regularly, especially after each therapeutic intervention has been given. A focused head-to-toe examination should be performed with particular emphasis on findings relevant to HF. Jugular venous distension, displaced point of maximal cardiac impulse, and a gallop are all highly specific for HF, but their absence does not rule out HF.[6,7] Pulmonary rales and dependent edema are supportive of a diagnosis of HF, but again their absence does not rule it out. Care should be taken to evaluate for any physical signs of shock, such as altered mental status, cool clammy skin, or oliguria. Even in the absence of physical findings, a strong suspicion for HF from the history is enough to warrant further work-up.

Differential diagnosis

Postoperative heart failure can present in a number of ways, ranging from mild peripheral edema to severe shortness of breath, hypoxia, or hypotension. Common cardiovascular causes for these heart-failure-like symptoms include HF, myocardial infarction (MI), unstable angina, and hypovolemia; pulmonary causes include atelectasis, laryngospasm, bronchospasm, obstructive sleep apnea, and chronic obstructive pulmonary disease.[8,9] Less common but equally important causes for these types of symptoms include pulmonary embolism, pleural effusion, negative pressure pulmonary edema, transfusion-related acute lung injury (TRALI), fat embolism, anemia, and anxiety.

Diagnostic work-up

A thorough history and physical exam should be supplemented by a pragmatic diagnostic work-up of postoperative HF that focuses on answering critically important questions first.

As such, the first studies to be done should assess for the adequacy of circulation. This should be done through the history/physical exam aspects discussed previously and by checking laboratory studies such as an arterial blood gas and a lactate level. Presence of a metabolic acidosis or elevated lactate, along with symptoms and signs of HF should prompt high suspicion for a shock state and aggressive treatment, possibly including placement of invasive hemodynamic monitors (arterial line, pulmonary artery [PA] catheter) and access lines if not already present from the prior surgical procedure.

After determining the patient's acid–base status, another early diagnostic step that should be taken is to evaluate for myocardial ischemia. Studies have found that patients with or at risk for cardiac disease undergoing non-cardiac surgery have an incidence of perioperative MI of 1.8% to 5.6%;[10–12] in studies looking at all patients – both high and low cardiac risk populations – the incidence was approximately 1%.[13] Pooled results of several large studies suggest that of patients experiencing a postoperative MI only 14% will have chest pain and only 53% will have a clinical symptom or sign suggestive of an MI.[5,10,11] Comparison of a new postoperative electrocardiogram (ECG) to a baseline preoperative ECG should be performed. Specific diagnostic ECG features for MI include new Q-wave changes ($\geq$30 ms) in any two contiguous leads; ST-segment elevation ($\geq$2 mm in leads V1–3 and $\geq$1 mm in other leads); ST-segment depression ($\geq$1 mm) in at least two contiguous leads; or symmetric inversion of T waves ($\geq$1 mm) in at least two contiguous leads.[14] In addition to the ECG, serial troponins should be followed; other biomarkers such as CK-MB and myoglobin are less helpful as surgical trauma can result in their release from skeletal muscle, leading to false-positive and false-negative values.[15,16] Standard hematological and chemistry panels should also be sent as part of a work-up for myocardial ischemia. Cardiac catheterization should be considered for diagnostic and/or therapeutic intervention, especially in the setting of unstable coronary syndrome (acute MI or unstable angina).

The next diagnostic steps should focus on investigating for other common precipitating factors for HF. Urine output and laboratory studies can be used to assess for acute or chronic renal insufficiency. The ECG should be reviewed for rate and rhythm abnormalities. A chest radiograph should be performed to assess for both gross volume overload and possibly undiagnosed prior pneumonia. If available, a two-dimensional ECG with Doppler should be performed to determine whether abnormalities of the myocardium, heart valves, or pericardium are present. This study should identify whether the left ventricular ejection fraction (LVEF) is preserved or reduced, whether the LV structure is normal or abnormal, and whether there are any other structural abnormalities (valvular, pericardial, RV) that may account for the clinical presentation. Right ventricular function and wall motion should also be assessed, as the presence or absence of right-sided HF has important management implications. Preload can be roughly estimated based on chamber filling volumes and pressure estimates. A summary of the diagnostic work-up is shown in Table 8.1.

The management of postoperative HF depends on the severity, acuity, and type of HF present, with manifestations ranging from mild HF symptoms to acute decompensated HF with cardiogenic shock.

Mild postoperative HF symptoms should be approached by quickly and accurately **determining the adequacy of perfusion**, the volume status, and the role of precipitating factors and/or co-morbid conditions. A work-up for myocardial ischemia should be performed early on in all cases of postoperative HF, and therapy initiated as appropriate.

Table 8.1 Summary of diagnostic work-up for postoperative heart failure

Assessment of heart failure		
Risk factors	Symptoms and signs	Diagnosis work-up
LV failure		
1. Prior HF 2. Coronary artery disease 3. Valvular disease 4. Intraoperative myocardial ischemia 5. Inadequate (diastolic HF) or excessive fluid administration 6. Loss of atrial kick due to tachyarrhythmia (diastolic HF) 7. Uncontrolled hypertension 8. Diabetes mellitus 9. Renal insufficiency 10. Age >70	1. Shortness of breath 2. Hypoxia 3. Hypotension 4. Peripheral edema 5. Rales	• Arterial blood gas and electrolytes, ECG, CX-ray, and serial troponins • ↑CVP, ↑MPAP, ↑PAD, ↑wedge • Decrease CO • Prominent "V" wave on wedge wave (MR) • Echo • SHF; full LV, low EF • DHF; empty LV, normal EF
RV failure		
Heart disease 1. Ischemic 2. Valvular 3. Congenital Respiratory disease 1. Obstructive 2. Restrictive 3. Morbid obesity 4. OSA 5. Pulmonary embolus 6. Chronic high altitude exposure 7. HIV	1. Dyspnea on exertion 2. Angina 3. Syncope 4. Hepatomegaly 5. Peripheral edema 6. Ascites	OR-panel, ECG, CX-rays, and serial troponins Pulmonary hypertension: 1. ↑ wedge 2. ↑ PVR usually MPAP-wedge >12 on PA cath Impaired RV: 1. ↑CVP, prominent "V" wave (TR) 2. Decrease CO 3. Full RV, empty LV, ↑RV–RA gradient on echo

OR, operating room; CVP, central venous pressure; MPAP, mean pulmonary artery pressure; PAD, pulmonary artery diastolic pressure; CO, cardiac output; SHF, systolic heart failure; DHF, diastotic heart failure; EF, ejection fraction; OSA, obstructive sleep apnea; PVR, peripheral vascular resistance.

Oxygen should be administered to avoid and/or treat hypoxia. For mild HF, intravenous loop diuretics with strict monitoring of input/output values should be used as a first-line pharmacological treatment of pulmonary congestion and peripheral edema symptoms. Other interventions should focus on treating other precipitating factors, such as rate or rhythm abnormalities, uncontrolled hypertension, or infections.

On the other end of the HF spectrum is acute decompensated HF. This represents the most severe form of HF and therefore requires the most aggressive intervention. Treatment should proceed in an orderly manner with reassessment performed after each intervention.

Establishment of a secured airway and adequate oxygenation/ventilation is the first step in treating all patients and is no different in acute HF. Whether establishing a secure airway and breathing involves airway maneuvers, non-invasive positive-pressure ventilation (NIPPV), or intubation will be based on the specific scenario.

Once airway and breathing has been established, the remaining management steps should focus on addressing issues of hemodynamics and inadequate circulation (i.e. shock). This should be done by first assessing the patient's current hemodynamic parameters (rate, rhythm, preload, contractility, pulmonary vascular resistance [PVR], and systemic vascular resistance [SVR]), then determining appropriate hemodynamic goals, and finally choosing the appropriate therapeutic intervention(s) (pharmacological, mechanical interventions) to achieve these goals. The remainder of this chapter discusses this approach, and a summary – with lists of potential therapeutic interventions – is shown in Table 8.2.

Assuming that the appropriate diagnostic steps discussed above were taken, an arterial blood gas and basic metabolic panel should be analyzed for hypoxia, hypercarbia, acidosis, and hyperkalemia. These abnormalities will need to be reversed to create a favorable "metabolic milieu." Next, ensure an adequate heart rate and rhythm; any bradycardia or tachycardia should be treated with the appropriate pharmacological or electrophysiological modality (i.e. pacing, cardioversion). Once rate and rhythm have been established, the adequacy of preload should be determined. In patients with existing invasive hemodynamic monitors, such as a central venous line or pulmonary artery (PA) catheter, this can be done by assessing central venous pressure (in the absence of significant structural heart or lung disease), pulmonary artery diastolic pressure, or pulmonary capillary wedge pressures. Calculated estimates of preload using arterial line tracings (i.e. pulse-pressure variability, stroke volume variability) can also be performed in select patients (intubated patients on positive pressure mechanical ventilation).[17] If not already present, appropriate hemodynamic monitors and central vascular access should be obtained at this point (i.e. arterial line, central venous catheter, or PA catheter). If preload is determined to be inadequate, especially in diastolic HF, it should be optimized by administering appropriate crystalloid or preferably colloid (to minimize total fluid volume); if it is excessive, then it should be treated using diuretics, venodilators, or inotropes.

The next step is to increase contractility. However, choosing an appropriate inotrope can be difficult. The first step in choosing is to determine whether SVR is excessively high (hypertension, cool clammy extremities in the absence of hypovolemia) or inappropriately low (hypotension, warm flushed extremities; i.e. vasoplegia). Current SVR will establish whether a patient would benefit more from an inoconstrictor or an inodilator.

Adrenergic inoconstrictors include norepinephrine, epinephrine, and dopamine. These agents all cause an increase inotropy via β_1 mechanisms as well as vasoconstriction via α_1. Norepinephrine is most useful in states of vasodilatory or distributive shock requiring a strong vasoconstrictor effect. Epinephrine is a powerful inotrope that has mixed α_1 vasoconstrictor and β_2 vasodilator effects, therefore producing a more unpredictable effect on SVR. Dopamine is an indirect β_1 adrenergic agent with differing effects based on the dosing level used – primarily dopaminergic at low doses (<3 mcg/kg/min), β-adrenergic at moderate doses (3 to 10 mcg/kg/min), and α adrenergic at high doses (>10 mcg/kg/min).

Adrenergic inodilators, which are all synthetic derivatives of dopamine, include dobutamine and isoproterenol. All of these agents have positive inotropic effects via β_1, as well as

Table 8.2 Summary of management algorithm for postoperative heart failure

Hemodynamic management	
Milieu (OR-panel): correct hypothermia, acidosis, hypercarbia, hypoxia, anemia, hypocalcemia, and hyper/hypokalemia	
Rhythm: Treat arrhythmia if possible	**SVR = (MAP – CVP) × 80/CO**
Rate: Low to normal rate, especially DHF High rate (90–100), especially SHF if not ischemic	**Low SVR:** 1. Phenylephrine 2. Norepinephrine 3. Vasopressin 4. Methylene blue
High preload: 1. Loop diuretic 2. Nitroglycerin 3. Inodilators (dobutamine, isoproterenol, milrinone) 4. Phlebotomy 5. Continuous venovenous hemofiltration	**High SVR:** 1. Nitroprusside 2. Nitroglycerin 3. Nesiritide 4. Inodilators (dobutamine, isoproterenol, milrinone)
Low preload: Volume, preferably colloid (albumin, blood)	
	PVR = (MPAP – LAP) × 80/CO
Contractility	
LV support	**RV support, hypertension, and high PVR**
1. Epinephrine 2. Dopamine 3. Milrinone 4. Dobutamine 5. Norepinephrine 6. Intra-aortic balloon pump 7. Left ventricular assist device	Avoid exacerbating factors, hypoxia acidosis, hypercarbia, hypothermia, pain 1. Nitroglycerin 2. Dobutamine 3. Milrinone 4. Nitric oxide 5. Prostacyclin
Extreme biventricular support	**RV support, hypotension**
1. Biventricular assist device 2. Extracorporeal membrane oxygenation	1. Volume 2. Epinephrine 3. Dopamine 4. Right ventricular assist device

CVP = central venous pressure; LAP = left atrial pressure; MAP = mean arterial pressure

β_2 vasodilatory effects. Dobutamine is a direct-acting β-adrenergic agent with a potent β_2-mediated dilatory effect; it even causes pulmonary artery dilation, which may be helpful in patients with a component of right ventricular HF. Isoproterenol has a potent positive chronotropic (i.e. heart rate increasing) effect that precedes its inotropic (contractility) effect and limits its usage to situations of profound bradycardia as a chemical pacemaker.

Other inotropic classes include the phosphodiesterase (PDE) inhibitors (i.e. milrinone). These agents work independently of the adrenergic receptor and thus are useful in patients with chronic HF and down-regulated β-receptors. PDE inhibitors are useful in both left- and right-sided HF, as well as diastolic dysfunction, because they enhance diastolic relaxation (known as a lusitropic effect).

Specialized **afterload** agents exist for use both in patients in whom contractility is adequate, but who have either an excessive or low SVR, and in patients on inotropes with persistently high or low SVR. Nitroglycerin and nitroprusside are two potent vasodilators with long-established use in management of HF. A newer agent, nesiritide (human recombinant B-type natriuretic peptide [BNP]) is a potent vasodilator with effects on reducing both afterload and preload, and relieving anasarca; its use has been limited primarily by cost.

The opposite situation may occur, in which SVR is inappropriately low, leading to a low perfusion state. This is typically seen in patients with an acute inflammatory syndrome (i.e. post-cardiopulmonary bypass, systemic inflammatory response syndrome, sepsis), which then leads to catecholamine (norepinephrine)-resistant vasodilatory shock. In these patients, low level infusions (1 to 4 units/hr) of arginine vasopressin (AVP) have been shown to reverse catecholamine-resistant vasoplegia.[18] Consider adding AVP when increasing doses of traditional inotropes fail to improve low SVR states. Additionally, a single dose of methylene blue (2 mg/kg) has also been reported to reverse vasoplegia in patients with an acute inflammatory syndrome.[19]

Most RV HF is due to LV dysfunction, but it can also be caused by either an increase in PVR or pure RV dysfunction because of myocardial ischemia. **RV function** could be improved by improving left-sided failure, lowering PVR (nitric oxide), and/or improving RV contractility (dobutamine, milrinone).

One final but critical point: HF or cardiogenic shock due to acute myocardial ischemia will likely not respond to standard inotropic agents (owing to worsening of the myocardial oxygen supply–demand balance). The most effective intervention for acute ischemic HF is insertion of an intra-aortic balloon pump (IABP). An IABP significantly improves the myocardial oxygen supply–demand balance via its counterpulsation mechanism – inflation during diastole and deflation during systole. Oxygen balance is improved by increasing coronary perfusion by forcing blood retrograde through the aorta during diastole (inflation) and decreasing afterload by creating a negative intra-aortic pressure during systole (deflation).[20] Contraindications to IABP use include aortic insufficiency, aortic aneurysm or dissection, and severe peripheral vascular disease. It is important to remember that an IABP is not a ventricular assist device and therefore does not pump blood through the circulation; if IABP insertion does not reverse the ischemic shock, more invasive mechanical circulatory support should be pursued such as extracorporeal membrane oxygenation (ECMO), cardiopulmonary bypass, or a ventricular assist device.

References

1. Y.O. Xu-Cai, D.J. Brotman, C.O. Phillips, et al. Outcomes of patients with stable heart failure undergoing elective noncardiac surgery. *Mayo Clin Proc* 2008; 83: 280–288.

2. B.G. Hammill, L.H. Curtis, E. Bennett-Guerrero, et al. Impact of heart failure on patients undergoing major noncardiac surgery. *Anesthesiology* 2008; 108: 559–567.

3. L. Goldman, D.L. Caldera, S.R. Nussbaum, et al. Multifactorial index of cardiac risk in noncardiac surgical procedures. *N Engl J Med* 1977; 297: 845–850.

4. M.E. Charlson, C.R. MacKenzie, J.P. Gold, et al. Risk for postoperative congestive

heart failure. *Surg Gynecol Obstet* 1991; 172: 95–104.

5. D.T. Mangano, W.S. Browner, M. Hollenberg, et al. Association of perioperative myocardial ischemia with cardiac morbidity and mortality in men undergoing noncardiac surgery. The Study of Perioperative Ischemia Research Group. *N Engl J Med* 1990; 323: 1781–1788.

6. S.A. Dosh. Diagnosis of heart failure in adults. *Am Fam Physician* 2004; 70: 2145–2152.

7. A. Nohria, E. Lewis, L. Stevenson. Medical management of advanced heart failure. *JAMA* 2002; 287: 628–640.

8. A.I. Arieff. Fatal postoperative pulmonary edema: pathogenesis and literature review. *Chest* 1999; 115: 1371–1377.

9. J. Timby, C. Reed, S. Zeilender, F.L. Glauser. "Mechanical" causes of pulmonary edema. *Chest* 1990; 98: 973–979.

10. C.M. Ashton, N.J. Petersen, N.P. Wray, et al. The incidence of perioperative myocardial infarction in men undergoing noncardiac surgery. *Ann Intern Med* 1993; 118: 504–510.

11. N.H. Badner, R.L. Knill, J.E. Brown, et al. Myocardial infarction after noncardiac surgery. *Anesthesiology* 1998; 88: 572–578.

12. P.J. Devereaux, L. Goldman, D.J. Cook, et al. Perioperative cardiac events in patients undergoing noncardiac surgery: a review of the magnitude of the problem, the pathophysiology of the events and methods to estimate and communicate risk. *CMAJ* 2005; 173: 627–634.

13. T.H. Lee, E.R. Marcantonio, C.M. Mangione, et al. Derivation and prospective validation of a simple index for prediction of cardiac risk of major noncardiac surgery. *Circulation* 1999; 100: 1043–1049.

14. J.S. Alpert, K. Thygesen, E. Antman, J.P. Bassand. Myocardial infarction redefined–a consensus document of The Joint European Society of Cardiology/ American College of Cardiology Committee for the redefinition of myocardial infarction. *J Am Coll Cardiol* 2000; 36: 959–969.

15. M.A. Costa, R.G. Carere, S.V. Lichtenstein, et al. Incidence, predictors, and significance of abnormal cardiac enzyme rise in patients treated with bypass surgery in the arterial revascularization therapies study (ARTS). *Circulation* 2001; 104: 2689–2693.

16. J.E. Adams, G.A. Sicard, B.T. Allen, et al. Diagnosis of perioperative myocardial infarction with measurement of cardiac troponin I. *N Engl J Med* 1994; 330: 670–674.

17. P.E. Marik, R. Cavallazzi, T. Vasu. Dynamic changes in arterial waveform derived variables and fluid responsiveness in mechanically ventilated patients: a systematic review of the literature. *Crit Care Med* 2009; 37: 2642–2647.

18. D.W. Landry, H.R. Levin, E.M. Gallant, et al. Vasopressin pressor hypersensitivity in vasodilatory septic shock. *Crit Care Med* 1997; 25: 1279–1282.

19. P. Yiu, J. Robin, C.W. Pattison. Reversal of refractory hypotension with single-dose methylene blue after coronary artery bypass surgery. *J Thorac Cardiovasc Surg* 1999; 118: 195–196.

20. D.A. Kontoyannis, J.N. Nanas, S.T. Toumanidis, S.F. Stamatelopoulos. Severe cardiogenic shock, after cardioversion, reversed by the intraaortic balloon pump. *Intensive Care Med* 2000; 26: 649.

Hypoxia

Gadi Arzanipour and James W. Heitz

- Hypoxia is very common after surgery.
- Hypoventilation and atelectasis are the most common sources of postoperative hypoxic episodes.
- Most causes of postoperative hypoxia respond to supplemental oxygen.
- Continuous pulse oximetry is necessary to detect most episodes of postoperative hypoxia.
- Most episodes of hypoxia occur more than 30 minutes into the recovery period.

Hypoxia (SpO_2 <90%) and arterial hypoxemia (PaO_2 <60) after surgery are very frequently observed in surgical patients.[1,2] General anesthesia and surgery both cause a variety of pathophysiological changes in the respiratory system that may promote the development of hypoxemia. These changes include hypoventilation, ventilation–perfusion (V/Q) mismatching, shunting, and atelectasis. Pain may cause respiratory splinting contributing to hypoxia depending upon the surgical site. Interference with the mechanics of breathing occurs with decreasing frequency among thoracoabdominal, upper abdominal, and peripheral surgeries.[1,2] Additionally, a number of patient risk factors, including advanced age, sex, weight, and pre-existing heart and lung disease predispose patients to postoperative hypoxemia.[3] Hypoxia may present with pulmonary (abnormal respiratory rate, tachypnea or hypopnea), cardiovascular (system or pulmonary hypertension, tachycardia, dysrhythmias), and neurological (confusion, restlessness, combativeness) manifestations. Obtundation, bradycardia, and hypotension are late signs that precede cardiac arrest.

The reported incidence of hypoxia varies widely in the medical literature and ranges from 0.3%[4] to 55%[5] or more. The incidence is dependent upon the surgical procedure, the co-morbidities of the surgical cohort, how hypoxia is defined, and how individual studies attempted to identify it. It is now acknowledged that pulse oximetry is necessary to recognize postoperative hypoxia. Attempts to diagnose hypoxia clinically prior to the advent of pulse oximetry were inefficient. In a large prospective trial of 20,802 surgical patients in the Post-Anesthesia Care Unit (PACU) randomized to either pulse oximetry monitoring or clinical observation only, there was an observed 19-fold increase in recognition of hypoxic episodes among the pulse oximetry group.[6] In a smaller prospective study in which surgical patients were monitored with pulse oximetry with the clinicians blinded to its readings, mild hypoxia ($SpO_2 < 90\%$) occurred in 55% of patients, and severe hypoxia ($SpO_2 < 80\%$) occurred in 13%.[5] Episodes of hypoxia recorded by pulse oximetry were not recognized clinically in 95% of episodes in that study. More recently, the advent of electronic databases has once again changed the clinical understanding of postoperative hypoxia. Since the residual effects of anesthesia dissipate after surgery, the risk of hypoxia would logically seem to diminish the longer the surgical patient is out of surgery. Indeed, it has been proposed that postoperative hypoxia is rare after the first 5 minutes in the PACU.[4] However, recent data culled from electronic databases would tend to dispute this accepted clinical axiom. A retrospective analysis of over 137,000 surgical patients in the tertiary care medical center PACU with electronically recorded pulse oximetry every 30 to 60 seconds revealed that the majority of hypoxia episodes (68.8%) occur more than 30 minutes after arrival.[7] Constant vigilance is necessary, since postoperative hypoxia may occur when clinically unexpected.

Most postoperative hypoxemia is mild and can be easily managed with supplemental oxygen to maintain a hemoglobin oxygen saturation of 92% or better. A variety of devices may be utilized to deliver the desired oxygen concentration. Nasal cannula can provide up to an FiO_2 of 40% with 8 liters/min of flow. A venturi mask provides a more precise amount of oxygen up to 60% oxygen. Partial and full non-rebreathing masks can provide upwards of 40% to 60% FiO_2. Non-invasive ventilatory support such as continuous positive airway pressure (CPAP), or bilevel positive airway pressure (BiPAP), should be considered in high-risk patients or those with persistent hypoxia requiring 50% oxygen or greater. If hypoxia persists in spite of these measures, endotracheal intubation and mechanical ventilation may be required.[8]

While pulse oximetry monitors oxygenation, this is only one component of ventilation. Direct arterial gas measurements are invaluable in evaluating blood oxygen content, alveolar–arterial (A–a) oxygen gradient, shunting, acid–base disturbances, and hypoventilation. An arterial catheter may be indicated if the patient is hemodynamically unstable or intubated, or if repeat blood sampling is anticipated.

Causes of postoperative hypoxemia

Upper airway obstruction: Upper airway obstruction can occur in the surgical patient, typically because of posterior displacement of the tongue and loss of airway muscular tone (see Table 9.1). Perioperative polypharmacy including opioids and sedatives is responsible for many cases of postoperative airway obstruction. Subclinical residual neuromuscular blockade may present with airway obstruction. As many as 31% of surgical patients arriving in the PACU have demonstrable residual neuromuscular blockade.[9] Residual neuromuscular blockade is implicated in a majority of hypoxic events in the PACU and many cases of upper airway obstruction.[10] Gauze throat packs are often used during surgical procedures to prevent the swallowing of blood to decrease the incidence of postoperative nausea and vomiting. Failure to remove the throat pack at the end of surgery may cause sudden airway obstruction in the early postoperative period. Upper airway edema from trauma, angioedema, vocal cord paralysis, and expanding neck hematoma after carotid endarterectomy are less common causes. Most upper airway obstructions may be managed with airway maneuvers including chin lift or jaw thrust. For refractory causes or when the patency of the airway is threatened, endotracheal intubation may be necessary. If endotracheal intubation is not successful in the presence of a postoperative neck hematoma, decompression of the hematoma may be life-saving and should not be delayed.

Table 9.1 Postoperative upper airway obstruction

Pharmacological	Opioids, sedatives, residual neuromuscular blockade, inhaled anesthetics
Vocal cord paralysis	Recurrent laryngeal nerve damage, thyroid, parathyroid, neck dissection
Trauma	Airway burn (hot air, steam), mandibular, maxillary fractures, hematoma (carotid endarterectomy, neck dissection)
Foreign body	Retained throat pack
Angioedema	Anaphylactic reactions, C1 inhibitor deficiency, angiotensin-converting enzyme inhibitors

Stridor: Causes of hypoxia which present with stridor are discussed separately in Chapter 10.

Atelectasis is the most common cause of postoperative hypoxemia (occurring in 45–90% of cases) and is the result of both mechanical and physiological pulmonary changes that accompany general anesthesia. Within 5 minutes of the induction of general anesthesia atelectasis develops and can persist days into the postoperative period.[11] Three mechanisms have been described that contribute to the development of atelectasis: compression, gas absorption, and surfactant impairment.[12]

Compression atelectasis results from a reduction in the transthoracic pressure leading to alveolar collapse. This is associated with patient positioning (supine, lithotomy), body habitus, surgical factors (retraction, packing), and surgical site (thoracic, abdominal). Gas absorption atelectasis can result from the use of high oxygen concentrations. Nitrogen makes up 80% of room air and is poorly absorbed, thereby serving to prevent alveolar collapse which may occur when nitrogen is displaced by oxygen. Anesthetic agents and low tidal volumes cause atelectasis by impairing surfactant action leading to increased surface tension. The physiological impact of the three mechanisms is to increase the shunt fraction.

Atelectasis is usually not visible on plain imaging unless severe; CT imaging is more sensitive but rarely necessary. Prevention begins intraoperatively with recruitment maneuvers, positive end-expiratory pressure (PEEP), and utilization of the minimal necessary oxygen concentration.[13] Supplemental oxygen corrects atelectasis-induced hypoxemia, but may exacerbate the atelectasis, so it should be administered with therapy directed at the atelectasis itself. Simple posture change from supine to upright may decrease atelectasis. Deep breathing maneuvers, including incentive spirometry, deep breathing exercises, intermittent positive pressure breathing, and chest physiotherapy, have been shown to improve atelectasis.[14]

Pulmonary embolism is more common in the perioperative period, and one must have a high level of suspicion in order to diagnose promptly. Multiple types of pulmonary emboli exist including venous thromboemboli (VTE), air, or fat.

VTE risk is elevated after surgery owing to a derangement in one or more of the components of Virchow's triad (hypercoagulability, venous stasis, and vessel injury). General anesthesia leads to a state of venous stasis due to immobility and vasodilation from the effect of anesthetic drugs. The surgical stress response leads to a hypercoagulable state, while the surgical intervention itself can lead to direct vessel injury. Major orthopedic procedures of the lower extremity or pelvis are especially high risk for VTE.

The clinical presentation of VTE can range from asymptomatic, to mild hypoxemia, to cardiovascular collapse, depending on the size and rapidity of embolism development. Typical non-specific signs and symptoms include tachypnea, tachycardia, dyspnea, hypoxia, chest pain, hypotension, and increased dead space ventilation. The latter manifests as an increased $PaCO_2$ to end-tidal CO_2 gradient as well as hypoxia uncorrected with supplemental oxygen. Signs of right ventricular dysfunction may also be present. Physical exam may demonstrate distended neck veins, increased pulmonic heart sound, and a tricuspid regurgitation murmur. Electrocardiogram (ECG) may demonstrate the classic S1Q3T3 pattern, but may also show T-wave inversion in leads V1–V4, or incomplete or complete right bundle-branch block.[15] However, it is important to note that the ECG is usually normal after pulmonary embolism, and the most common ECG abnormality is sinus tachycardia, so the more specific signs of acute right heart strain may be absent. Laboratory studies are of limited utility in the postoperative period,[16] and the diagnosis of pulmonary embolism can be confirmed by imaging studies. CT angiography is the study of choice because of its rapidity and ability to also evaluate the veins of the legs and pelvis for embolic sources. Treatment consists of supportive therapy and anticoagulation is usually administered to prevent further progression of clot formation. If anticoagulation is contraindicated, an inferior vena cava filter should be placed. In hemodynamically unstable patients, thrombolytic therapy as well as catheter or surgical based embolectomy may be considered.[17]

Venous air embolism (VAE) is associated with surgeries in which air enters the venous circulation via an incision or cannulated vein above the level of the heart. Small air emboli resolve spontaneously, but large quantities of air may cause respiratory embarrassment. Intracardiac air may be associated with a "mill-wheel" murmur. Air embolism may present after surgery and may be associated with central line (CVP) insertion or vascular catheter open to air. Preventing further air entrainment is crucial. Transesophageal echocardiography, pulmonary artery catheters, or precordial Dopplers have a high yield in diagnosis.[18] Placing the patient in the Trendelenburg position, left side down, to prevent paradoxical cerebral embolism through a patent foramen ovale, and aspiration of intracardiac air from a CVP placed into the right ventricle may be necessary.

Fat emboli and emboli of surgical debris are most commonly seen in orthopedic procedures where fat from bone marrow or debris from cement enters the venous system owing to elevated medullary pressure or surgical manipulation from placement of rods or nails. Symptoms of fat embolism are protean because of the diffuse effect of numerous emboli. Mental status changes are common, and a petechial rash may be observed in about one-half of affected patients. Treatment is supportive with intravenous steroids possibly demonstrating benefit in some trials. Heparin, aspirin, alcohol, hypertonic glucose with insulin, surfactant, clofibrate, α-blockers, corticosteroids, albumin, dextran, and aprotinin have all been advocated in therapy, but none have been shown to improve outcome.[19]

Pneumothorax is an uncommon but potentially fatal complication after surgery. Pneumothorax can occur spontaneously or iatrogenically from a surgical or barotrauma related to mechanical ventilation. It should be considered in the setting of central line placement (risk: subclavian > internal jugular vein), rib fracture, regional anesthesia (neuraxial, brachial plexus, and intercostal blocks), neck dissections, tracheostomy, nephrectomies, or other retroperitoneal or intraabdominal procedures. Patients with history of emphysema, subpleural blebs, or large bullae can develop pneumothorax with positive pressure ventilation. Pneumothorax can also result from anesthesia machine malfunction or a patient coughing or bucking during positive pressure ventilation.

The clinical presentation of pneumothorax is based on the underlying etiology, but includes chest pain, shortness of breath, and possibly hemoptysis. Physical exam will demonstrate hyperresonance and decreased breath sounds on auscultation and decreased chest excursion on the affected side. Chest radiography and computed tomography can aid in the diagnosis of pneumothorax. If the size of the pneumothorax is relatively small (15% to 20%) it can be managed conservatively with 100% oxygen and radiological follow-up to ensure resolution.[20] However, if the pneumothorax is larger or the patient is symptomatic, a chest tube should be inserted. Tension pneumothorax can develop if a one-way valve exists in the lungs or pleura such that air enters the pleural space but cannot exit. Needle decompression and chest tube insertion may be necessary.

Pleural effusion causes hypoxia by compression of lung parenchyma by fluid accumulation in the thoracic cavity. Pleural effusions may be exacerbated by fluid shifts after surgery, but rarely have first presentation postoperatively. Exceptions include hemothorax, which may occur after surgical trauma or CVP, and urinothorax, very rarely reported after urinary tract procedures. It is important to remember that hemothorax may occur after unsuccessful attempt at CVP, so the postoperative patient with hemothorax may not have an indwelling CVP.

Bronchospasm is caused by a contraction of the smooth muscles surrounding the bronchial tree. It may present as a component of an allergic reaction, but more commonly it is an isolated non-allergy event. Bronchospasm is more common and more severe in patients with a history of reactive airway disease such as asthma or chronic obstructive pulmonary disease, but can occur in patients with no such history. Other risk factors include history of tobacco exposure, recent respiratory infection, endotracheal intubation, airway manipulation, mechanical or chemical airway irritation, or pulmonary edema.[19] Clinical presentation may include expiratory wheezing, prolonged expiration, reduced breath sounds, and increased airway pressures during positive pressure ventilation.

The mainstay of treatment is inhaled short-acting β-agonist, such as albuterol, administered via a metered dose inhaler (MDI; 6 to 8 puffs repeated as needed) or nebulizer (5 mg). In the intubated patient, only 10% of the MDI administered reaches the airway while 90% condenses in the circuit; therefore treatment should be based on the clinical response (or appearance of side effects) rather than a set dose. In severe bronchospasm, inhaled agents may be ineffective owing to limited air movement. Important second-line agents include: epinephrine (10–100 mcg IV) titrated to effect, ipratropium bromide (0.5 mg q 6 hr), magnesium sulphate (50 mg/kg IV over 20 min, max 2 g), hydrocortisone 200 mg IV q 6 hr, and ketamine bolus 10–20 mg.[20]

Pulmonary edema can be classified as either cardiogenic or non-cardiogenic. Cardiogenic pulmonary edema (increased hydrostatic pressure) results from acute left ventricular failure from fluid overload (>1.5 liter), myocardial ischemia or infarction. Patients often carry a history of cardiopulmonary dysfunction such as congestive heart failure, coronary artery disease, cardiomyopathy, arrhythmia, or valvular dysfunction. Non-cardiogenic pulmonary edema (increased permeability) occurs in the setting of acute respiratory distress syndrome, SIRS, sepsis, transfusion, trauma, burns, and aspiration. Damage to the alveolar cells allows fluid to enter the alveolar space, leading to pulmonary edema. Non-cardiac pulmonary edema occurring within 6 hours of the transfusion of blood products should raise suspicion for transfusion-related lung injury (TRALI). TRALI occurs after 1:3,000 transfusions of red cells and is the most common cause of transfusion-related mortality.[21]

Patients usually present with hypoxemia, tachypnea, dyspnea, tachycardia, or airway secretions ("pink frothy" secretions). Chest auscultation may reveal rales, and chest radiography will demonstrate pulmonary cephalization. Troponin levels and ECG may suggest cardiac ischemia or infarction. Echocardiography can evaluate myocardial function and valvular anatomy. Left ventricular apical ballooning syndrome (Takotsubo cardiomyopathy) is increasingly recognized by the characteristic chest pain, ECG abnormalities indicative of cardiac ischemia, pulmonary edema, and transient echocardiographic abnormalities including ballooning of the ventricular apex with relative sparing of the wall motion at the base of the heart. When there is diagnostic uncertainty, a wedge pressure may aid in the diagnosis. Pulmonary occlusion pressure is usually elevated in cardiogenic pulmonary edema but normal in non-cardiogenic edema. Management is guided by the underlying etiology. In the case of cardiogenic pulmonary edema, treatment consists of diuresis and afterload reduction with further intervention specific to the underlying etiology. In non-cardiogenic edema, lung protective measures should be undertaken in the intubated patient with low peak pressures and low tidal volume ventilation (6 ml/kg of ideal body weight).[21]

Hypoventilation with severe hypercapnia can lead to hypoxemia by necessarily lowering the alveoral oxygen content. Hypoventilation in the recovery period is common, but usually mild and undiagnosed. Signs usually become apparent at a $PaCO_2$ above 60 mmHg and include somnolence, slow respiratory rate, labored breathing, tachypnea, and shallow breaths. Mild to moderate hypercapnia leads to sympathetic activation with tachycardia, hypertension, and cardiac irritability, but cardiac depression when hypercapnia becomes severe.

Hypoventilation is usually a result of the depressant effects of the anesthetic agents on respiratory drive. These agents include opioids, benzodiazepines, and anesthetic gases, as well as residual neuromuscular blockade and/or inadequate reversal. In addition to anesthetic drugs, other causes of hypoventilation include splinting, airway obstruction, bronchospasm, and restrictive conditions such as abdominal binders and abdominal distension.

Arterial blood gas tensions will allow one to assess the severity of hypoventilation and respiratory acidosis, and will guide management. Management should target the underlying cause. Patients with severe hypoventilation, obtundation, severe respiratory acidosis, or circulatory depression require intubation. Naloxone can be used to antagonize the respiratory depressant effects of opioids, remembering that most opioids have a longer duration of action than naloxone and will require careful monitoring. Flumazenil may reverse the sedative effects of benzodiazepines, but the reversal of respiratory depression is less reliable. Residual neuromuscular blockade can be ruled out with a sustained head-lift or observation of a train-of-four twitches elicited by a peripheral nerve stimulator in intubated patients, and further anticholinesterase can be given. Respiratory splinting can be mitigated with analgesics.

Hypoxia due to competitive binding to hemoglobin is a rare cause of postoperative hypoxia. Carbon monoxide may be produced when volatile anesthetics contact desiccated baralyme used to scrub carbon dioxide from the system.[22] Desiccation occurs from air flow through the circuit, so this complication may occur on Monday morning (from a machine running over the weekend) or if anesthesia is conducted in infrequently used outpost locations. Oxygen administration is therapeutic. Methemoglobinemia may occur because of exposure to a variety of medications that may be administered during surgery, but is most often reported after exposure to benzocaine. Cyanosis that does not respond to supplemental oxygen in a patient having received a precipitating medication should raise suspicion for methemoglobinemia. Treatment with methylene blue may be curative.

Right-to-left shunting of pulmonary blood returning poorly oxygenated blood into systemic circulation is a cause of hypoxia refractory to supplemental oxygenation. This may occur in individuals with known intracardiac defects or may occur *de novo* after surgery. Patients with pulmonary hypertension may experience shunting through a patent foramen ovale or other pathway when systemic pressure falls. Even in the absence of pre-existing pulmonary hypertension, new right-to-left shunts may occur rarely after surgical procedures. Pulmonary resections including pneumonectomy or lobectomy may precipitate right-to-left shunts which develop gradually over months, but on very rare occasions these have occurred acutely in the PACU.[23] The normal 5% of intrapulmonary shunting may be exaggerated in conditions in which mixed venous oxygen falls, including severe anemia. Treatment of right-to-left shunting is directed at correction of the underlying cause.

Factitious hypoxemia from pulse oximeter failure can occur. Patient movement, interference from ambient light, poor tissue perfusion, or the use of vasopressors may lead to inaccurate readings. The incidence of pulse oximeter failure in the PACU setting is about 1 in every 150 patients.[24] Poor plethysmography waveform may suggest this etiology, and rotation of the probe to another site may correct this problem.

References

1. F.S. Xue, Y.G. Huang, S.Y. Tong, et al. A comparative study of early postoperative hypoxemia in infants, children, and adults undergoing elective plastic surgery. *Anesth Analg* 1996; 83:709–715.

2. J. Canet, M. Ricos, F. Vidal. Early postoperative arterial oxygen desaturation determining factors and response to oxygen therapy. *Anesth Analg* 1989; 69:207–212.

3. F.S. Xue, B.W. Li, G.S. Zhang, et al. The influence of surgical sites on early postoperative hypoxemia in adults undergoing elective surgery. *Anesth Analg* 1999; 88:213–219.

4. M.K. Kim, J.Y. Kim, B.N. Koo, K.Y. Cho, Y-S Shin. The incidence of low saturation by pulse oximetry in the postanesthesia care unit. *Korean J Anesthesiol* 2005; 4930:360–364.

5. J.T. Møller, M. Wittrup, S.H. Johansen. Hypoxemia in the postanesthesia care unit: an observer study. *Anesthesiology* 1990 73;890–895.

6. J.T. Møller, N.W. Johannessen, K. Espersen. Randomization evaluation of pulse oximetry in 20,802 patients: II. *Anesthesiology* 1993; 78:445–453.

7. R.H. Epstein, F. Dexter, M.G. Lopex, J.M. Ehrenfeld. Anesthesiologist staffing considerations consequent to the temporal distribution of hypoxemic episodes in the postanesthesia care unit. *Anesth Analg* 2014; 119:1322–1333.

8. S. Jaber, J.M. Delay, G. Chanques, et al. Outcomes of patients with acute respiratory failure after abdominal surgery treated with noninvasive positive pressure ventilation. *Chest* 2005; 128:2688–2695.

9. P.C. Yip, J.A. Hannam, A.J. Cameron, D. Campbell. Incidence of residual neuromuscular blockade in a post-anaesthetic care unit. *Anaesth Intensive Care* 2010; 38:91–95.

10. G.S. Murphy, J.W. Szokol, J. Marymont, et al. Residual neuromuscular blockade and critical respiratory events in the postanesthesia care unit. *Anesth Analg* 2008; 107:130–137.

11. M. Duggan, B.P. Kavanagh. Pulmonary atelectasis: a pathogenic perioperative entity. *Anesthesiology* 2005; 102:838–854.

12. L. Magnusson, D.R. Spahn. New concepts of atelectasis during general anaesthesia. *Br J Anaesth* 2003; 91:61–72.

13. C.J. Joyce, A.B. Baker, R.R. Kennedy. Gas uptake from an unventilated area of lung: computer model of absorption atelectasis. *J Appl Physiol* 1993; 74:1107–1116.

14. J.A. Thomas, J.M. McIntosh. Are incentive spirometry, intermittent positive pressure breathing, and deep breathing exercises effective in the prevention of postoperative pulmonary complications after upper abdominal surgery? A systematic overview and meta-analysis. *Phys Ther* 1994; 74:3–10.

15. S.Z. Goldhaber, C.G. Elliott. Acute pulmonary embolism. Part II: Risk stratification, treatment, and prevention. *Circulation* 2003; 108:2834–2838.

16. C.W. Whitten, P.E. Greilich, R. Ivy, D. Burkhardt, P.M. Allison. D-dimer formation during cardiac and noncardiac thoracic surgery. *Anesth Analg* 1999; 88:1226–1231.

17. D.C. Gulba, C. Schmid, H.G. Borst, et al. Medical compared with surgical treatment for massive pulmonary embolism. *Lancet* 1994; 343:576–577.

18. M.A. Mirski, A.V. Lele, L. Fitzsimmons, T.J. Toung. Diagnosis and treatment of vascular air embolism. *Anesthesiology* 2007; 106:164–177.

19. P. Glove, L.I.G. Worthley. Fat embolism. *Crit Care Resusc* 1999; 1:276–284.

20. M. Noppen, T. De Keukeleire. Pneumothorax. *Respiration* 2008; 76:121–127; 2009; 103(Suppl. 1):i57–i65.

21. A.P.J. Vlaar, N.P. Juffermans. Transfusion-related acute lung injury: a clinical review. *Lancet* 2013; 382:984–994.

22. E. Holak, D.A. Mei, M.B. Dunning, et al. Carbon monoxide production from sevoflurane breakdown: modeling of exposures under clinical conditions. *Anesth Analg* 2003; 96:757–764.

23. F. Godart, H.L. Porte, C. Rey, J-M. Lablanche, A. Wurtz. Postpneumonectomy interatrial right-to-left shunt: successful percutaneous treatment. *Ann Thorac Surg* 1997; 64:834–836.

24. B.S. Gillies, K. Posner, R. Freund, F. Cheney. Failure rate of pulse oximetry in the postanesthesia care unit. *J Clin Monit* 1999; 9:326–329.

Chapter

10

Wheezing and stridor

Michelle McMaster and James W. Heitz

- The presence of stridor after surgery is an airway emergency.
- Supportive care for stridor includes humidified supplemental oxygen.
- The causes of stridor are protean, and definitive therapy should be directed at the underlying cause.
- Stridor management may require continuous positive airway pressure or endotracheal intubation.

Stridor is a high-pitched sound produced when the normally laminar airflow through the larynx, trachea, or bronchi is replaced by turbulent airflow. Stridor may be inspiratory, expiratory, or both. It must be distinguished clinically from either stertor or wheezing. Stertor is a lower-pitched sound created from turbulent airflow in the nasopharynx or pharynx. Wheezing is also a high-pitched sound with a whistling character caused by airflow through narrowed bronchial airways. The tonal quality of stridor may be highly variable and may cause clinical confusion with stertor or wheezing in some patients.

There is a paucity of literature on postoperative stridor and, although common, the true incidence is unknown. While the etiology of stridor in a medical patient population has a wide differential diagnosis, the likely causes are less numerous for the surgical patient population and include laryngospasm, foreign body, anaphylaxis, nerve injury secondary to surgical manipulation, nerve palsy secondary to local anesthetic infiltration, post-thyroidectomy tracheomalacia, post-thyroidectomy hypocalcemia-induced laryngospasm, external compression from a hematoma, and laryngeal edema. Evaluation of the stridor needs to be performed promptly, as it can be a sign of impending respiratory failure.

Review of laryngeal anatomy

Since many causes of stridor in the postoperative patient relate to vocal cord dysfunction, a quick review of laryngeal anatomy, including muscle innervation, is warranted. The larynx in an adult is located between the C3 and C6 vertebrae, whereas in an infant it is located at the level of the C2–C3 vertebrae. The larynx connects the hypopharynx to the trachea. The muscles of the larynx can be categorized as intrinsic or extrinsic, and it is the intrinsic muscles of the larynx that control phonation (see Table 10.1). All of the intrinsic muscles of the larynx are innervated by the recurrent laryngeal nerve (a branch of the vagus nerve), with the exception of the cricothyroid muscle, which is innervated by the external branch

Post-Anesthesia Care: Symptoms, Diagnosis, and Management, ed. James W. Heitz. Published by Cambridge University Press. © Cambridge University Press 2016.

Table 10.1 Function of laryngeal muscles

Muscle	Function
Cricothyroid	Lengthen and stretch the vocal folds
Posterior cricoarytenoid	Abduct and externally rotate the arytenoid cartilages, resulting in abducted vocal folds
Lateral cricoarytenoid	Adduct and internally rotate the arytenoid cartilages, which can result in adducted vocal folds
Transverse arytenoid	Adduct the arytenoid cartilages, resulting in adducted vocal folds
Oblique arytenoid	Narrow the laryngeal inlet by constricting the distance between the arytenoid cartilages
Vocalis	Increase the thickness of the cords, changing the tone
Thyroarytenoid	Sphincter of vestibule, narrowing the laryngeal inlet

of the superior laryngeal nerve (also a branch of the vagus nerve). Sensory innervation of the glottis is also a function of the internal branch of the superior laryngeal nerve.[1]

Etiology of stridor after surgery

Laryngospasm: Laryngospasm is a serious complication of anesthesia. It involves spasm of all the muscles of the larynx and can lead to hypoxia, hypercarbia, and cardiac arrhythmias. Inspiratory stridor often precedes true laryngospasm, which involves complete occlusion of the larynx. Laryngospasm is a protective reflex, preventing aspiration of foreign objects, secretions, or blood into the trachea. One large retrospective study examining nearly 140,000 patients found the highest incidence of perioperative laryngospasm among children with bronchial asthma and/or a recent respiratory infection. An elevated incidence of stridor was also identified among patients in the age range of 50 to 59 years, women who underwent an inhalational induction of general anesthesia, and when the procedure was esophagoscopy or hypospadias correction.[2]

Procedure-related stridor: Injury to the recurrent laryngeal nerve causes the vocal cord on the side of the injury to be fixed in a semi-closed position (also called the cadaveric position) which produces hoarseness and can result in stridor. If bilateral injury occurs, the voice may not be preserved and breathing may become difficult. Injury to the external laryngeal nerve causes weakened phonation because the vocal folds cannot be adducted. Injury to the recurrent laryngeal nerve and/or the external laryngeal nerve is a well-established risk associated with neck dissections, with procedures of thyroid or parathyroid imparting the greatest risk. The incidence of temporary and permanent (>1 year) nerve palsies following thyroid surgeries was found to be 5.4% and 1.2%, respectively, and patients with thyroid cancer or requiring surgery for recurrent substernal goiters were at increased risk.[3] There are also several reports of severe stridor after infiltration of local anesthesia during brachial plexus blocks performed by varying anatomical approaches.[4–6] In each of these cases, transient anesthetic-induced unilateral vocal cord paresis became clinically significant because of pre-existing contralateral vocal cord palsy (related to previous surgery or radiation), underscoring the importance of recognizing this prior to performing a nerve block of the brachial plexus.

Hypocalcemia may occur following thyroidectomy or parathryoidectomy. Although acute postoperative hypocalcemia may more typically present as paresthesia, perioral numbness, neuromuscular irritability, and tetany, laryngospasm, or stridor may rarely be the initial presenting sign. Hypocalcemia in this setting is the result of surgical disturbance or removal of the parathyroid gland.[7] Parathyroid hormone production becomes inadequate to maintain calcium at normal levels, and hypocalcemia results. Osteopenia from sustained hyperparathyroidism exacerbates both the severity and duration of acute hypocalcemia (hungry bone syndrome), and patients with both hyperparathyroidism and radiographic evidence of bone loss appear to be at greatly increased postoperative risk for hypocalcemia after parathyroidectomy.[8] Among thyroidectomy patients, substernal thyroid disease, Graves' disease, thyroid cancer, and reoperative thyroidectomy appear to be risk factors for acute postoperative hypocalcemia.[7] The nadir of serum calcium levels usually occurs between 48 and 72 hours following surgery, but hypocalcemia should be considered throughout the early postoperative time frame for any patient with stridor after central neck dissections.

Hematoma formation with airway compromise is a more common and often more difficult to manage cause of stridor among patients after neck procedures. Tracheal deviation from the hematoma may be discernable, but compression typically occurs when the hematoma extends to the posterior and membranous portion of the trachea. Therefore, significant airway compromise may occur without obvious deviation of the trachea. Carotid endarterectomy and thyroidectomy carry the greatest risk for airway compromise from hematoma, but one case series of 27 airway hematomas with one mortality after stellate ganglion block underscores that surgical trespass as seemingly insignificant as needle puncture may incur risk.[9] Airway management is challenging in the setting of an expanding neck hematoma. Attempts at direct laryngoscopy and endotracheal intubation may be unsuccessful, and deaths have been reported. When hematoma makes airway management ineffective, removal of the sutures and hematoma decompression may be necessary. This crucial and potentially life-saving intervention must not be overlooked. Clinical fear of uncontrolled bleeding is secondary to the need for airway control when hypoxia develops. Even after carotid endarterectomy, only a small minority of patients with neck hematomas have an arterial source of bleeding identified on surgical reexploration, so decompression of the hematoma in the post-anesthesia care unit (PACU) should not be delayed if respiratory distress is profound and endotracheal intubation impossible.[10]

Other etiologies of postoperative stridor related to procedure include post-thyroidectomy tracheomalacia as well as retained instruments, throat packs, and foreign bodies including aspirated teeth. These can be serious, but are generally uncommon.

Airway management-related stridor: Laryngeal edema is an accepted risk associated with endotracheal intubation and can be the source of post-extubation stridor. If endotracheal intubation requires repeated attempts or is traumatic, the risk of post-extubation stridor is increased. Laryngeal mask airways appear to have a lower incidence of postoperative laryngeal edema.[11] Although it is common practice to use intravenous steroids to prevent post-extubation stridor, most of the literature on this topic relates to patients in intensive care units and may not be applicable to a perioperative population.[12,13]

Paradoxical vocal cord movement (PVCM) occurs from bilateral adduction of the vocal folds on inspiration, with resultant inspiratory stridor. Historically, this condition was believed to be exclusively psychogenic in origin, and the condition has been referred to as hysterical croup or Munchausen's stridor.[14] More recently, the role of laryngeal irritation has been recognized, and the condition is observed after endotracheal intubation. Diagnosis is confirmed by flexible laryngoscopy and observation of vocal fold movement. If vocal fold movement is not observed clinically, PVCM may be mistaken for stridor of another etiology, or for bronchospasm. Knowledge of postoperative PVCM is limited primarily to a few case reports, but the condition is most likely underdiagnosed.[15]

Anaphylactic and anaphylactoid reactions: Anaphylactic and anaphylactoid reactions, although different in their mechanism, are clinically indistinguishable. Patients present with airway edema (stridor or wheezing), hypotension, and tachycardia. Other symptoms include urticaria, flushing, nausea, vomiting, diarrhea, and abdominal pain. These signs and symptoms can occur anytime during perioperative course. Neuromuscular blockers, latex proteins, and antibiotics are the most often implicated allergens in the surgical patient.[16]

Other etiologies: Most, but not all, perioperative stridor is associated with perioperative interventions. Many cases of stridor will be associated with underlying disease. Neurological diseases such as myasthenia gravis and bulbar palsy can lead to stridor. Reactive airway disease, in its most severe form, can present as stridor. Infectious or neoplastic processes affecting the airway may present as stridor. A myriad of pre-existing conditions such as laryngeal candidiasis[17] or subglottic stenosis[18] have been implicated in the incidental development of stridor after procedures.

Assessment of stridor in the PACU

History and physical exam are the most important components of evaluating stridor. Reviewing the chart for pertinent data, including type of surgery and anesthesia, can give valuable clues to the cause.

Auscultation of the airway is imperative. An inspiratory stridor usually suggests airway obstruction above the glottis while an expiratory stridor is indicative of obstruction in the lower trachea. A biphasic stridor suggests a glottic or subglottic lesion. Injury to the larynx may also present with voice changes. A positive Chvostek's sign (twitching of facial muscles when the facial nerve is tapped) or Trousseau's sign (tetany of the arm when a blood pressure cuff is inflated and held for 3 minutes) is suggestive of hypocalcemia. Flexible fiber-optic bronchoscopy is invaluable and relatively safe when assessing the stridor. In the evaluation of over 1,000 pediatric patients with stridor, flexible bronchoscopy or laryngoscopy helped establish a diagnosis in over 75% of the cases, with minimal associated risk.[19] Rigid bronchoscopy with general anesthesia may be helpful and necessary to remove foreign bodies. Diagnostic roentgenograms may be useful in identifying retained operative instruments. Blood calcium levels may confirm the diagnosis of hypocalcemia.

Treatment: Treatment of stridor is both supportive and etiology-specific. Administering supplemental oxygen via nasal cannula or facemask carries minimal risks and should be instituted without delay. Humidified oxygen, helium–oxygen mixtures to restore laminar airflow, continuous positive airway pressure, and endotracheal intubation may benefit some patients.

Most nerve palsies associated with thyroid surgeries are transient and may simply require observation. Laryngospasm induced by airway irritants is treated by removing the offending stimulus (suctioning the airway for secretions or blood) and by administration of oxygen with positive pressure. If this fails, a small dose of a muscle relaxant and intubation may be necessary. If laryngospasm is induced by hypocalcemia, intravenous calcium gluconate should be administered. Anaphylaxis and anaphylactoid reactions are treated with small doses of epinephrine, fluids, nebulized beta-adrenergic agonists (albuterol), steroids, and histamine blockers. Some etiologies, e.g. hematoma, may require decompression if the airway obstruction significantly compromises ventilation.

Signs of impending respiratory failure including restlessness, hoarseness, cyanosis, nasal flaring, hypoxia, and use of accessory muscles should prompt an immediate assessment of the need for endotracheal intubation.

The treatment of PVCM requires special mention. Historically considered psychogenic and treated with anxiolytics in medical patient populations, there are anecdotal reports of similar successful therapy for postoperative PVCM. PVCM after extubation has been successfully treated with midazolam[14,20] and fentanyl[21] in small doses. It must be emphasized that these reports are both anecdotal and occurred after visual conformation of PVCM. The decision to sedate a patient with stridor must be made with great caution and only if other etiologies have been reliably excluded.

References

1. C.T. Sasaki, G. Isaacson. Functional anatomy of the larynx. *Otolaryngol Clin North Am* 1988; 21:595–612.

2. G.L. Olsson, B. Hallen. Laryngospasm during anesthesia. A computer aided incidence study in 136,929 patients. *Acta Anaesthesiol Scand* 1984; 28:567–575.

3. J. Fewins, C. Simpson, F. Miller. Complications of thyroid and parathyroid surgery. *Otolaryngol Clin North Am* 2003; 36:189–206.

4. S.L. Solanki, A. Jain, J.K. Makkar, S.A. Nikhar. Severe stridor and marked respiratory difficulty after right-sided supraclavicular brachial plexus block. *J Anesth* 2011; 25:305–307.

5. M. Rollins, W.R. McKay, R.E. McKay. Airway difficulty after a brachial plexus subclavian perivascular block. *Anesth Analg* 2003; 96:1191–1192.

6. M.L. Plit, P.N. Chhajed, P. Macdonald, et al. Bilateral vocal cord palsy following interscalene brachial plexus nerve block. *Anaesth Intensive Care* 2002; 30:499–501.

7. T. Wang, S. Roman, J. Sosa. Postoperative calcium supplementation in patients undergoing thyroidectomy. *Curr Opin Oncol* 2012; 24:22–28.

8. J.E. Witteveen, S. van Thiel, J.A. Romijn, N.A. Hamdy. Hungry bone syndrome: still a challenge in the post-operative management of primary hyperparathyroidism: a systematic review of the literature. *Eur J Endocrinol* 2013; 168:R45–R53.

9. K. Higa, H. Kazuhiko, N. Kazunori, et al. Retropharyngeal hematoma after stellate ganglion block: analysis of 27 patients reported in the literature. *Anesthesiology* 2006; 105:1238–1245.

10. W.A. Shakespeare, W.L. Lanier, W.J. Perkins, J.J. Pasternak. Airway management in patients who develop neck hematomas after carotid endarterectomy. *Anesth Analg* 2010; 110:588–593.

11. A. Tanaka, S. Isono, T. Ishikawa, J. Sato, T. Nishino. Laryngeal resistance before and after minor surgery: endotracheal tube versus laryngeal mask airway. *Anesthesiology* 2003; 99:252–258.

12. L.I. Ho, H.J. Harn, T.C. Lien, P.Y. Hu, J.H. Wang. Postextubation laryngeal edema in adults. Risk factor evaluation and prevention by hydrocortisone. *Intensive Care Med* 1999; 22:933–936.

13. R.J. Roberts, S.M. Welch, J.W. Devlin. Corticosteroids for prevention of postextubation laryngeal edema in adults. *Ann Pharmacother* 2008; 42:686–691.

14. W.H. Ibrahim, H.A. Gheriani, A.A. Almohamed, T. Raza. Paradoxical vocal cord motion disorder: past, present and future. *Postgrad Med J* 2007; 83:164–172.

15. B. Larsen, L.J. Caruso, D.B. Villariet. Paradoxical vocal cord motion: an often misdiagnosed cause of postoperative stridor. *J Clin Anesth* 2004; 16:230–234.

16. D.L. Hepner, M.C. Castells. Anaphylaxis during the perioperative period. *Anesth Analg* 2003; 97:1381–1395.

17. O.I. Kocyigit, S. Celebi, H. Gonen, et al. Laryngeal candidiasis: an uncommon cause of postoperative stridor. *Internet J Anesthesiol* 2009; 21. https://ispub.com/IJA/21/2/12068#.

18. V. Talwar, S.G. Raheja, M. Pawar. Post intubation stridor in a child with unsuspected congenital subglottic stenosis – a case report. *Indian J Anaesth* 2002; 46:61–63.

19. Wood, R. The diagnostic effectiveness of the flexible bronchoscope in children. *Pediatr Pulmonol* 1985; 1:188–192.

20. M.K. Baldwin, J.I. Benumof. Paradoxical vocal cord movement: a unique case of occurrence and treatment. *Anesthesiology* 2007; 107:359.

21. S.M. Neutstein, L.M. Taitt-Wynter, M.A. Rosenblatt. Treating stridor with opioids: a challenging case of paradoxical vocal cord movement. *J Clin Anesth* 2010; 22:130–131.

Chapter

11

Tachypnea and hypopnea

Erika Davis and Marc Fisicaro

- Tachypnea or hypopnea after surgery is common.
- Postoperative tachypnea may be secondary to hypoxia or non-hypoxic causes.
- Most hypopnea is secondary to pharmacological causes.
- Opioids, benzodiazepines, and neuromuscular blockers contribute to hypopnea.
- Bedside capnography or arterial blood gas sampling is needed to rule out serious hypoventilation which may occur in patients receiving supplemental oxygen without overt hypoxia.

Respiratory issues are some of the most common and challenging problems encountered in a Post-Anesthesia Care Unit (PACU). Anesthesia and surgical manipulation disrupt normal pulmonary physiology and can also exacerbate underlying pulmonary pathophysiology. Changes in respiratory rate, such as tachypnea or hypopnea, can herald the onset of major physiological derangement. In the PACU, respiratory compromise may also present as cardiac or neurological dysfunction, making expeditious recognition and treatment paramount.

Respiratory function is largely controlled by subcortical structures on the unconscious level. The brainstem is responsible for basic respiratory function, with the medulla oblongata acting as the "pacemaker" for respiration and the pons housing the pneumotaxic and apneustic centers which control the depth of inspiration.[1] Higher cortical centers may adjust respiration in response to information received from peripheral chemoreceptors, peripheral stretch receptors, and central nervous system receptors. Chemoreceptors, found in the carotid and aortic bodies, trigger changes in respiration due to fluctuations in PaO_2 and $PaCO_2$. In general, derangements in respiratory rate are due to conscious effort by the patient, physiological disturbance, or pharmacologic effect.[1] This chapter will review the commonly encountered causes of tachypnea and hypopnea in the PACU.

Tachypnea

Tachypnea means "rapid breathing." In an adult this can be defined as a respiratory rate above 20 breaths/min.[1] Young children have a much higher resting respiratory rate, especially during the first three years of life.[2] The initial evaluation of the tachypneic

Post-Anesthesia Care: Symptoms, Diagnosis, and Management, ed. James W. Heitz. Published by Cambridge University Press. © Cambridge University Press 2016.

postoperative patient should always include an immediate assessment of all vital signs and a focused history and physical exam, with attention to surgical procedure, type of anesthetic, and anesthetic course. Causes of tachypnea can be divided into two main categories, hypoxic and non-hypoxic (see Tables 11.1 and 11.2). When evaluating a postoperative patient, it is important to make this distinction rapidly. A decreased pulse oximetry reading (less than 90%) is probably the most efficient method of determining whether or not hypoxia is the cause.

Causes of hypoxic tachypnea include atelectasis, pulmonary embolism, pneumothorax, hemothorax, carbon monoxide poisoning from inhalational anesthetics delivered through closed or semi-closed circuits with desiccated CO_2 absorbents, fluid overload/congestive heart failure, transfusion-related acute lung injury, asthma, acute coronary syndrome, and anemia. In contrast, causes of non-hypoxic tachypnea include pain, anxiety, dehydration, acidosis, and malignant hyperthermia.

Postoperative hypoxia due to hypoventilation and/or atelectasis is commonly seen in the postoperative patient. It is important to note that hypoxia itself can cause tachypnea. Successful treatment may be as simple as supplying supplemental oxygen via nasal cannula or facemask, sitting the patient upright, encouraging deep breathing and the use of incentive spirometry. If hypoxia is not relieved by these simple maneuvers, then investigation into one of the other listed causes must be sought. Vital sign assessment along with history and physical examination should help direct the clinical approach. Hypoxia is discussed in detail in Chapter 9.

Hypopnea

Hypopnea is defined as either low tidal volumes or slow respiratory rate. Risk factors for postoperative hypopnea or apnea include residual anesthetic and/or opioids, extremes of age, obstructive sleep apnea (OSA), residual neuromuscular blockade, chronic obstructive pulmonary disease (COPD), and neurological causes. Preterm infants are at an increased risk for postoperative hypopnea and apnea.[2] A relationship has been described between an infant's risk of postoperative apnea and young postconceptional age as well as history of necrotizing enterocolitis.[3]

Inhaled anesthetics simultaneously increase respiratory rate and decrease tidal volume.[1] Although minute ventilation is preserved, the smaller tidal volumes lead to an increased proportion in dead space ventilation which results in a net increase in the $PaCO_2$.[1] Additionally, volatile anesthetics blunt the normal physiological response to hypercarbia and diminish hypoxic drive.[1] Therefore the effect of residual anesthesia may confuse the diagnostic picture.

OSA is a disorder characterized by repetitive episodes of apnea or reduced inspiratory airflow due to upper airway obstruction during sleep. The incidence of postoperative complications in patients with sleep apnea is increased over that of the general population.[4] Volatile anesthetics, intravenous anesthetics, and opioid analgesics all compromise upper respiratory muscle tone and have the potential to induce or worsen upper airway collapse. The combination of OSA and long-acting opioids is extremely dangerous. Patients with OSA may require continuous pulse oximetry monitoring, especially for opioid administration, owing to an increased risk of apnea. Simple maneuvers such as supplemental oxygen, placing the patient in a sitting upright position, and the use of a nasal airway or continuous positive airway pressure (CPAP) can relieve obstructive symptoms. Having the patient bring in his/her CPAP machine to hospital the day of surgery so that it is available in the immediate postoperative period is an effective strategy. Upon discharge from the PACU, continuous pulse oximetry should be maintained.

Table 11.1 Hypoxic causes of tachypnea

Cause	Additional signs and symptoms	Diagnostic tests	Initial treatment
Atelectasis	Decreased breath sounds, crackles, wheezes, narrowed intercostal spaces	Chest X-ray	Deep breathing exercises, incentive spirometry, analgesics if incisional pain contributing to hypoventilation
Pulmonary embolism	Chest pain, hypoxia, sinus tachycardia, right heart strain on electrocardiogram (ECG)	Spiral computed tomography scan, ventilation–perfusion scan	Systemic anticoagulation
Pneumothorax	Chest pain, cyanosis, confusion, hypotension, diminished breath sounds, hyperresonance to chest percussion, tracheal deviation, subcutaneous emphysema, narrowed pulse pressure	Chest X-ray, arterial blood gas	Increase FiO_2, immediate needle decompression prior to imaging if tension pneumothorax is suspected, consult surgical service for chest tube placement, use caution with positive pressure ventilation
Hemothorax	Chest pain, cyanosis, confusion, hypotension, diminished breath sounds, tracheal deviation, narrowed pulse pressure	Chest X-ray, arterial blood gas, complete blood count, coagulation studies	Consult surgical service for chest tube placement, search for and treat underlying cause of hemorrhage
CO poisoning	Lightheadedness, confusion, headache, vertigo	Blood spectrophotometry or chromatography	Deliver 100% FiO_2, may consider hyperbaric O_2 in extreme cases
Congestive heart failure (fluid overload, transfusion-associated circulatory overload)	Respiratory distress, rales and crackles, gallop rhythm, peripheral edema, jugular venous distention, cyanosis, dullness to percussion	ECG, chest X-ray, arterial blood gas	Discontinue IV fluids, administer diuretics
Transfusion-related acute lung injury (TRALI)	Hypoxia, hypotension, pulmonary edema, recent (within 6 hours) transfusion	Chest X-ray	Supplemental oxygen, mechanical ventilation, supportive care, avoid diuresis

Table 11.1 (*cont.*)

Cause	Additional signs and symptoms	Diagnostic tests	Initial treatment
Asthma	Wheezing, coughing, bronchospasm, use of accessory muscles, chest tightness	Arterial blood gas	Administer β_2-agonist via nebulizer such as albuterol, consider adrenergic agonist such as epinephrine and emergent intubation in extreme cases
Acute coronary syndrome	Chest pain, jaw pain, chest pressure, nausea, diaphoresis, feeling of impending doom	ECG, complete blood count, cardiac enzymes, chest roentgenogram, urine drug screen	Morphine, oxygen, nitroglycerin, aspirin, immediate cardiology consultation
Anemia	Weakness, fatigue, malaise, dyspnea, palpitations, chest pain	Hemoglobin and hematocrit, blood glucose	Transfusion of packed red blood cells for acute symptomatic anemia

Table 11.2 Non-hypoxic causes of tachypnea

Cause	Additional signs and symptoms	Diagnostic tests	Initial treatment
Pain	Tachycardia, hypertension, agitation, delirium, diaphoresis	Pain score assessment	Analgesics
Anxiety	Tachycardia, hypertension, agitation, delirium, diaphoresis	Pain score assessment	Anxiolytics (e.g. benzodiazepines)
Dehydration	Tachycardia, hypotension, pulse pressure variation on pulse oximeter/arterial line, decreased urinary output	Hemoglobin and hematocrit	Fluid bolus, reassess for improved hemodynamics and urine output, search for underlying cause
Acidosis	Confusion, lethargy, hyperventilation (compensatory in metabolic acidosis) in response to hypercarbia or hypoventilation (respiratory acidosis)	Arterial blood gas	Determine underlying cause as respiratory or metabolic in nature and treat accordingly
Malignant hyperthermia	Increased temperature, tachycardia, muscle rigidity	Arterial blood gas, assess for hyperkalemia and acidemia	Dantrolene

Neuromuscular blocking agents are used as an adjuvant to anesthetic care by causing muscle paralysis of all skeletal muscles. These drugs are helpful during intubation to relax the vocal cords and enhance surgical exposure during the case. All muscle relaxants act at the neuromuscular endplate of skeletal muscles and block the action of acetylcholine. Non-depolarizing muscle relaxants may be reversed by anticholinesterases such as neostigmine or edrophonium. An incomplete reversal may lead to residual weakness, and the patient may not be able to take satisfactory tidal volumes. The use of nerve stimulation to assess the state of neuromuscular blockade will be painful for an awake patient. Instead, simply asking the patient to perform a 5 second head lift may be sufficient to assess the degree of reversal. If reversal is incomplete, an additional dose of anticholinesterase may be given.

Over-sedation and opioid overdose commonly cause hypopnea and, in extreme cases, overt apnea. All opioids produce a dose-dependent depression of ventilation by acting on receptors located on the brainstem ventilation centers.[1] The decrease in ventilation caused by opioids is characterized by a blunted normal physiological response to carbon dioxide. Hence, patients undergoing opioid therapy may have an increased resting $PaCO_2$.[1] Opioid overdose is typically characterized by a low respiratory rate, small tidal volumes, and pinpoint pupils. Physical arousal will temporarily increase the respiratory rate, but as soon as the stimulus is removed, patients will become hypopneic. Naloxone reverses opioid-induced hypopnea, but postoperatively may also carry the undesirable side effect of reversing analgesia. In severe cases, naloxone can be titrated to reverse respiratory depression while preserving analgesia. To reverse postoperative hypopnea, naloxone should be titrated in small doses (20–40 mcg).[1] The clinical effects of naloxone do not last as long as some commonly prescribed opioids such as morphine. Therefore, it is important to continue to monitor the patient after a therapeutic dose of naloxone has been administered.[5] Opioid withdrawal symptoms may be seen when large doses of naloxone are given to chronic opioid users. Other side effects that may be seen with naloxone administration include hypertension, hypotension, cardiac arrhythmias, dyspnea, and pulmonary edema.

Benzodiazepines can be used for anxiolysis and sedation, as premedication for surgery, or as part of the anesthetic in monitored anesthesia care. Typical preinduction doses of benzodiazepines will have negligible effect on respiration during recovery in the PACU for most patients. However, a dose-dependent respiratory depression is well described and can be exacerbated by co-administration of opioids. Flumazenil is a short-acting benzodiazepine competitive antagonist that may be used to reverse over-sedation associated with benzodiazepine overdose. Flumazenil acts quickly and has a short half-life, often much shorter than the drug it is being used to antagonize; therefore, continuous monitoring should remain in place after it has been given.[5] Subsequent doses may be needed. Flumazenil does not reliably reverse respiratory depression due to benzodiazepines.[6] Patients who are chronic benzodiazepine users may be at risk for benzodiazepine withdrawal, which includes the onset of seizures. It is important to remember that other medications used in the perioperative period, including some anti-emetics and antihypertensives, may have sedating side effects that are synergistic with other sedatives causing hypopnea.

Patients with COPD are at an increased risk for postoperative pulmonary complications including hypopnea and apnea. General anesthetic agents, opioids, and muscle relaxants combined with intubation and mechanical ventilation interfere with normal respiratory physiology. These effects along with supine positioning and thoracic or abdominal incisions produce an immediate decline in lung volumes with resultant atelectasis formation in the most dependent parts of the lung. Surgical procedures that are closer to the diaphragm put patients at a higher risk for atelectasis and poor respiratory effort in the PACU owing to pain and splinting. These effects are exaggerated in patients with COPD because of their increased airway inflammation after airway manipulation, and the blunted response to hypercarbia and hypoxia. These patients may present in the PACU in respiratory distress due to an exacerbation of their underlying illness. They may require supplemental oxygen and bronchodilators. If pulmonary status continues to deteriorate, then intubation and mechanical ventilation may be necessary. Pain management is extremely important in patients with COPD.[7] Splinting and pain with breathing may reduce tidal volumes and cause increased dead space, which may prove catastrophic in patients with compromised pulmonary function. Preoperatively, these patients should be optimized and regional anesthetic techniques used when appropriate to avoid airway manipulation and maximize postoperative pain control.

Neurological injury can be a devastating cause of abnormal respiratory patterns. Risk factors for postoperative intracranial hemorrhage include hypertension, coagulopathies, hematological abnormalities, intraoperative hypertension, blood loss, tumors, and chronic subdural hematomas. Patients may present in the PACU with impaired respiration and can deteriorate rapidly to an unconscious state. Patients may also exhibit the classic signs of a stroke: one-sided weakness, slurred speech, facial drooping, and decreased level of consciousness. A CT scan may be necessary to rule out an intracranial bleed.

Patients who have had neck surgery, including but not limited to carotid endarterectomy, thyroidectomy, and parathyroidectomy, are at risk for postoperative respiratory compromise due to mass effect from a surgical hematoma or airway edema. Immediate surgical decompression and exploration for the cause of ongoing bleeding is indicated. Intubation of the trachea should not be delayed in these cases to avoid impending respiratory collapse. Tracheal intubation may prove difficult because of altered airway anatomy; therefore, the decision to intubate should be made sooner rather than later, and back-up airway equipment including a bronchoscope should be available.

When treating a hypoxic patient after surgery, the decision to assist ventilation or intubate and mechanically ventilate should be made rapidly. The decision to intubate the trachea may be clinical based upon accessory muscle usage for ventilation and impending respiratory embarrassment, or based upon arterial blood gas sampling (pH <7.25, PaO_2 <60, $PaCO_2$ >50). Correction of hypercarbia and hypoxia, and restoration of acid–base status will decrease patient morbidity and provide time necessary to determine the etiology and begin appropriate treatment.

References

1. M.A. Fowler, B.D. Spiess, Post anesthesia recovery. In P.G. Barash, B.F. Cullen, R.K. Stoelting, eds. *Clinical Anesthesia* 6th edition. Lippincott Williams & Wilkins; 2009:1421–1443.

2. C. Cote, J. Lerman, I. Todres. *Practice of Anesthesia in Infants and Children* 4th edition. Saunders/Elsevier; 2009.

3. C.D. Kurth, A.R. Spitzer, A.M. Broennle, J.J. Downes. Postoperative apnea in preterm infants. *Anesthesiology* 1987; 66:483–488.

4. J.B. Gross, K.L. Bachenberg, J.L. Benumof, et al. Practice guidelines for the perioperative management of patients with obstructive sleep apnea: a report by the American Society of Anesthesiologists Task Force on Perioperative Management of Patients with Obstructive Sleep Apnea. *Anesthesiology* 2014; 120:268–286.

5. A.F. Ghouri, M.A. Ramirez, P.F. White. Effect of flumazenil on recovery after midazolam and propofol sedation. *Anesthesiology* 1994; 81:333–339.

6. http://labeling.pfizer.com/ShowLabeling .aspx?id=684 accessed March 7, 2013.

7. M. Licker, A. Schweizer, C. Ellenberger, et al. Perioperative medical management of patients with COPD. *Int J Chron Obstruct Pulmon Dis* 2007; 2:493–515.

Dyspnea

Erika Davis and Marc Fisicaro

12

- The differential diagnosis of dyspnea in the surgical patient is broad.
- Focused physical examination is necessary to distinguish between pulmonary, cardiac, and other etiologies of dyspnea.
- Although dyspnea may be due to benign causes, prompt investigation to exclude life-threatening causes is warranted.

Dyspnea is defined as shortness of breath or "air hunger." The main causes of dyspnea are usually cardiac or pulmonary issues; however, neurological, musculoskeletal, endocrine, psychological, and surgical causes must also be considered in the Post-Anesthesia Care Unit (PACU) setting. Dyspnea should be promptly evaluated and treated as it can lead to impaired ventilation and oxygenation. The initial assessment of the dyspneic patient in the PACU begins with an evaluation of the airway, breathing, and circulation, followed by a focused medical history including the surgical procedure and anesthetic course. Additionally, a physical exam that focuses on, but is not limited to, pulmonary function should be performed. The presence of hypotension, hypoxia, tachycardia, tracheal deviation, stridor, use of accessory muscle, or cyanosis may indicate severe pulmonary compromise necessitating emergent ventilatory support and possible tracheal intubation.

Cardiac

Common cardiac causes of dyspnea in the PACU include acute coronary syndrome (ACS) and an acute exacerbation of congestive heart failure. Postoperative patients are at an increased risk for ACS given the hypercoagulable state following surgical intervention. An electrocardiogram (ECG), cardiac enzymes, and a chest X-ray can aid in the diagnosis of cardiogenic causes of dyspnea. Treatment for ACS involves increasing the oxygen supply to the heart while decreasing myocardial oxygen demand. Treatment for congestive heart failure involves decreasing lung congestion through fluid restriction and diuresis. The PACU provider should have a clear understanding of intraoperative and postoperative fluid administration, as well as preoperative cardiac function, while assessing these patients. Careful consideration should also be paid to chronic medications that may or may not have been administered preoperatively.

Post-Anesthesia Care: Symptoms, Diagnosis, and Management, ed. James W. Heitz. Published by Cambridge University Press. © Cambridge University Press 2016.

Pulmonary

Dyspnea due to pulmonary etiology in the PACU may be attributed to many conditions ranging from pre-existing pulmonary pathophysiology such as asthma and chronic obstructive pulmonary disease (COPD) to acute postoperative issues such as anaphylaxis, pulmonary embolism (PE), pneumothorax, mechanical obstruction, or inability to efficiently clear mucus. A focused physical exam and medical history can lead to the diagnosis.

Underlying pulmonary pathophysiology may be exacerbated and present as dyspnea in the PACU. Patients may arrive for surgery with pulmonary disease that has not been medically optimized. Endotracheal intubation and manipulation of the trachea and larynx during intubation are risk factors for bronchospasm especially among patients with a prior history of asthma and COPD. These patients may present in the PACU with dyspnea, cyanosis, cough, wheeze, and increasing oxygen requirements. Arterial blood gas may reveal an increased $PaCO_2$ and a decreased PaO_2. Patients with chronic COPD may have an elevated $PaCO_2$ at baseline, making extubation criteria complicated. Nebulized bronchodilators such as albuterol and ipratroprium should be administered during an acute COPD exacerbation along with supplemental O_2 to maintain adequate blood oxygenation levels as measured by pulse oximetry or serial arterial blood gas samples. Inhaled corticosteroids have not proven to be effective in an acute exacerbation of COPD.[1] To decrease postoperative pulmonary complication, patients should be advised to stop smoking at least 4 to 8 weeks preoperatively.[2] In addition, early ambulation and deep breathing, combined with incentive spirometry, intermittent positive-pressure breathing, and effective analgesia, may decrease postoperative complications.[3]

During an acute asthma attack, wheezing may or may not be heard depending upon the severity of the exacerbation. Patients will typically rely on accessory muscles of respiration and may present with tachycardia and tachypnea. Treatment involves delivering oxygen via nasal cannula or facemask until a SaO_2 greater than 90% is achieved.[1] β_2 agonists such as albuterol and inhaled agents such as ipratropium should be administered via metered dose inhaler or nebulizer. In refractory cases, inhaled or intravenous (IV) epinephrine may be administered, and intubation and mechanical ventilation should be considered.

PE commonly results from lower-extremity deep venous thrombosis, stressing the importance of preventative measures throughout the perioperative period. In addition to dyspnea, common signs and symptoms of PE include chest pain, tachycardia, cyanosis, acute desaturation, and a decrease in end-tidal CO_2 ($ETCO_2$) in an intubated patient. Imaging studies offer definitive diagnosis with the gold standard being a pulmonary angiogram. However, CT offers a non-invasive alternative and should be used as first-line study in most patients.[2]

Pneumothorax presents with absent breath sounds on the ipsilateral side. Signs and symptoms also include chest pain, cyanosis, confusion, hypotension, hyperresonance to chest percussion, tracheal deviation, subcutaneous emphysema, and narrowed pulse pressure. Immediate treatment depends on the hemodynamic status of the patient. For a simple pneumothorax in a spontaneously breathing patient, increasing the inspired FiO_2 often allows for adequate tissue oxygenation until chest X-ray can be obtained and surgical consultation can be performed to determine the necessity of a tube thoracostomy. In the case of tension pneumothorax in a hemodynamically compromised patient, immediate needle decompression prior to imaging is indicated. Should pneumothorax be suspected in the PACU, extreme caution should be taken with positive pressure ventilation as a simple pneumothorax can rapidly convert to tension pneumothorax resulting in hemodynamic collapse.

Airway obstruction

Dyspnea in the PACU may also be caused by a mechanical upper airway obstruction. Most commonly the tongue is the culprit. More rarely, retained surgical throat packs, surgical gauze occasionally placed in the posterior oropharynx during dental and ENT cases, may be inadvertently left in place, causing mechanical upper airway obstruction. Other causes of obstruction that may present in the PACU include acute laryngeal injury, hemorrhage, mucous plug, and vocal cord paralysis. Also, extrinsic compression from a pre-existing tumor or an expanding hematoma may result in acute dyspnea and signal impending complete airway obstruction. Factors contributing to airway edema include head and neck surgery, procedures in the prone position, and large intraoperative volume resuscitation. In addition to dyspnea, patients with upper airway obstruction may present with stridor, tachypnea, cyanosis, and use of accessory muscles of respiration. Careful examination of the oral cavity should be performed and assistance provided to relieve the obstruction, i.e. chin lift or jaw thrust maneuvers. If oxygenation and ventilation are compromised despite efforts to relieve the obstruction, tracheal intubation may be indicated.

Vocal cord injury or dysfunction may also present as dyspnea in the PACU. Although rare, it can be a catastrophic injury. Patients will present with hoarseness, dyspnea, dysphagia, and coughing. Risk factors include vocal cord surgery, extended intubation (greater than 100 hours), traumatic intubation, aortic surgery, and laryngeal nerve damage.[4] Patients with vocal cord injury are at an increased risk for aspiration pneumonia, which will increase surgical morbidity and mortality. A nasal pharyngeal laryngoscopy allowing direct visualization of vocal cord motion may be required to make an affirmative diagnosis. If the patient has had thyroid or parathyroid surgery, hypocalcemia should also be considered as a cause for dyspnea, although typically patients will not develop clinically relevant hypocalcemia until 24 to 72 hours postoperatively.[5]

Laryngospasm is a frightening cause of dyspnea in the PACU which is especially common in the pediatric population. Laryngospasm may be triggered by stimulation of pharynx or vocal cords by secretions, blood, foreign body, or extubation. Treatment is immediate and includes 100% oxygen delivered by positive pressure, followed by a small dose of succinylcholine and/or propofol to deepen sedation if the condition persists. Emergent intubation after resolution of laryngospasm may be necessary if spontaneous respiration does not resume and attempts at bag mask ventilation are inadequate.

Neuromuscular weakness

Weakness of respiratory musculature can lead to dyspnea in the PACU. Residual neuromuscular blockade should be assessed clinically, and careful consideration should be given to the type and total dose of neuromuscular blocking agent used. The anesthesia record will reflect the extent of neuromuscular blockade at the conclusion of surgery as well as the dose of reversal agent administered. The incidence of residual block, defined as a train-of-four (TOF) ratio <0.7, and postoperative pulmonary complications have been found to be significantly higher in a group who received the long-acting non-depolarizing muscle relaxant pancuronium versus the intermediate-acting atracurium or vecuronium.[6] Weakness of respiratory muscles may also be due to pre-existing conditions such as myasthenia gravis and myasthenic syndromes. These patients may present with dyspnea in addition to ptosis, diplopia, and dysphagia. Ideally, a diagnosis will be made prior to surgery and communicated to the PACU physician, who can make informed management decisions based on the severity of the disease, surgical procedure, and recent anesthetic.

Disturbances of respiratory drive

Inadequate respiratory drive due to residual anesthetic and postoperative opioids is common in the PACU. Recovery from most anesthetics can blunt physiological responses to hypercarbia and hypoxia. Immediately following arrival in the PACU is a critical time for hypercarbia and hypoventilation to occur.[7] It is common for patients to receive opioid narcotics after emergence in the operating room (OR), with the peak effect occurring during transport to the PACU. Patients with morbid obesity, COPD, age greater than 60 years, diabetes, or obstructive sleep apnea (OSA) are at particular risk for abnormal response to hypercarbia and respiratory acidosis.[8] Treatment involves increasing the inspired FiO_2, verbal and physical stimulation to improve the level of consciousness, lateral positioning, oral or nasal airways, and simple chin lift to prevent upper airway obstruction. In severe cases, naloxone (a pure opioid antagonist) may be administered in small doses to treat respiratory depression associated with opioid overdose.

Patients are at increased risk of aspiration in both the OR and PACU setting. Major risk factors include decreased level of consciousness which can compromise the cough reflex and endotracheal intubation or tracheostomy. Aspiration pneumonitis may present as dyspnea in the PACU. It should be noted that aspiration pneumonitis differs from aspiration pnuemonia in the constitution of the aspirate and rapidity of symptoms. Chemical pneumonitis refers to aspiration of substances that are toxic to the lower airways, not necessarily related to bacteria. Common toxins causing pneumonitis are gastric secretions, blood, and bile. Aspiration pneumonia refers to a bacterial infection caused by the aspiration of microorganisms from the oral/nasal pharynx or from microorganisms in the gut. The clinical course of aspiration pneumonia may take a few days and present with fever, productive cough, crackles, wheezes, and a loculated infiltrate seen on X-ray a few days later. The patient may also have increasing oxygen demands. Because of its time course, it is unlikely that aspiration pneumonia will be seen in the acute PACU setting. On the other hand, aspiration pneumonitis has a much more rapid and fulminate course. Within 2 hours of aspiration, patients may appear in respiratory distress. Common symptoms include cyanosis, increased oxygen demand, low-grade fever, and crackles upon auscultation. A chest X-ray will likely show unilateral or bilateral infiltrates in dependent pulmonary lobes. Keep in mind that if aspiration occurred while the patient was in the supine position, dependent portions of the lungs involve superior segments of the lower lobes and/or posterior segments of upper lobes. Bronchoscopy may reveal erythema of the involved bronchus. Despite its ominous course, most patients recover within a few days. A minority of patients, however, will go on to develop acute respiratory distress syndrome, which can be diagnosed with characteristic findings on arterial blood gas and chest X-ray.

The treatment of aspiration pneumonitis is mainly supportive, with oxygen as needed to maintain adequate pulse oximetry. Bronchial lavage or antibiotics are not indicated unless a specific species is cultured. If the patient is critically ill, empiric antibiotics may be started, but if no infiltrate is seen in 48 to 72 hours, then they should be stopped. Corticosteroids are not indicated. Mechanical ventilation is indicated in patients with respiratory failure.

Dyspnea may also be a symptom of a psychological impairment such as anxiety. Panic attacks are characterized by periods of intense fear that may last minutes to hours. The majority of symptoms are due to overactivity of the sympathetic nervous system causing dyspnea, tachycardia, diaphoresis, tachypnea, and subsequent respiratory alkalosis. Panic attack may be mistaken for ACS in the PACU. Symptomatic treatment involves anxiolysis with benzodiazepines.

The approach to the dyspneic patient should begin by ruling out the most life-threatening situations and performing life-saving procedures in a timely fashion. The PACU physician should then be able to identify impending airway compromise and provide preventative care. Finally, all non-life-threatening causes of dyspnea should be considered and systematically ruled out or treated. A focused history and physical exam along with surgical and postoperative history must be obtained in a timely fashion, and good communication with perioperative colleagues including surgeons, nurses, laboratory technicians, and radiologists cannot be overemphasized.

References

1. C. Karner, C.J. Cates. The effect of adding inhaled corticosteroids to tiotropium and long-acting beta(2)-agonists for chronic obstructive pulmonary disease. *Cochrane Database Syst Rev* 2011; 9:CD009039.

2. I.C. Mos, F.A. Klok, L.J. Kroft, A. de Roos, M.V. Huisman. Imaging tests in the diagnosis of pulmonary embolism. *Semin Respir Crit Care Med* 2012; 33:138–143.

3. B.R. Celli, W. MacNee for the ATS/ERS Task Force. Standards for the diagnosis and treatment of patients with COPD: a summary of the ATS/ERS position paper. *Eur Respir J* 2004; 23:932–946.

4. M. Kikura, S. Sato. Incidence and risk factors of postoperative vocal cord paralysis in 987 patients after cardiovascular surgery. *Ann Thorac Surg* 2007; 83:2147–2152.

5. M. Fowler, B.D. Spiess. Post anesthesia recovery. In P.G. Barash , B.F. Cullen, R.K. Stoelting, eds. *Clinical Anesthesia* 6th edition. Philadelphia: Lippincott Williams & Wilkins; 2009:1421–1443.

6. H. Berg, J. Rode, J. Viby-Mogensen, et al. Residual neuromuscular block is a risk factor for postoperative pulmonary complications. A prospective, randomized, and blinded study of postoperative pulmonary complications after atracurium, vecuronium and pancuronium. *Acta Anaesthesiol Scand* 1997; 41:1095–1103.

7. D.K. Rose, M.M. Cohen, D.F. Wigglesworth, D.P. Deboer. Critical respiratory events in the postanesthesia care unit. Patient, surgical, and anesthetic factors. *Anesthesiology* 1994; 81:410–418.

8. W.J. DePaso. Aspiration pneumonia. *Clin Chest Med* 1991; 12:269–284.

Chapter 13

Dysphonia and airway trauma

Megan J. Sharpe and Julie P. Ma

- Dental injury accounts for the majority of post-anesthetic airway injuries.
- Mild sore throat is a common and usually self-limited complaint after endotracheal intubation or laryngeal mask airway placement.
- Severe sore throat is very uncommon and should raise suspicion for airway injury.
- Postoperative hoarseness and changes in phonation should raise suspicion for possible arytenoid cartilage dislocation.

Airway trauma is a well-known potential complication of anesthesia that can result in significant morbidity and mortality. According to the American Society of Anesthesiologists Closed Claims Database, approximately 6% of the 4,460 claims analyzed were recorded as "airway injury" with the most frequent sites of injury consisting of the larynx (33%), pharynx (19%), and esophagus (18%).[1] Injury results from a combination of instrumentation of the airway with rigid equipment (laryngoscope, endotracheal tube [ETT], laryngeal mask airway), skill level of the anesthesia provider, and patient anatomy (i.e. micrognathia, inadequate neck extension or mouth opening, airway mass).

The most common symptoms of airway trauma in the postoperative patient include pain, bleeding, dysphonia, stridor, dysphagia, and/or odynophagia. Review of the anesthetic record and physical examination of the patient are important in diagnosis of airway injuries in the postoperative setting. In this chapter we review different types of airway trauma, mechanism, presentation, diagnosis, and management.

Nerve injuries

- Mechanisms:
  - Endotracheal intubation: injury to hypoglossal nerve, laryngeal nerve, or internal branch of the superior laryngeal nerve due to direct pressure with laryngoscope blade, rupture of piriform recess by an ETT, malposition of endotracheal tube cuff, or improper ETT size.[2]
  - Facemask ventilation: injury to the mandibular branch of the facial nerve, or mental branch of the trigeminal nerve from direct mechanical compression with the mask.[2]

Post-Anesthesia Care: Symptoms, Diagnosis, and Management, ed. James W. Heitz. Published by Cambridge University Press. © Cambridge University Press 2016.

- Laryngeal mask airway (LMA): injury to lingual, hypoglossal, or recurrent laryngeal branch of the vagus nerve from direct mechanical compression (specific cause unknown but could be overinflated LMA, too small sized LMA, use of nitrous oxide, or prolonged LMA use).[2,3]

- Presentation: within 48 hours of surgery and depends on the nerve injured.
  - Lingual nerve injury: loss of taste, and of sensation over the anterior tongue.
  - Hypoglossal nerve injury: difficulty in swallowing.
  - Mandibular branch of the facial nerve: facial nerve palsy.
  - Mental nerve injury: lower lip numbness.
  - Recurrent laryngeal nerve injury: dysarthria, stridor, postoperative aspiration, hoarseness (unilateral injury), respiratory obstruction (bilateral injury).[2,3] Hoarseness is a common postoperative complication with an incidence of 14.4% to 50%.[4]
  - Superior laryngeal nerve injury: numbness of the upper surface of the larynx.

- Diagnosis: clinical based on exam and patient symptoms. Direct visualization of vocal cords (e.g. with fiber-optic scope) may help to diagnose recurrent laryngeal nerve injury.
- Management: reassurance for most nerve injuries as they usually resolve spontaneously over a period of days to months.[3] If recurrent laryngeal nerve is injured, patient may be at risk for aspiration.[5] An otolaryngology consult should be considered.

Dislocations

- Temporomandibular joint (TMJ) dislocation
  - Mechanism: pressure applied to the angle of the mandible during facemask ventilation, or during routine tracheal intubations when excessive force is applied to the joint when opening the mouth. Patient with facial skeletal abnormalities are at an increased risk.[6]
  - Presentation: pain, trismus.
  - Diagnosis: history of dislocation in OR, clinical symptoms.
  - Treatment: soft diet for 2 weeks. If symptoms persist after 2 weeks, an oral surgery consult should be considered.[6]

- Arytenoid dislocation
  - Mechanism: tearing of cricoarytenoid ligaments resulting in vocal cord immobility on affected side. Occurs during direct laryngoscopy with inadequate visualization, use of a large ETT, or rarely with an LMA. Risk factors include elderly, systemic joint diseases (i.e. rheumatoid arthritis), difficult airway, use of blind intubation technique.[6]
  - Presentation: persistent hoarseness after extubation, "breathy" voice, odynophagia, weak cough, aspiration.[7]
  - Diagnosis: direct visualization or CT scan.
  - Management: otolaryngology consult for reduction of dislocation as soon as possible to avoid permanent damage.

Nasopharyngeal injuries

Types of injuries include false passage of tube into posterior pharyngeal wall, dislodgement of nasal polyps or turbinates, adenoidectomy, injury of the nasal septum, or mucosal lacerations.

- Mechanisms: placement of rigid/semirigid devices such as nasogastric and nasotracheal tubes, as well as nasal trumpets, in the nasopharynx.
- Presentation: epistaxis, pain, edema, hyposmia, or anosmia (reduced ability or inability to detect odors).[2]
- Diagnosis: direct visualization.
- Management: reassurance, otolaryngology consult for persistent epistaxis that may require nasal packing.

Injuries of oral cavity/pharynx/larynx

Injuries can range from superficial mucosal lacerations to internal carotid artery thrombosis or pseudoaneurysm, thrombosis of the internal jugular vein, or pharyngoesophageal perforation which can result in mediastinitis.[8] Other injuries include dental injuries (incidence greater than 1 in 4,500 anesthetics[9]), tongue lacerations, perforation of the piriform recess or epiglottic vallecula, hematoma of vocal cord (usually on left).[2,10] The most frequent injury of the larynx is to the recurrent laryngeal nerve, causing vocal cord paralysis (see "Nerve injuries" above). Most commonly, however, patients complain of a sore throat: 7% to 12% of patients whose airway was maintained with an LMA, 14.4% to 90% of patients who had an ETT, and 15% to 22% who had a plastic oral airway and facemask report a sore throat in the postoperative period.[9,11,12] Women tend to report sore throat more often than men do.[11]

- Mechanisms:
    . Videolaryngoscope injuries: insertion of ETT and/or stylette into soft tissues of pharynx/larynx causing laceration likely due to placement of tube without a period of direct visualization until the tip comes into view on video screen.
    . Laryngoscope blade, ETT, stylette, tube exchanger, bougie, Yankauer suction, naso or orogastric tube, oral or nasal airway, transesophageal echo probe, temperature probe, LMA can all cause trauma with routine insertion/use.

- Presentation: depends on location and severity of injury but can include pain, bleeding, odynophagia, hematoma, mediastinitis, subcutaneous crepitus, pneumothorax, and chest pain.[6,8]
- Diagnosis: history, direct visualization, radiologist consultation for advice on imaging. Diagnosis of perforations may be delayed, as early symptoms, such as sore throat, deep cervical neck pain, chest pain, and cough, are non-specific.[1]
- Treatment:
    . Sore throat: reassurance as it usually resolves spontaneously. Ice chips or a gargle with a topical drug such as benzydamine hydrochloride can provide symptomatic relief.[13]
    . Dental injuries: avulsed teeth should be placed in saline and an oral surgery consult should be called, as the tooth should be re-implanted within one hour. A partial or complete dental fracture should be evaluated by an oral surgeon postoperatively for consideration of restoration.[2,6]

. Minor lacerations: usually self-limited and do not require surgical intervention. For deeper lacerations patients should remain NPO for 48 hours and be placed on broad spectrum antibiotics. Otolaryngology consult is suggested for more severe injuries that may need to be surgically repaired. Those patients necessitating surgical repair should be NPO for at least one week. If a hematoma is present, antibiotics should be administered, and it should be drained if it is large.[6]

. Pharyngoesophageal perforations: the high mortality associated with these perforations warrants early intervention. If a perforation is suspected a surgical consult should be made, the patient should remain NPO, and broad spectrum intravenous antibiotics should be started.[14]

Tracheal injuries

Risk is increased for patients with difficult airway, emergency situations, repetitive attempts, inexperience of the operator, inappropriate choice of ETT size, double lumen tube, cuff overinflation, misuse of the stylette, poor tube positioning, excessive coughing, female sex, elderly, corticosteroid use, compromised medical condition, inflammatory diseases, tracheomalacia, and congenital tracheal malformations.[15]

- Mucosal injury

  . Mechanism: direct injury to mucosal surface of trachea by ETT or overinflation of ETT cuff causing necrosis or ulceration of the mucosa. Hypotensive patients are at increased risk for mucosal necrosis.[2]

  . Presentation: bleeding; may be asymptomatic if injury is small.

  . Diagnosis: direct visualization via fiber-optic bronschoscopy.

  . Management: superficial lacerations typically produce an ulcer that will heal over several days without any intervention; otolaryngology consultation for more severe injuries/lacerations.

- Tracheal rupture: extremely rare after orotracheal intubation, but serious complication.

  . Mechanism: direct injury to trachea. Lesions are usually longitudinal and frequently located in the pars membranosa, the posterior part of the trachea that lacks support from the cartilaginous rings.[16]

  . Presentation: cough, hemoptysis, subcutaneous emphysema, respiratory distress, pneumothorax, dysphonia, and pneumoperitoneum.

  . Diagnosis: direct visualization via fiber-optic bronchoscopy, chest CT, and chest X-ray, which can show focal defects of tracheal wall, pneumomediastinum, pneumothorax, progressive extrapulmonary soft tissue air and should raise suspicion of tracheal rupture.[17]

  . Treatment: thoracic surgery consult. Consensus has not yet been reached on the management of PiTR (post-intubation tracheal rupture). Early surgical repair has traditionally been advocated, with supporters considering that surgery has good results with prognosis depending more upon the patient's underlying disease than on the actual tracheal injury. However, there are others who are in favor of conservative treatment with small rupture, less than 2 cm, and in certain patients with benign symptoms and no air leakage with spontaneous ventilation.[18]

References

1. K.B. Domino, K.L. Posner, R.A. Caplan, F.W. Cheney. Airway injury during anesthesia. *Anesthesiology* 1999; 91: 1703–1711.

2. C. Hagberg, R. Georgi, C. Krier. Complications of managing the airway. *Best Pract Res Clin Anaesthesiol* 2005; 19: 641–659.

3. J. Brimacombe, G. Clarke, C. Keller. Lingual nerve injury associated with the ProSeal laryngeal mask airway: a case report and review of the literature. *Br J Anaesth* 2005; 95: 420–423.

4. T. Mencke, M. Echtemach, S. Kleinschmidt, *et al.* Laryngeal morbidity and quality of tracheal intubation. *Anesthesiology* 2003; 98: 1049–1056.

5. Y. Kawauchi, K. Nakazawa, S. Ishibashi, *et al.* Unilateral recurrent laryngeal nerve neuropraxia following placement of a ProSeal laryngeal mask airway in a patient with CREST syndrome. *Acta Anaesthesiol Scand* 2005; 49: 576–578.

6. K.S. Loh, J.C. Irish. Traumatic complications of intubation and other airway management procedures. *Anesthesiol Clin North Am* 2002; 20: 953–969.

7. E.J. Frink, B.D. Pattison. Posterior arytenoid dislocation following uneventful endotracheal intubation and anesthesia. *Anesthesiology* 1989; 70: 358–360.

8. R.D. Vincent, M.P. Wimberly, R.C. Brockwell, J.S. Magnuson. Soft palate perforation during orotracheal intubation facilitated by the GlideScope videolaryngoscope. *J Clin Anesth* 2007; 19: 619–621.

9. M.E. Warner, S.M. Benefeld, M.A. Warner, *et al.* Perianesthetic dental injuries. *Anesthesiology* 1999; 90: 1302–1305.

10. F.E. McHardy, F. Chung. Postoperative sore throat: cause, prevention and treatment. *Anaesthesia* 1999; 54: 444–453.

11. C.A. Alexander, A.B. Leach. Incidence of sore throats with the laryngeal mask. *Anaesthesia* 1989; 44: 791.

12. P.C. Stride. Postoperative sore throat: topical hydrocortisone. *Anaesthesia* 1990; 45, 968–971.

13. R.S. Turnbull. Benzydamine hydrochloride (Tantum) in the management of oral inflammatory conditions. *J Can Dental Assoc* 1995; 61: 127–134.

14. B.L. Bufkin, J.I. Miller Jr, K.A. Mansour. Esophageal perforation: emphasis on management. *Ann Thorac Surg* 1996; 61:1447–1452.

15. E.H. Chen, Z.M. Logman, P.S. Glass, T.V. Bilfinger. A case of tracheal injury after emergent endotracheal intubation: a review of the literature and causalities. *Anesth Analg* 2001; 93: 1270–1271.

16. E.B. Lobato, W.P. Risley, D.P. Stoltzfus. Intraoperative management of distal tracheal rupture with selective bronchial intubation. *J Clin Anesth* 1997; 9: 155–158.

17. J.D. Chen, K. Shanmuganathan, S.E. Mirvis, K.L. Killeen, R.P. Dutton. Using CT to diagnose tracheal rupture. *Am J Roentgenol* 2001; 176: 1273–1280.

18. E. Minambres, J. Buron, M.A. Ballesteros, *et al.* Tracheal rupture after endotracheal intubation: a literature systematic review. *Eur J Cardiothorac Surg* 2009; 35: 1056–1062.

Chapter

14

Fever, hyperpyrexia, and hyperthermia

Andrea M. Hages and James W. Heitz

- Fever is rare during surgery, but common afterwards.
- Most low-grade postoperative fever is due to inflammatory response to surgical insult.
- Fewer than 1% of surgical patients develop postoperative sepsis, and fewer than 10% of postoperative fevers are caused by infection.
- The association between atelectasis and postoperative fever is unproven.
- Malignant hyperthermia presenting after surgery is very rare.

A variety of physiological and behavioral mechanisms work to maintain human body temperature at a thermostatic setting determined in the preoptic area of the anterior hypothalamus. Perioperative disturbances in thermoregulation are common. Fever, hyperpyrexia, and hyperthermia are all terms that designate an elevation in core body temperature above normal. Fever (>38.0 °C, 100.4 °F) and hyperpyrexia (>41.5 °C, 106.7 °F) are increases in body temperature caused by elevation of the hypothalamic set-point. Hyperthermia is an increase in body temperature caused by heat production which exceeds the ability of the body to dissipate heat without a change in the hypothalamic set-point.[1]

Fever in the immediate postoperative setting has been variously reported to have an incidence between 14% and 91%.[2] Although some version of the "Wind, Water, Walking, Wound" mnemonic* has been recited by medical students for decades to remember the causes and time course of postoperative fever, little evidence supports atelectasis (wind) as a cause of early postoperative temperature elevations.[3] The broad differential diagnosis of fever narrows considerably when confined to the early postoperative setting (see Table 14.1). Rectal, esophageal, and tympanic measurements best reflect actual core body temperature; oral temperatures average 0.3 °C and axillary skin 0.3 °C to 0.6 °C below core temperature. In most instances, history and physical examination can significantly narrow the differential diagnosis.

---

* Wind = atelectasis on day 1–2; Water = urinary tract infection on day 3–5; Walking = deep vein thrombosis on day 4–6; and Wound = incisional infection on day 5–7. Wonder or Weird Drug is sometimes included for drug fevers after day 7.

Post-Anesthesia Care: Symptoms, Diagnosis, and Management, ed. James W. Heitz. Published by Cambridge University Press. © Cambridge University Press 2016.

Table 14.1 Differential diagnosis of early postoperative fever

Non-infectious etiologies	Drug associated	Other iatrogenic	Endocrine disorders	Infectious
Elevated thermostatic set-point Aspiration pneumonitis	Drug-induced hyperthermia Drug/alcohol withdrawal Malignant hyperthermia Central anticholinergic syndrome Neuroleptic malignant syndrome Serotonin syndrome	Febrile transfusion reaction Active overwarming	Thyroid storm Adrenal crisis Pheochromocytoma	Aspiration pneumonia Sepsis Toxic shock syndrome Necrotizing fasciitis

Non-infectious

Elevated thermostatic set-point: An elevated thermostatic set-point after surgery is a frequent and benign cause of a 0.5 °C to 1.0 °C elevation past preoperative baseline measures, resulting from the release of cytokines and interleukins associated with perioperative stress. In a prospective study of 271 patients followed for 24 hours after vascular, abdominal, and thoracic procedures, longer surgical duration and extensive surgical incision was related to a higher postoperative rise in core body temperature, supporting the hypothesis that tissue injury and an inflammatory response is accountable for this rise.[4]

The majority of postoperative fevers occurring within the first 48 hours following surgery are attributable to this stress response.[4] This rise in body temperature is true fever, and the body may employ regulatory mechanisms including vasoconstriction and shivering to raise core body temperature. Although the pyrogenic mediators are released during the surgery, fever is seldom seen until the postoperative setting. General anesthesia and regional anesthesia both suppress fever. In a study of 10 healthy volunteers given a pyrogenic challenge with IL-2 prior to desflurane inhalation anesthesia, a minimum alveolar concentration (MAC) of desflurane of 1.0 completely suppressed fever during the anesthetic, while 0.6 MAC incompletely suppressed fever, with both groups quickly spiking fevers equal to the control group after the anesthesia was discontinued (Figure 14.1).[5]

Management: Fever may be commonly observed in the Post-Anesthesia Care Unit (PACU) and early postoperative period owing to inflammatory mediators released by surgical trauma. An acute postoperative fever caused by an elevated thermostatic set-point requires no treatment. The routine use of laboratory and radiological tests to work-up postoperative fevers may not be cost effective. Diagnostic work-ups for early postoperative fever rarely discover treatable causes.[6,7] Multiple studies over the past three decades have concluded that positive blood cultures in the first 48 hours after surgery do not change outcome when obtained for the evaluation of fever among adult patients without other constitutional symptoms consistent with infection,[8] and more recent data suggest this may also be true for pediatric patients.[9]

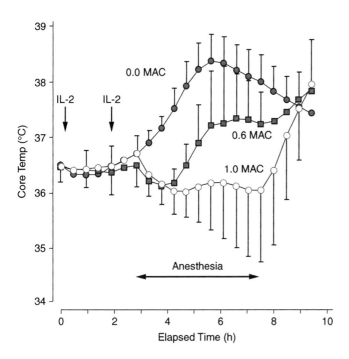

Figure 14.1 Fever during anesthesia.

Aspiration pneumonitis: The aspiration of gastric contents into the trachea and lower respiratory tract may occur if regurgitation occurs while protective airway reflexes are depressed. The acidity of the gastric contents may induce chemical injury of the tracheo-bronchial tree and pulmonary parenchyma with a subsequent inflammatory reaction. Clinically, this may be referred to by the eponym "Mendelson syndrome" after the author of the classic description in obstetrical patient populations.[10] Larger volumes and lower pH of the aspirate and the presence of particulate matter are correlated with more severe lung injury. Aspiration pneumonitis is rare, with an incidence of 1:895 emergency and 1:3,688 elective surgeries.[11]

Most perioperative aspiration is subclinical and asymptomatic. In one large retrospective study, 62% of witnessed perioperative aspiration displayed no clinical sequelae.[11] Hypoxia and dyspnea are the cardinal symptoms of severe cases, but fever may also be present owing to the inflammatory response. The fever of aspiration pneumonitis is typically low grade. Arterial blood gas may demonstrate hypoxia with increased alveolar–arterial gradient, and chest X-ray may show infiltrates in the posterior segment of the upper lobes or apical segments of the lower lobes if the aspiration occurs while the patient is supine.[12,13]

Unfortunately, efforts to prevent perioperative aspiration are not universally successful. The prohibition against eating before elective surgery does not ensure an empty stomach, nor does it reduce gastric acid content. In fact, the ingestion of clear liquids 2 hours prior to surgery may promote gastric emptying and reduce gastric residual volumes.[14] While the risk may be highest during airway manipulation, regurgitation and leakage around an endotracheal cuff may occur at any point during the anesthetic. Cricoid pressure has been used for decades during endotracheal intubation to lessen the risk of regurgitation by compressing and occluding the esophagus between the trachea and the vertebrae, but recent magnetic resonance imaging studies have suggested that the esophagus actually lies lateral to the trachea in more than half the population and cricoid pressure may shift it laterally in over 90%.[15] It is also important to emphasize that aspiration may occur after surgery, particularly if emesis occurs while mental status and protective airway reflexes are diminished. As much as 10% of perioperative aspiration occurs more than 5 minutes after tracheal extubation.[11]

Management: The acidity of gastric contents generally renders them sterile and treatment is supportive. If an aspiration event is witnessed, fiber-optic bronchoscopy may be useful to remove gastric contents or particulate matter from the airway by suctioning. Patients taking H_2-antagonists or proton pump inhibitor medications may have less gastric acidity, lessening the chemical pneumonitis, but increasing the likelihood of gastric colonization with bacteria. However, empiric antibiotic therapy has not been shown to improve outcome after aspiration and may select for subsequent infection with more virulent pathogens.[12]

Iatrogenic: Medication associated

Central anticholinergic syndrome: This complication occurs with the administration of medications with centrally acting anticholinergic effects. "Anti" medications including antidepressants, antihistamines, antipsychotics, and anticholinergics may precipitate the syndrome. Anticholinergics may be administered during the anesthetic for a variety of reasons. Atropine and scopolamine have been implicated in causing central anticholinergic syndrome. Glycopyrrolate does not cross the blood–brain barrier and should not contribute to the syndrome. Clinical manifestations can include fever, variable central nervous system disturbances ranging from delirium and agitation to coma, tachycardia, and hypertension with a wide pulse pressure. While mild fever is more common, hyperpyrexia occurs in approximately 25% of patients with this syndrome.[16]

Management: There are no clinical tests to verify this diagnosis; however, the rapid resolution of symptoms, including defervescence, with the administration of physostigmine 1–2 mg IV is both therapeutic and diagnostic.[16] Physostigmine has been associated with both severe bronchospasm and profound bradycardia and should not be administered more quickly than 1 mg/min.

Drug-induced fever: Many medications may induce fever due to hypersensitivity reactions. Penicillins and cephalosporins administered for wound prophylaxis are the perioperative medications most frequently implicated in causing hypersensitivity-mediated fever.[17] The preoperative use of psychotropic medications and illicit drug use may cause temperature elevation in the postoperative period for the trauma patient or surgical patient undergoing emergency procedures. Cocaine may cause temperature elevation. The mechanism appears to be impairment of thermoregulatory mechanisms rather than increased heat production by the body and occurs primarily in warm environments.[18] Methylenedioxymethamphetamine (ecstasy) is also implicated in hyperpyrexia with acute intoxication, but the mechanism appears to be increased heat production.[19] Similarly, phencyclidine[20] and amphetamine[21] may cause fever.

Management: Identification and cessation of the causative medication is the treatment of drug-induced fever. This may be challenging with the polypharmacy of the perioperative period. A preoperative urine drug screen, if available, may provide evidence of illicit drug use.

Alcohol withdrawal syndrome: Abrupt cessation of chronic alcohol intake can produce an alcohol withdrawal syndrome which begins within 5–10 hours of the decreased intake and may present in the early postoperative period. Severely affected individuals may begin to experience withdrawal while plasma ethanol levels are still measurable. Signs and symptoms include tremors, agitation, anxiety, tachycardia, tachypnea, and an increased core body temperature. More than two-thirds of affected patients display only low-grade temperature elevations (37–37.9 °C). Among the one-fifth of patients who experience temperature greater than 38.0 °C, most do not experience the fever spike until 48 hours of abstinence, and three-quarters of these patients have an infectious source (catheter phlebitis, urinary tract infection, or pneumonia).[22] The most severe form of withdrawal, delirium tremens, refers to the mental confusion and fluctuating levels of consciousness associated with the above symptoms. Delirium tremens occurs most commonly in males over the age of 30 years. Most will have a prior history of alcohol withdrawal syndrome.

Management: Benzodiazepines are used for prophylaxis and treatment of alcohol withdrawal syndrome. Diazepam 5 to 10 mg IV or lorazepam 2 to 4 mg IV may be used for the treatment of mild alcohol withdrawal syndrome. Both need to be titrated to effect, with considerable inter-patient variability in effect. Clinical caution must be exercised to avoid over-sedation in patients who may also have concurrent hepatic insufficiency related to alcoholism. Oxazepem 15 to 30 mg by mouth every 6 to 8 hours may be administered for prophylaxis or treatment of mild cases in patients able to tolerate oral medications. While most withdrawal syndromes are managed with return of withdrawn medication, administering ethanol for alcohol withdrawal syndrome is a historical practice now considered inferior to benzodiazepine therapy.[23] Benzodiazepines are the mainstay of treatment for delirium tremens as well, but propofol, dexmedetomidine, and barbiturates are also infrequently employed as adjuvant therapy.

Malignant hyperthermia (MH): MH is triggered by one of a variety of mutations of the ryanodine receptor that have been identified as causing a rise in intracellular calcium levels in response to the administration of succinylcholine and/or inhalational anesthetics. This initiates a hypercatabolic state which presents as tachycardia, tachypnea, muscle rigidity, acidosis, increased oxygen consumption, increased carbon dioxide production, and hyperthermia. An increase in carbon dioxide production may be the first clinical sign if end-tidal carbon dioxide exhalation is being monitored. Hyperthermia is a late sign, and the syndrome derives its name from a historical era when early diagnosis was not possible.

MH occurs with an incidence of 1 in 15,000 anesthetics administered to children and 1 in 50,000 anesthetics administered to adults in North America.[24] MH is one of the most feared diagnoses in a patient with an acute rise in body temperature in the perioperative setting, but it rarely presents *de novo* after surgery. In a recent review of the 528 cases reported to the North America Malignant Hyperthermia Registry, less than 2% occurred after surgery and in none of these cases was fever the presenting symptom.[25] However, recrudescence of MH occurs in nearly 25% of episodes and the diagnosis must be considered if the patient received treatment intraoperatively.

Management: If MH is suspected after surgery, immediate consultation with the anesthesiologist is mandatory. Prompt treatment with dantrolene 2.5 mg/kg IV can be life-saving. Dantrolene should be repeated until signs of MH are reversed and may require a cumulative dose of 30 mg/kg. Each 20 mg vial of dantrolene must be dissolved in 60 ml of sterile water for injection, which is a labor intensive process that may take 20 minutes or more to prepare the initial bolus dose. In July 2014, the US Food and Drug Administration approved a new formulation of dantrolene (*Ryanodex®*, Eagle Pharmaceuticals, Woodcliff Lake, NJ), which is packaged in a 250 mg vial that requires reconstitution in only 5 ml sterile water and can be prepared in under 1 minute. Dantrolene 1 mg/kg may be administered every 6 to 8 hours for 2 to 3 days to prevent recrudescence. Sodium bicarbonate may be administered intravenously to treat hyperkalemia and metabolic acidosis, and to alkalinize the urine if myoglobinuria is present. Other supportive measures include vigorous aggressive hydration, control of dysrhythmia (but avoidance of calcium channel blockers), and aggressive total body cooling to 38 °C. A urinary catheter will aid in diagnosis of myoglobinuria and allow for accurate measures of urine output and guide fluid resuscitation. Serial mixed venous blood gases and potassium measurements are necessary as aggressive treatment of hyperkalemia with glucose, insulin, bicarbonate, and hyperventilation should be employed. Baseline laboratory values including creatinine, coagulation tests, creatinine kinase, and liver function tests should also be obtained. The MH Hotline is available to assist with the diagnosis and treatment of possible cases.

24-hour MH Hotline
800-644-9737
Outside the US: 1-209-417-3722
www.mhaus.org

Neuroleptic malignant syndrome (NMS): NMS is characterized by increased heat generation and decreased heat dissipation caused by the inhibition of central dopamine receptors in the hypothalamus with the use of neuroleptic agents or the withdrawal of dopaminergic drugs. Older neuroleptic drugs are most often associated with NMS, but perioperative antidopaminergic agents including phenothiazines, haloperidol, prochlorperazine, and metoclopramide may precipitate NMS. NMS has clinical features similar to MH, but is a pharmacologically distinct entity which typically has a much more indolent onset. Unlike MH which typically occurs near the time of the triggering agent, the signs and symptoms of NMS generally occur over days to weeks with chronic therapy. NMS presenting in the early postoperative setting is very rare, but is occasionally reported.[26-32]

Management: Treatment is supportive and includes active cooling, antipyretic medications, and aggressive intravenous hydration to promote diuresis and reduce the risk of rhabdomyolysis-induced acute kidney injury. Dantrolone may be administered with good effect. For patients able to take oral medications, bromocriptine 2.5 mg by mouth every 6–8 hours and amantadine 100 mg by mouth every 12 hours may be prescribed.

Serotonin syndrome: Serotonin syndrome is believed to result from the hyperstimulation of central $5-HT_{2A}$ receptors. Monoamine oxidase inhibitors (MAOIs), tricyclic antidepressants (TCAs), selective serotonin reuptake inhibitors (SSRIs), and serotonin-norepinephrine reuptake inhibitors (SNRIs) may trigger serotonin syndrome either individually or more frequently when administered in combination with other serotonergic medications. This hyperstimulation results in the triad of altered mental status, autonomic dysfunction, and neuromuscular excitability.[33] The clinical manifestations include myoclonus, agitation, abdominal cramping, hyperpyrexia, hypertension, rhabdomyolysis, and potentially death. Symptoms may be present in various combinations or severity, making the clinical presentation variable and confounding diagnosis. Fever or hyperpyrexia may be a prominent sign. The Hunter Criteria require both a history of serotonergic agent

Serotonergic opioids
Fentanyl
Oxycodone
Methadone
Meperidine
Codeine
Dextromethorphan
Buprenorphine
Tramadol

use and one or more of the following symptoms to make the diagnosis of serotonin syndrome: clonus (spontaneous, inducible, ocular), agitation, autonomic dysfunction (including fever), tremor, or hyperreflexia.[34] However, the Hunter Criteria must be applied cautiously in the perioperative period, since most surgical patients will have received at least one agent with serotonin effects, but many of these agents, including methylene blue,[35] and some opioids,[36–38] are only weakly serotonergic. Serotonin syndrome has been reported following the administration of ondansetron, palonosetron, dolasetron, and ganisetron either as sole agents or in combination with SSRIs, SNRIs, or MOAIs. Most reports to the Food and Drug Administration regarding serotonin syndrome and anti-HT$_3$ have occurred in the PACU, so the clinician should have awareness of this possibility in the early postoperative course.[39]

Management: If serotonin syndrome is suspected clinically, serotonergic medications should be discontinued. Mild to moderate serotonin syndrome will usually resolve with discontinuation of the precipitating medications. Severe serotonin syndrome, characterized by muscular rigidity, temperature >41.5 °C, seizures, or coma requires aggressive therapy. Cyproheptadine blocks serotonin production and should be administered orally (4 mg PO every 4 hours as needed, up to 20 mg in 24 hours). Chlorpromazine IV may be substituted if patients are unable to take oral medications. Seizures may be treated with benzodiazipines or antiepileptics.[33] Endotracheal intubation and mechanical ventilation may be necessary for extreme cases. Lipid rescue therapy has recently been reported in the treatment of serotonin syndrome.[40]

Iatrogenic: Not medication associated

Febrile non-hemolytic transfusion reaction: Febrile transfusion reactions are a result of antibody activation to donor leukocytes. Patients who have received multiple transfusions of red blood cells or platelets develop antibodies to the human leukocyte antigens in these products. Clinically, it is typically seen as a temperature rise of 1 °C within 4 hours, and patients usually defervesce within 48 hours.[41] Oral acetaminophen may alleviate discomfort associated with the fever, although treatment is not necessary.

Iatrogenic overwarming: Avoidance of unintended hypothermia is a component of modern anesthetic care. Many anesthetic agents cause vasodilation and redistribution of the heat from the body core to the periphery. This heat is ultimately lost through convection to the colder atmosphere in the operating room. Evaporation of skin preparations and insensible fluid loss from surgical incisions exposing the interior of the body to ambient temperature also have an important role in heat loss. Unintended hypothermia can have adverse effects upon wound perfusion and oxygenation and coagulation, cause patient discomfort and shivering postoperatively, precipitating myocardial ischemia, prolong anesthetic drug action, and increase length of stay in the PACU.[4] Forced air heating devices, increasing the ambient air temperature, fluid warming devices, and warming blankets are used to prevent hypothermia in the operating room. Inadvertent "overshooting" may increase body temperature beyond the normal range. In contradistinction to malignant hyperthermia, this anesthesia-related increase in body temperature has been whimsically termed "malignant heating pad."[42]

Endocrine abnormalities

A variety of endocrine abnormalities may cause perioperative fever by activation of the sympathetic nervous system.

Pheochromocytoma: The typical location for a pheochromocytoma is the adrenal medulla, but it may develop extra-adrenally as well. Pheochromocytomas produce and secrete catecholamines, causing their clinical manifestations. Severe hypertension, not controlled by conventional measures, is the hallmark of a pheochromocytoma. Fever is commonly present with pheochromocytoma.[43] Tachycardia and fever may also be present, but unexplained hypotension or shock in association with surgery or trauma may develop because of diminished plasma volume and blunted sympathetic reflexes. Fever is consistently present in pheochromocytoma multisystem crisis, which presents with hyperpyrexia, multi-organ system failure, and hemodynamic instability.[43,44]

Thyroid storm: Thyrotoxicosis can result from any condition causing excess circulating thyroid hormone, including Graves' disease, toxic multinodular goiter, toxic adenomas, thyroiditis, and excess administration of thyroid hormone. This syndrome is less common today as early diagnosis and treatment typically occurs before the disease process progresses to this point. The clinical picture is that of excessive sympathetic stimulation and can include arrhythmias, shock, vomiting, liver failure, dehydration, hypertension or hypotension, fever, tachycardia, agitation, and delirium. There are also well-known triggers including trauma, burns, pregnancy, and the postoperative state.[45] Patients should be monitored in the intensive care unit (ICU) setting with an arterial catheter and aggressive fluid management.

Management: Pharmacological interventions are aimed at reducing fever, inhibiting thyroid production and release, addressing any precipitating illness, and reduction of the hyperadrenergic state; propylthiouracil, potassium iodide, propranolol, esmolol, and acetaminophen are some of the pharmacological interventions that may be employed.[45]

Adrenocortical insufficiency: Surgical patients may develop postoperative adrenocortical insufficiency due to pharmacological inhibition of β-11-hydroxylase with etomidate, intrinsic adrenal malfunction, or suppression from exogenous steroid therapy. The incidence of symptomatic adrenal suppression in surgical patients on exogenous steroids without stress dose steroids is 1% to 2%.[46,47] Continuation of the maintenance steroid dose throughout the perioperative course is adequate for most surgical patients to prevent adrenal insufficiency.[48] Acute adrenal insufficiency in the early postoperative setting would more typically manifest as hypotension than fever. If suspected, hydrocortisone 100 mg IV every 8 hours may be life-saving.

Infectious

Aspiration pneumonia: The term "aspiration pneumonia" is frequently applied incorrectly to the syndrome of aspiration pneumonitis.[49] However, the chemical pneumonitis is a nidus for secondary infection which may develop around 48 hours after the aspiration event. The use of H_2-antagonists or proton pump inhibitors may raise gastric pH, allowing for bacterial colonization, making subsequent infection for aspiration more likely. If true aspiration pneumonia is suspected, cultures including sputum should be obtained, and antimicrobial therapy consistent with the policy of the hospital for treatment of hospital-acquired pneumonia should be initiated.

Bacteremia/sepsis: Fever is a non-specific marker of infection in the immediate post-operative setting, and the severity does not provide any further indication as to its etiology.[3] The literature suggests that without signs of sepsis, blood cultures in the perioperative patient are unlikely to be revealing and therefore are not routinely used to evaluate causes of postoperative fever during the initial 3 days following surgery.[3,8] A recent retrospective study demonstrated that the incidence of severe postoperative sepsis has increased following elective surgery from 0.3% to 0.9% over a 10-year period.[50] There are various theories as to why this increase has occurred, including an increase in the number of nosocomial infections caused by resistant organisms and the increase in patients undergoing elective surgery who are more ill with more complicated co-morbidities. Postoperative bacteremia may be more common with nasotracheal intubation during surgery.[51,52]

Although unlikely to be recognized in the early postoperative period, two important infectious etiologies are worthy of special mention here since fever is prominent and each requires immediate intervention. **Necrotizing fasciitis** may present with fever, pain, skin blistering, multi-organ system failure, and confusion as early as postoperative day 2 and requires surgical debridement and broad spectrum antibiotics. **Toxic shock syndrome** arises because of enterotoxin type B secretion by *Staphylococcus aureus*. High fever, rash (typically a truncal sunburn appearance), confusion, and multi-organ system failure are prominent signs. Typically occurring 4 or more days postoperatively, toxic shock syndrome has rarely been reported within the first 48 hours after surgery.[53,54]

References

1. D. Kasper, A. Fauci, D. Longo, et al., eds. *Harrison's Principles of Internal Medicine.*16th edition. 2005. New York: McGraw-Hill Medical Publishing Division.

2. J.C. Pile. Evaluating postoperative fever: a focused approach. *Cleve Clin J Med* 2006; 73:S62–S66.

3. M.N. Mavros, G.C. Velmahos, M.W. Falagas. Atelectasis as a cause of postoperative fever: where is the clinical evidence? *Chest* 2011; 140:418–424.

4. S.M. Frank, M.J. Kluger, S.L. Kunkel. Elevated thermostatic setpoint in postoperative patients. *Anesthesiology* 2000; 93:1426–1431.

5. C. Negishi, R. Lenhardt. Fever during anaesthesia. *Best Pract Res Clin Anaesthesiol* 2003; 17:499–517.

6. J.E. Kendrick, T.M. Numnum, J.M. Estes, et al. Conservative management of postoperative fever in gynecologic patients undergoing major abdominal or vaginal operations. *J Am Coll Surg* 2008; 207:393–397.

7. R. Lesperance, R. Lehman, K. Lesperance, D. Cronk, M. Martin. Early postoperative fever and the "routine" fever work-up: results of a prospective study. *J Surg Res* 2011; 171:245–250.

8. C.P. Theurer, F.S. Bongard, S.R. Klein. Are blood cultures effective in the evaluation of fever in perioperative patients? *Am J Surg* 1991; 162:615–619.

9. A.W. Kiragu, J. Zier, D.N. Cornfield. Utility of blood cultures in postoperative pediatric intensive care unit patients. *Pediatr Crit Care Med* 2009;10:364–368.

10. C.L. Mendelson. The aspiration of stomach contents into the lungs during obstetric anesthesia. *Am J Obstet Gynecol* 1946; 52:191–200.

11. M.A. Warner, M.E. Warner, J.G. Weber. Clinical significance of pulmonary aspiration during the perioperative period. *Anesthesiology* 1993: 78:56–62.

12. P.E. Marik. Aspiration pneumonitis and aspiration pneumonia. *N Engl J Med* 2001; 344:665–671.

13. P.E. Marik. Pulmonary aspiration syndromes. *Curr Opin Pulm Med* 2011; 17:148–154.

14. J.L. Afelbaum, R.A. Caplan, R.T. Connis et al. for the American Society of Anesthesiologists Committee on Standards and Practice Parameters. Practice guidelines for preoperative fasting and the use of pharmacologic agents to reduce the risk of pulmonary aspiration: application to healthy patients undergoing elective procedures. An updated report by the American Society of Anesthesiologists Committee on Standards and Practice Parameters. *Anesthesiology* 2011; 49:495–511.

15. K.J. Smith, J.Y. Dobranowski, D. Gordon, C. Alezandre, T.L. Peter. Cricoid pressure displaces the esophagus: an observational study using magnetic resonance imaging. *Anesthesiology* 2003; 99:60–64.

16. R.L. Torline. Extreme hyperpyrexia associated with central anticholinergic syndrome. *Anesthesiology* 1992; 76:470–471.

17. P.A. Tabor. Drug-induced fever. *Drug Intell Clin Pharm* 1986; 20:413–420.

18. C.G. Crandall, W. Vonopatanasin, R.G. Victor. Mechanism of cocaine-induced hyperthermia in humans. *Ann Intern Med* 2002; 36:785–791.

19. H. Kalant. The pharmacology and toxicology of "ecstasy" (MDMA) and related drugs. *CMAJ* 2001; 165:917–928.

20. T. Bey, A. Patel. Phencyclidine intoxication and adverse effects: a clinical and pharmacological review of an illicit drug. *Cal J Emerg Med* 2007; 8:9–14.

21. A.R. Bodenham, A. Mallick. New dimensions in toxicology: hyperthermic syndrome following amphetamine derivatives. *Intensive Care Med* 1996; 22:622–624.

22. E. Otero-Antón, A. González-Quintela, J. Saborido et al. Fever during alcohol withdrawal syndrome. *Eur J Int Med* 1999; 10:112–116.

23. B. Hodges, J.E. Mazur. Intravenous ethanol for the treatment of alcohol withdrawal syndrome in critically ill patients. *Pharmacotherapy* 2004; 24:1578–1585.

24. N. Monnier, R. Krivosic-Horber, J.F. Payen et al. Presence of two different genetic traits in malignant hyperthermia families: implication for genetic analysis, diagnosis, and incidence of malignant hyperthermia susceptibility. *Anesthesiology* 2002; 97:1067–1074.

25. R.S. Litman, C.D. Flood, R.F. Kaplan, Y.L. Kim, J.R. Tobin. Malignant hyperthermia: an analysis of cases from the North American Malignant Hyperthermia Registry. *Anesthesiology* 2008; 109:825–829.

26. P. Adnet, P. Lestavel, R. Krisvosic-Horber. Neuroleptic malignant syndrome. *Br J Anaesth* 2000; 85:129–135.

27. P. Patel, G. Bristow. Postoperative neuroleptic malignant syndrome. A case report. *Can J Anaesth* 1987; 34:515–518.

28. C.C. Young, B.S. Kaufmann. Neuroleptic malignant syndrome postoperative onset due to levodopa withdrawal. *J Clin Anesth* 1995; 7:652–656.

29. P.C. So. Neuroleptic malignant syndrome induced by droperidol. *Hong Kong Med J* 2001; 7:101–103.

30. N. Tsuchiya, E. Morimura, T. Hanafusa, T. Shinomura. Postoperative neuroleptic malignant syndrome that occurred repeatedly in a patient with cerebral palsy. *Paediatr Anaesth* 2007; 17:281–284.

31. R.P. Ambulkar, V.P. Patil, A.V. Moiyadi. Neuroleptic malignant syndrome: a diagnostic challenge. *J Anaesthesiol Clin Pharmacol* 2012; 28:517–519.

32. S. Kishimoto, K. Nakamura, T. Arai, O. Yukimasa, N. Fukami. Postoperative neuroleptic malignant syndrome-like symptoms improved with intravenous diazepam: a case report. *J Anesth* 2013; 27:768–770.

33. D. Jones, D.A. Story. Serotonin syndrome and the anaesthetist. *Anaesth Intensive Care* 2005; 33:181–187.

34. E.J.C. Dunkley, G.K. Isbister, D. Sibbritt, A.H. Dawson, I.M. Whyte. The Hunter Serotonin Toxicity Criteria: simple and accurate diagnostic decision rules for serotonin toxicity. *QJM* 2003; 96:635–642.

35. S. Izdes, N.D. Altintas, C. Soykut. Serotonin syndrome caused by administration of methylene blue to a patient receiving selective serotonin reuptake inhibitors. *Anesth Analg* 2014; 2:111–112.

36. S.T. Rang, J. Field, C. Irving. Serotonin toxicity caused by an interaction between fentanyl and paroxetine. *Can J Anaesth* 2008; 55:521–525.

37. R. Rastogi, R.A. Swarm, T.A. Patel. Case scenario: opioid association with serotonin syndrome: implication to the practitioners. *Anesthesiology* 2011; 115:1291–1298.

38. S.C. Stanford, B.J. Stanford, P.K. Gillman. Risk of severe serotonin toxicity following co-administration of methylene blue and serotonin reuptake inhibitors: an update on a case report of postoperative delirium. *J Psychopharmacol* 2010; 24:1433–1438.

39. http://www.fda.gov/Safety/MedWatch/SafetyInformation/ucm418818.htm. Accessed 12/7/2014.

40. O. Dagtekin, H. Marcus, C. Müller, B.W. Böttiger, F. Spöhr. Lipid therapy for serotonin syndrome after intoxication with venlafaxine, lamotrigine and diazepam. *Minerva Anestesiol* 2011; 77:93–95.

41. K.E. Ponnusamy, T.J. Kim, H.S. Khanuja. Perioperative blood transfusions in othopaedic surgery. *J Bone Joint Surg Am* 2014; 96:1836–1844.

42. R.E. Johnstone. Malignant heating pad. *Anesthesiology* 1974; 41:307.

43. D.L. Gordon, S.D. Atamian, M.H. Brooks. Fever in pheochromocytoma. *Arch Intern Med* 1992; 152:1269–1272.

44. F.M. Browers, G. Eisenhofer, J.W. Lenders, K. Pacak. Emergencies caused by pheochromocytoma, neuroblastoma, or ganglioneuroma. *Endocrinol Metab Clin North Am* 2006; 35:699–724.

45. J.N. Wilkinson. Thyroid storm in a polytrauma patient. *Anaesthesia* 2008; 63:1001–1005.

46. H. Kehlet, C. Binder. Adrenocortical function and clinical course during and after surgery in unsupplemented glucocorticoid-treated patients. *Br J Anaesth* 1973; 45:1043–1048.

47. L. Knudsen, L.A. Christiansen, J.E. Lorentzen. Hypotension during and after operation in glucocorticoid-treated patients. *Br J Anaesth* 1981; 51:295–301.

48. P.E. Marik, J. Varon. Requirement of perioperative stress doses of corticosteroids: a systematic review of the literature. *Arch Surg* 2008; 143:1222–1226.

49. R.L. Jurado, C. Franco-Paredes. Aspiration pneumonia: a misnomer. *Clin Infect Dis* 2001; 33:1612–1613.

50. B.T. Batement, U. Schmidt, M.F. Berman, E.A. Bittner. Temporal trends in the epidemiology of severe postoperative sepsis after elective surgery: a large, nationwide sample. *Anesthesiology* 2010; 112:917–925.

51. F. Berry, W. Blankenbaker, C. Ball. A comparison of bacteremia occurring with nasotracheal and orotracheal intubation. *Anesth Analg* 1973; 6:873–876.

52. M. Dinner, M. Tjeuw, J.F. Artusio. Bacteremia as a complication of nasotracheal intubation. *Anesth Analg* 1987; 66:460–462.

53. R. Wagner, J.M. Toback. Toxic shock syndrome following septoplasty using plastic septal splints. *Laryngoscope* 1986; 96:609–610.

54. R.T. Younis, C.W. Gross, R.H. Lazar. Toxic shock syndrome following function endonasal sinus surgery: a case report. *Head Neck* 1991; 13:247–248.

Chapter 15

Hypothermia

Min J. Chun and Lisa Luyun

- Unintentional postoperative hypothermia is common.
- Anesthesia impairs normal thermoregulatory mechanisms and promotes heat loss.
- Forced air warming is the most effective intervention to correct postoperative hypothermia.

Human body temperature is tightly regulated to within 0.4 °C. Thermoregulation is controlled through the body's regulatory action and can be characterized by three general phases: (1) afferent sensory input, (2) central regulation mainly through the hypothalamus, and (3) efferent responses. Aδ and C fibers act as thermal receptors and can be found throughout the body, including the skin, spinal cord, and hypothalamus. Efferent responses to reduction of body temperature include behavior change (seeking warmer environment, donning more clothing), vasoconstriction, non-shivering thermogenesis, and shivering thermogenesis. The administration of anesthetics impairs these efferent responses and promotes the development of unintentional hypothermia. Mild hypothermia may be defined as a body temperature between 33.0 °C and 36.4 °C.

The administration of general anesthetics decreases the threshold for response to hypothermia from 37 °C to between 33 °C and 35 °C. With the induction of anesthesia, the body's voluntary behavioral defenses are lost, and involuntary autonomic compensatory mechanisms are activated in a predictable pattern as core temperature decreases, beginning with vasoconstriction, then non-shivering thermogenesis, and finally shivering thermogenesis.[1] The initial decrease in core body temperature by 0.5 °C to 1.5 °C after anesthesia-induced vasodilation results from redistribution of heat from central compartment to peripheral tissues down the temperature gradient.[2] Exposure of the patient to a cold operating room environment further contributes to the development of intraoperative hypothermia.

Mechanisms of heat loss include radiation, conduction, convection, and evaporation. Radiation constitutes the largest portion of heat lost and occurs through the emission of infrared rays. Conductive heat loss occurs through direct skin transfer by the loss of kinetic energy, while convective loss occurs through the removal of heat by air currents. Evaporative heat loss occurs through the vaporization of water.[3] About 90% of heat loss can be accounted for by cutaneous heat loss, which is proportional to the exposed body surface

Post-Anesthesia Care: Symptoms, Diagnosis, and Management, ed. James W. Heitz. Published by Cambridge University Press. © Cambridge University Press 2016.

area. The remaining 10% of metabolic heat loss is thought to be from respiration when patients are ventilated with dehumidified gas.

Clinical stages of hypothermia

Unintentional perioperative hypothermia occurs when heat loss to the environment exceeds metabolic heat production. Mild hypothermia (between 33.0 °C and 36.4 °C) is associated with mild central nervous system depression. Peripheral vasoconstriction and tachycardia may ensue. Vasoconstriction decreases cutaneous heat loss and conserves heat in the core. Post-anesthetic shivering is another common presentation of hypothermia in the Post-Anesthesia Care Unit (PACU), especially in young patients who have mild hypothermia.[4] Shivering is a potentially serious complication, which can double or even triple oxygen consumption and carbon dioxide production. Shivering results from hypothalamic regulation to increase endogenous heat production during emergence from general anesthesia.[3] In patients with pre-existing cardiopulmonary conditions such as coronary artery disease, low cardiac output, intrapulmonary shunts, or respiratory derangement, increases in metabolic requirement due to shivering may predispose to myocardial ischemia or respiratory failure.[5]

Moderate hypothermia (31 °C to 32.9 °C) results in further depression in the central nervous system and decreased motor activity. Patients may have depressed consciousness and unstable vital signs. Cardiac dysrhythmias may follow. Unintentional perioperative hypothermia is rarely this severe, but when it occurs, surgical patients with moderate hypothermia are generally kept intubated and mechanically ventilated until the body temperature is corrected.

Severe hypothermia (<30.9 °C) is associated with significantly depressed vital signs and cardiac impulse conduction. Ventricular fibrillation and asystole generally occur in core temperature below 23 °C. Respiratory arrest usually follows cardiac arrest. Patients may be comatose and areflexic at this point. If left untreated, such a profound level of hypothermia will soon lead to death.

Adverse effects of hypothermia

Postoperative hypothermia is a common complication after surgery and it prolongs PACU length of stay by an average of 40 to 90 minutes.[6,7] Although mild hypothermia of brief duration is usually well tolerated by patients, it can represent a significant clinical risk if it remains unrecognized and uncorrected. Postoperative hypothermia increases sympathetic nervous system activity. Levels of circulating epinephrine and norepinephrine rise, resulting in tachycardia, hypertension, and systemic vasoconstriction. Imbalance between oxygen demand and supply may lead to a higher incidence of postoperative myocardial ischemia. Unintentional hypothermia on arrival to PACU is associated with a significantly higher incidence of myocardial ischemia, angina, and PaO_2 less than, 80 mmHg during the early postoperative period.[8] Tissue hypoperfusion may occur and can lead to metabolic acidemia. This acidemia can worsen tissue hypoperfusion by shifting the oxygen–hemoglobin dissociation curve to the left and, therefore, compromise tissue oxygen unloading.

Coagulopathy may ensue even from mild hypothermia causing platelet sequestration and platelet function impairment. Enzymes of the coagulation cascade are directly attenuated by hypothermia.[9,10,11] Many randomized trials and subsequent meta-analysis report increased blood loss and transfusion requirements in hypothermic patients.[12]

Adverse consequences of postoperative hypothermia	
Altered medication metabolism	Decreased enzymatic function
Delayed emergence	Decreased drug metabolism, CNS depression
Electrolyte abnormalities	Transcellular shift causing hypokalemia
Hemorrhage	Coagulopathy, increased fibrinolysis
Hyperglycemia	Insulin resistance, decreased insulin secretion
Hypoglycemia	Increased glucose utilization (shivering)
Hypoxia	Blunted ventilatory response to hypoxia, left shift in hemoglobin–oxygen dissociation curve
Hypertension	Increased norepinephrine; increased SVR
Hyperthermia	Vigorous shivering
Myocardial ischemia	Increased SVR, HR, norepinephrine
Patient discomfort	Decreased satisfaction with perioperative care
Tachycardia	Increased norepinephrine
Ventricular dysrhythmia	Severe hypothermia
Wound infection	Decreased macrophage mobility, phagocytosis, decreased tissue oxygenation

CNS = central nervous system, SVR = systemic vascular resistance, HR = heart rate

Surgical wound infection is a major cause of postoperative morbidity. Perioperative hypothermia contributes to the development of surgical wound infections by directly impairing immune function. As stated above, hypothermia also triggers systemic and tissue vasoconstriction, decreasing wound oxygen delivery, which impairs proper healing.[13] Moderate hyperglycemia resulting from hypothermia also contributes to increased postoperative infection rates.

Hypothermia may lead to decreased hepatic perfusion and metabolism as well as decreased renal blood flow and clearance, therefore prolonging drug effects. Residual sedation may be accentuated from a decrease in the minimal alveolar concentration of inhalation anesthetics, which is shown to be 5% to 7% per 1 °C decrease in core body temperature. Durations of neuromuscular relaxants and sedatives are increased because of impaired biotransformation and low perfusion. Given the multitude of adverse physiological effects that result from hypothermia, it is prudent to pay close attention to monitoring its development, its adverse implications, and management.

Management

Management of postoperative hypothermia starts from intraoperative monitoring and maintenance of normal body temperature. Prevention is preferable to treatment.

Three standard core temperature measurement sites include the pulmonary artery, nasopharynx, and distal esophagus. The tympanic membrane is thought to be the most accurate location to obtain core body temperature because of its proximity to the internal carotid artery (approximates blood flow through the hypothalamus), but it may not be reliable secondary to interference by ambient temperature. Less reliable, but less invasive sites include oral and rectal, given that they constitute areas of highly perfused tissues. Skin temperature is not as dependable because readings are easily affected by surrounding environment.

To maintain perioperative normothermia, pre-emptive warming prior to the surgical procedure is crucial. Prewarming minimizes the redistribution of heat that occurs after anesthesia induction. It has been found that active warming for 30 to 60 minutes during the pre-induction period sufficiently increases body heat content of the peripheral thermal compartment, and core temperature decreases less in patients who were pre warmed.[14] Operating room temperature plays a crucial role in determining the rate of heat loss by radiation, convection, and evaporation. Aside from increasing room temperature to a comfortable point to all operating room personnel, passive insulation and active warming throughout available body surface during the operation are effective methods of preventing perioperative hypothermia. Forced air heating device is currently the safest and most effective active warming system, which can prevent and treat most cutaneous heat loss, and is widely used intraoperatively as well as postoperatively.[15]

Postoperatively, it is important to identify the presence of hypothermia as the patient arrives in PACU. Forced air warming is the most effective method for rewarming the surgical patient. One hour of forced air warming results in as much increase in core body temperature as the application of three cotton blankets for 4 hours or a single cotton blanket for 10 hours.[1] Fluid warmers are ineffective in rewarming surgical patients unless very large volumes of fluid are infused. However, each liter of crystalloid infused at room temperature decreases core body temperature of the average size adult by 0.25 °C, so fluid warmers should be utilized to avoid exacerbating unintentional postoperative hypothermia.[1]

Hypothermic-induced postoperative shivering should be treated to prevent adverse effects. Supplemental oxygen should be administered to increase myocardial oxygen supply in the face of increased demand. In addition to actively warming the patient, pharmacological interventions to abolish shivering include a number of opioids including alfentanil, meperidine, tramadol, and α-agonists such as clonidine and dexmedetomidine. Among these, meperidine, 12.5 to 25 mg IV (0.35 to 0.4 mg/kg), is most efficacious, with its proposed action being reduction in a shivering threshold.[16]

References

1. D.I. Sessler. Mild perioperative hypothermia. N Engl J Med 1997; 336:1730–1737.

2. T. Matsukawa, D.I. Sessler, A.M. Sessler, et al. Heat flow and distribution during induction of general anesthesia. Anesthesiology 1995; 82:662–673.

3. M. Diaz, D.E. Becker. Thermoregulation: physiological and clinical consideration during sedation and general anesthesia. Anesth Prog 2010; 57: 25–32.

4. L.H. Eberhart, F. Doderlein, G. Eisenhardt, et al. Independent risk factors for postoperative shivering. Anesth Analg 2005; 101:1849–1857.

5. J. De Witte, D.I. Sessler. Perioperative shivering: physiology and pharmacology. Anesthesiology 2002; 96:467–484.

6. S.M. Frank, L.A. Fleisher, M.J. Breslow, et al. Perioperative maintenance of normothermia reduces the incidence of morbid cardiac events. A randomized clinical trial. *JAMA* 1997; 277:1127–1134.

7. D.I. Sessler. Complication and treatment of mild hypothermia. *Anesthesiology* 2001; 95:531–543.

8. F.M. Frank, C. Beattie, R. Christopherson, et al.; The Perioperative Ischemia Randomized Anesthesia Trial Study Group. Unintentional hypothermia is associated with postoperative myocardial ischemia. *Anesthesiology* 1993; 78:468–476.

9. R. Lenhardt, E. Marker, V. Goll, et al. Mild intraoperative hypothermia prolongs postanesthetic recovery. *Anesthesiology* 1997; 87:1318–1323.

10. C.R. Valeri, H. Feingold, G. Cassidy, et al. Hypothermia-induced reversible platelet dysfunction. *Ann Surg* 1987; 205:175–181.

11. D.B. Staab, V.J. Sorensen, J.J. Fath, et al. Coagulation defects resulting from ambient temperature-induced hypothermia. *J Trauma* 1994; 36:634–648.

12. S. Rajagopalan, E. Mascha, J. Na, D.I. Sessler. The effects of mild perioperative hypothermia on blood loss and transfusion requirement. *Anesthesiology* 2008; 108:71–77.

13. C. Wenisch, E. Narzt, D.I. Sessler, et al. Mild intraoperative hypothermia reduces production of reactive oxygen intermediates by polymorphonuclear leukocytes. *Anesth Analg* 1996; 82:810–812.

14. J.M. Hynson, D.I. Sessler, A. Moayeri, J. McGuire, M. Schroeder. The effects of pre-induction warming on temperature and blood pressure during propofol/nitrous oxide anesthesia. *Anesthesiology* 1993; 79:219–228.

15. J. Hynson, D.I. Sessler. Intraoperative warming therapies: a comparison of three devices. *J Clin Anesth* 1992; 4:194–199.

16. E. Kelsaka, S. Baris, D. Karakaya, B. Sarihasan. Comparison of ondansetron and meperidine for prevention of shivering in patients undergoing spinal anesthesia. *Reg Anesth Pain Med* 2006; 30:40–45.

Chapter

Hypoglycemia

16

Brian Hipszer, James W. Heitz, and Jeffrey I. Joseph

- Most episodes of postoperative hypoglycemia occur in known diabetics owing to alterations in activity, oral intake, and diabetic therapy.
- Drug–drug interactions are significant for oral hypoglycemic agents and may occur perioperatively as new medications are initiated.
- Effective treatment of hypoglycemia requires rapid recognition and correction, as well as continued monitoring to avoid recurrence.

Hypoglycemia is a condition that primarily occurs in individuals with diabetes mellitus. In the outpatient setting, the diagnosis pairs the observation of clinical symptoms associated with hypoglycemia (e.g. sweating, arrhythmia, hunger, confusion, etc.) with the measurement of plasma glucose concentration. However, in the inpatient setting, the clinical symptoms are often masked, and hypoglycemia is simply defined as a plasma glucose concentration in the blood below 70 mg/dl. It can be further categorized as moderate or severe with severe hypoglycemia defined as a glucose concentration less than 40 mg/dl.[1] The clinical impact of the glucose concentration relates to the ability to effectively deliver glucose to the cells of the body to support metabolism more than to an arbitrarily derived number; therefore, individuals may experience symptoms of hypoglycemia at differing serum glucose levels.

Hypoglycemia has been associated with increased mortality in the hospital setting.[2–4] There is evidence that this association is related to spontaneous, as opposed to drug-induced, hypoglycemia.[3] And, although causality has not been established, the stress attributed to the counter-regulatory response to a hypoglycemic event is a likely candidate for increased acute cardiovascular complications in an already compromised patient population.[5,6]

High-risk populations

Diabetic individuals typically use insulin (administered subcutaneously through multiple daily injections or continuous infusion) or oral medications to manage their glucose levels in the outpatient setting. Improper transition of these therapies upon admission to the hospital can increase the likelihood of a hypoglycemic event. Elderly and pediatric populations also need special consideration. Aging can blunt the counter-regulatory response, the mechanism that enables the body to avoid hypoglycemia by decreasing insulin secretion

Post-Anesthesia Care: Symptoms, Diagnosis, and Management, ed. James W. Heitz. Published by Cambridge University Press. © Cambridge University Press 2016.

and increasing glucose production, while an intact and vigorous counter-regulatory response can stress the cardiovascular system during a hypoglycemic episode.[6] In young children, inadequate stores of glycogen or gluconeogenic precursors may interfere with the maintenance of euglycemia if challenged, especially after a prolonged fast.[7,8]

Causes

In the hospital, hypoglycemia is associated with altered nutritional state, heart failure, renal or liver disease, malignancy, infection, or sepsis. The administration of insulin and/or other anti-diabetic agents often precedes the onset of hypoglycemia. These agents either increase the glucose uptake into the insulin-sensitive tissues or inhibit hepatic glucose production.[9] When there is not enough glucose available (via endogenous production and/or exogenous delivery) to offset its uptake, hypoglycemia will result. The risk of hypoglycemia may increase with the transition of care to the Post-Anesthesia Care Unit (PACU). Thrashing and shivering, which may accompany emergence from anesthesia, can increase muscle work and body temperature, both of which increase the effectiveness of circulating insulin to promote glucose uptake.

Postoperative-specific etiologies of hypoglycemia

Continuation of long-acting hypoglycemics in known diabetics in association with peri-operative fasting is the most common cause of perioperative hypoglycemia. This risk is well-known and anticipated. However, postoperative hypoglycemia can develop unexpectedly in both diabetic and non-diabetic individuals.

The perioperative period is frequently associated with polypharmacy. Newly introduced medications by themselves or in combination with pre-existing oral hypoglycemic therapy may cause clinical hypoglycemia (Table 16.1; Figure 16.1). Anesthetic agents are rarely implicated in causing hypoglycemia, with the exception of a few anecdotal reports. Dexmedetomidine was reported to cause hypoglycemia in a child, but only when inadvertently administered in 60 times the intended dose.[10] Hypoglycemia has not been reported with typical clinical doses of dexmedetomidine, but has been rarely reported with clinical doses of clonidine, also an α_2-agonist. Etomidate may cause adrenal suppression for 24 to 48 hours and therefore may be associated with symptoms and signs of hypoadrenalism including hypoglycemia on postoperative days 1 and 2. However, one anecdotal report implicates etomidate with acute-onset hypoglycemia after bolus administration; the mechanism of this phenomenon was not identified.[11]

Many non-anesthetic pharmaceuticals have the potential to cause hypoglycemia in susceptible individuals; many more have drug–drug interactions that may potentiate the action of oral hypoglycemic agents and indirectly cause hypoglycemia. For example, many medications compete for plasma protein binding sites, displacing sulfonylurea medications and increasing the free fraction within the plasma, while others inhibit metabolism by competing for hepatic enzymes responsible for metabolism. Some of these medications are often initiated around the time of surgery. Fortunately, the hypoglycemic effect of most medications initiated perioperatively is weak and resultant hypoglycemia rarely clinically encountered.[12,13]

Postoperative hypoadrenalism may feature hypoglycemia along with the other clinical features, usually including hypotension, hypothermia, confusion, myalgias, and diarrhea. Hypoadrenalism may have a pharmacological cause for patients on chronic exogenous steroid therapy with suppression of pituitary–adrenal axis or patients receiving etomidate

Table 16.1 Pharmacological causes of perioperative hypoglycemia

Medication	Sole agent hypoglycemia	Drug–drug interactions with oral hypoglycemics causing hypoglycemia
ACE inhibitors	Rare	Glibenclamide, gliclazide
β-blockers	Rare	No, but may mask signs of hypoglycemia
Disopyramide	Yes	Gliclazide
Nicardipine	Not reported	Gliclazide
Salicylates	Rare	Tolbutamide, chlorpropamide, glibenclamide
NSAIDs	Not reported	Tolbutamide, chlorpropamide, glibenclamdie
Acetaminophen	Not reported	Some sulphonylureas
Quinolones	Rare	Gibenclamide, glimepiride, glipizide
Sulfonamides	Not reported	Chlorpropamide, glibenclamide, gliclazide, tolbutamide
Macrolides	Not reported	Glibenclamide, glipizide, tolbutamide
H$_2$-receptor blockers	Not reported	Gliclazide, glibenclamide
Heparin calcium	Not reported	Glipizide

ACE, angiotensin-converting enzyme; NSAIDs, non-steroidal anti-inflammatory drugs.

for induction of general anesthesia. The incidence of hypoadrenalism among surgical patients whose chronic exogenous steroids are abruptly interrupted appears to be about 1% to 2%.[14,15] Adrenalectomy may produce hypoadrenalism, as may other adrenal procedures. Hypoadrenalism has very rarely been observed after resection of pheochromocytoma.[16] Hypoadrenalism may also be a part of panhypopituitarism, seen most frequently after procedures near the sella turcica or after sustained hypotension from hemorrhage causing pituitary apoplexy (Sheehan's syndrome).

Postoperative hypoglycemia may be caused by gastric dumping syndrome, frequently observed after esophageal, gastric, or bariatric surgery. Gastric dumping syndrome may cause hypoglycemia when large food particles are prematurely delivered to the small bowel, resulting in poor glucose absorption and a relative excess of endogenous insulin. Although clinically important, this typically presents after feeding has resumed and relatively late in the postoperative course.[17]

Technical limitations of glucose meters also contribute to hypoglycemia. Most meter errors are due to operator errors or calibration errors, but meter design may influence performance under clinical conditions. Acetaminophen, dopamine, and mannitol, all of which may be administered perioperatively, interfere with the performance of meters which employ a peroxide reduction detection method for glucose measurements, leading to pseudohypoglycemia, while meters using an amperometric technique are unaffected by these medications.[18] Hypotension may also lead to pseudohypoglycemia as poor perfusion of the extremities allows for greater utilization of glucose and lower measured levels. This pseudohypoglycemia is not a failure of the meter to measure the sample accurately, but rather a discrepancy between capillary and venous samples. Glucose meters utilizing a glucose–oxygen-based measurement may be affected by blood oxygenation. Supplemental

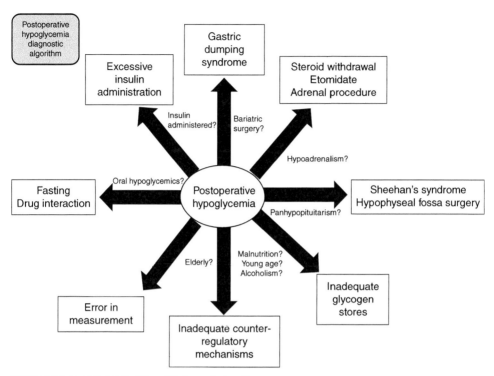

Figure 16.1 Hypoglycemia differential diagnosis algorithm.

oxygen can cause false depressed glucose readings and hypoxia can cause falsely elevated measurements. Severe acidosis (pH <6.95) may also lead to spuriously low glucose readings with many types of meters.[18]

A root cause analysis of severe hypoglycemia (40 mg/dl) recognized during surgery among 80,379 patients at a large tertiary care hospital identified preventable errors in 47% of cases.[19] Ineffective communication (such as providers being unaware that the patient received/administered insulin that morning), circulatory shock, failure to monitor, and excessive insulin administration were the four most commonly identified contributing factors. This serves to underscore the importance of communication among the various providers of different disciplines in the postoperative period in order to avoid preventable hypoglycemic episodes due to miscommunication or failure of vigilance. In one tragic case of inadequate communication, there was a failure to report the use of icodextrin peritoneal dialysate in the postoperative period. Icodextrin falsely elevates glucose readings on some glucose dehydrogenase-based meters and contributed to excessive insulin therapy in an attempt to treat factious hyperglycemia, resulting in death.[20]

Prevention

Prevention of hypoglycemia is preferred over detection and treatment. It requires that patients at risk for hypoglycemia be identified prior to or upon admission to the hospital. For these patients, glucose monitoring should start at admission and continue in the intraoperative period. The Society for Ambulatory Anesthesia recommends a monitoring frequency of every one to two hours.[9] Considering not only the current glucose measurement, but also the rate of change will allow you to anticipate an impending hypoglycemic event and make proactive adjustments in therapy (e.g. reduction of intravenous [IV] insulin infusion or administration of an IV bolus/infusion of dextrose) to avoid it. Recognition of other precipitating factors such as discontinuation of dextrose-containing infusions, recent administration of exogenous insulin, or the presence of predisposing co-morbidities is also helpful in prevention. If a hypoglycemic event does occur, it must be treated promptly with appropriate follow-up. Care should be taken to avoid overtreatment to avoid hyperglycemia. Treatment protocols should be established and disseminated. Adequate oversight can increase adherence to, and identify deficiencies in, established hypoglycemia treatment protocols.

With proper staff education, and patient monitoring and care, hypoglycemia can be avoided. Educated staff should be able to quickly identify at-risk patients and, coupled with proper monitoring, recognize and treat a patient before clinically significant hypoglycemia develops.

Management

Treatment of hypoglycemia in the immediate postoperatively period is unique (see Figure 16.2). Here, it is common for the patient to be unresponsive and have IV access. Whereas treatment with oral glucose is often the first recommendation if it can be tolerated, administration of an IV bolus or infusion of dextrose should be considered the first option in the PACU.

To avoid mistreatment, aberrant glucose measurements should be scrutinized. Blood obtained from a catheter, especially a central venous catheter, is susceptible to pre-analytical error due to contamination with dextrose-containing solutions or dilution with dextrose-free solutions.[21] In addition, poor perfusion, interfering substances, and hematocrit abnormalities have been known to produce erroneous glucose readings when using portable glucose meters.[22–24] When a critical glucose value does not appear to be physiologically possible, a new sample should be drawn and/or repeat testing should be performed to confirm results.

Whether administered via an IV bolus or taken by mouth as simple or complex carbohydrates, the default amount of glucose to deliver in response to hypoglycemia is 15g. However, to avoid overtreatment, this amount should be calculated. If the body is taken as a single pool for the distribution of glucose, a simple calculation provides the estimated amount of glucose to deliver to regain euglycemia. First, the distribution volume (V_d) [in dl/kg] is estimated to be between 1.0 and 3.0.[25–27] Given the patient's weight (Wt) [in kg], desired glucose concentration ($G_{desired}$) [in mg/dl], and current glucose concentration (G_{actual}) [in mg/dl], the amount of dextrose to administer [in g] as an IV bolus is:

$$\text{Rescue dose [in grams]} = \frac{(G_{desired} - G_{actual}) \times \text{Wt} \times V_d}{1000}$$

Using the glucose distribution volume of 2 dl/kg, for a 70 kg patient with a measured glucose concentration of 50 mg/dl, the appropriate rescue dose is 7 g to achieve a desired glucose value of 100 mg/dl. It is recommended that this dose is delivered as a bolus and, if no contraindication for IV fluids exists, a dextrose infusion should also be started until

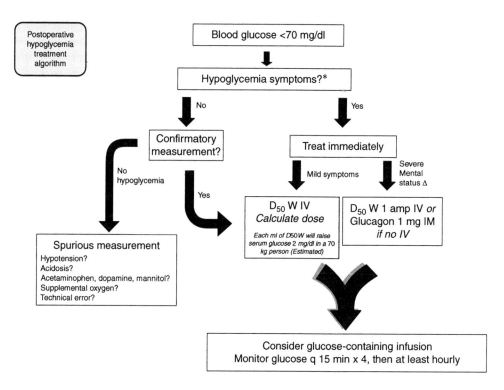

*Hypoglycemic symptoms require treatement even if blood glucose >70 mg/dl

Figure 16.2 Hypoglycemia treatment algorithm.

stable euglycemia is established. Moreover, more frequent monitoring (q 15 min) is recommended for at least one hour following the IV bolus. Here, the time taken for complete distribution of the glucose bolus from the vascular space to the interstitial space and intracellular space can be at least one hour for glycemic response to IV glucose tolerance tests, so glucose measurements following an IV bolus should be evaluated accordingly. While each ml of $D_{50}W$, dextrose 50% in water raises serum glucose by approximately 2 mg/dl in the average 70 kg adult, wide variation in clinical effect of $D_{50}W$ has been observed in euglycemic volunteers, necessitating clinical evaluation of response to therapy and vigilant post-treatment monitoring.[28]

Summary

To successfully mitigate hypoglycemic events, follow the four steps illustrated in Figure 16.3:

Step 1. Identify patients at risk for hypoglycemia prior to or at admission. Continually reassess patients for risk. Proper education will allow staff to quickly identify high-risk patients.

Step 2. Monitor at-risk patients frequently. Measure the plasma glucose concentrations throughout the patient's entire length of stay. It is important to make frequent measurements (every 1 to 2 hours) when the patient is anesthetized or sedated,

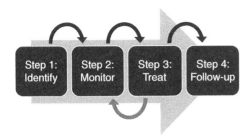

Figure 16.3 Steps to prevent and treat hypoglycemia.

as clinical signs and symptoms can be masked by these agents. Proactively adjust therapy to avoid a hypoglycemic event.

Step 3. Treat the hypoglycemia appropriately to regain euglycemia and avoid overtreatment.

Step 4. Follow up on the hypoglycemic event to determine the root cause and recommend any adjustment to the patient's current therapy.

References

1. C. Ichai, J. Preiser for the Societe Fd, Societe de Reanimation de langue Francaise (SRLF) and the Experts group. International recommendations for glucose control in adult non diabetic critically ill patients. *Crit Care* 2010; 14(5):R166. doi: 10.1186/cc9258.

2. M. Egi, R. Bellomo, E. Stachowski, *et al.* Hypoglycemia and outcome in critically ill patients. *Mayo Clin Proc* 2010;85(3): 217–224.

3. L. Boucai, W.N. Southern, J. Zonszein. Hypoglycemia-associated mortality is not drug-associated but linked to comorbidities. *Am J Med* 2011; 124(11):1028–1035.

4. The NICE-SUGAR Study Investigators. Hypoglycemia and risk of death in critically ill patients. *N Engl J Med* 2012; 367(12):1108–1118.

5. C.V. Desouza, G.B. Bolli, V. Fonseca. Hypoglycemia, diabetes, and cardiovascular events. *Diabetes Care* 2010; 33(6):1389–1394.

6. B.M. Frier, G. Schernthane, S.R. Heller. Hypoglycemia and cardiovascular risks.

Diabetes Care 2011; 34(Suppl 2): S132–S137.

7. A.N. Lteif, W.F. Schwenk. Hypoglycemia in infants and children. *Endocrinol Metab Clin North Am* 1999; 28(3):619–646.

8. J. Chaussain, P. Georges, L. Calzada, J. Job. Glycemic response to 24-hour fast in normal children: III. Influence of age. *J Pediatr* 1977; 91(5):711–714.

9. G.P. Joshi, F. Chung, M.A. Vann, *et al.* Society for Ambulatory Anesthesia consensus statement on perioperative blood glucose management in diabetic patients undergoing ambulatory surgery. *Anesth Analg* 2010; 111(6):1378–1387.

10. P.A. Bernard, C.E. Makin, H.A. Werner. Hypoglycemia associated with dexmedetomidine overdose in a child? *J Clin Anesth* 2009; 21(1):50–53.

11. A. Banerjee, W.E. Rhoden. Etomidate-induced hypoglycaemia. *Postgrad Med J* 1996; 72(850):510.

12. C.B. Salem, N. Fathallah, H. Hmouda, K. Bouraoui. Drug-induced hypoglycaemia: an update. *Drug Saf* 2011; 34(1):21–45.

13. M.H. Vue, S.M. Setter. Drug-induced glucose alterations. Part 1: Drug-induced hypoglycemia. *Diabetes Spectr* 2011; 24(3):171–177.

14. H. Kehlet, C. Binder. Adrenocortical function and clinical course during and after surgery in unsupplemented glucocorticoid-treated patients. *Br J Anaesth* 1973; 45(10):1043–1048.

15. L. Knudsen, L.A. Christiansen, J.E. Lorentzen. Hypotension during and after operation in glucocorticoid-treated patients. *Br J Anaesth* 1981; 53(3):295–301.

16. D. Kastelan, K.G. Ravic, M. Cacic, *et al.* Severe postoperative hypoglycemia in a patient with pheochromocytoma and preclinical Cushing's syndrome. *Med Sci Monit* 2007; 13(3):CS34–CS37.

17. J. Tack, J. Arts, P. Caenepeel, D. De Wulf, R. Bisschops. Pathophysiology, diagnosis and management of postoperative dumping syndrome. *Nat Rev Gastroenterol Hepatol* 2009; 6(10):583–590.

18. K. Tonyushkina, J.H. Nichols. Glucose meters: a review of technical challenges to obtaining accurate results. *J Diabetes Sci Technol* 2009; 3(4):971–980.

19. E.S. Schwenk, B. Mraovic, R.P. Maxwell, *et al.* Root causes of intraoperative hypoglycemia: a case series. *J Clin Anesth* 2012; 24(8):625–630.

20. H.R. Kroll, T.R. Maher. Significant hypoglycemia secondary to icodextrin peritoneal dialysate in a diabetic patient. *Anesth Analg* 2007; 104(6):1472–1474.

21. P.P. Nayak, K. Morris, H. Lang, *et al.* Lack of agreement between arterial and central venous blood glucose measurement in critically ill children. *Intensive Care Med* 2009; 35(4):762–763.

22. A. Desachy, A.C. Vuagnat, A.D. Ghazali, *et al.* Accuracy of bedside glucometry in critically ill patients: influence of clinical characteristics and perfusion index. *Mayo Clin Proc* 2008; 83(4):400–405.

23. S.B. Chakravarthy, B.A. Markewitz, C. Lehman, J.F. Orme. Glucose determination from different vascular compartments by point-of-care testing in critically ill patients. *Chest* 2005; 128(Suppl):220S–221S.

24. M.E. Lyon, J.A. DuBois, G.H. Fick, A.W. Lyon. Estimates of total analytical error in consumer and hospital glucose meters contributed by hematocrit, maltose, and ascorbate. *J Diabetes Sci Technol* 2010; 4(6):1479–1494.

25. R. Hovorka, F. Shojaee-Moradie, P.V. Carroll, *et al.* Partitioning glucose distribution/transport, disposal, and endogenous production during IVGTT. *Am J Physiol Endocrinol Metab* 2002; 282(5):E992–E1007.

26. F. Sjöstrand, L. Edsberg, R.G. Hahn. Volume kinetics of glucose solutions given by intravenous infusion. *Br J Anaesth* 2001; 87(6):834–843.

27. E. Ferrannini, J.D. Smith, C. Cobelli, *et al.* Effect of insulin on the distribution and disposition of glucose in man. *J Clin Invest* 1985; 76(1):357–364.

28. J.R. Balentine, T.J. Gaeta, E. Bagiella, T. Lee. Effect of 50 milliliters of 50% dextrose in water administration on the blood sugar of euglycemic volunteers. *Acad Emerg Med* 1999; 5(7):691–694.

Chapter

17

Hyperglycemia

Boris Mraovic and Jeffrey I. Joseph

- Hyperglycemia commonly occurs in the Post-Anesthesia Care Unit (PACU) owing to type 1 or type 2 diabetes (T1DM, T2DM), gestational diabetes, metabolic stress, rapid glucose infusion, steroids, catecholamines, anesthetics, and hypothermia.
- Hyperglycemia, hypoglycemia, and glycemic variability are markers of unstable physiology and metabolism, and have been strongly associated with increased morbidity, mortality, length of stay, and cost.
- The concentration of blood glucose (BG) should be controlled in the desired target range (for example 80 to 110 mg/dl; 100 to 140 mg/dl; 100 to 180 mg/dl; or 140 to 180 mg/dl) according to the unique physiology of each hospitalized patient.
- The BG concentration of all patients being treated with insulin should be monitored frequently using an accurate laboratory or point-of-care (POC) glucose analyzer.
- Whole blood sampled from a peripheral arterial catheter provides the most accurate BG measurement for clinical management.
- Samples of fingerstick capillary blood may produce an erroneous BG measurement because of poor tissue perfusion, dilution with edema fluid, or contamination from glucose on the skin surface.
- Whole blood samples obtained from a central venous catheter (CVC) or a peripheral venous catheter may be contaminated or diluted by adjacent infusions.
- The most effective way to control the concentration of BG requires an intravenous (IV) infusion of regular insulin and frequent adjustments in the rate of insulin delivery, based upon a validated dosing protocol and frequent BG measurements.
- Patients with T1DM need to receive a continuous supply of insulin to avoid ketosis that may lead to diabetic ketoacidosis (DKA).
- Sliding-scale dosing protocols that use subcutaneous (SC) tissue injections of regular insulin do not provide effective BG control.
- Stable patients are commonly managed with one SC dose of long-acting insulin each day (basal dose insulin); a SC dose of rapid-acting insulin prior to each meal (prandial dose insulin); and one or more additional SC doses of rapid-acting insulin to correct for post-prandial hyperglycemia (correction dose insulin).

Post-Anesthesia Care: Symptoms, Diagnosis, and Management, ed. James W. Heitz. Published by Cambridge University Press. © Cambridge University Press 2016.

- Hyperglycemia can be avoided by matching the pharmacokinetic and dynamic (PK-PD) actions of delivered insulin to the amount of glucose that enters the bloodstream from an IV catheter, from the intestines after a meal, and from the liver and kidneys (gluconeogenesis).
- Hyperglycemia and glycemic variability occur most commonly in patients who develop an acute change in insulin sensitivity, renal function, metabolic rate, carbohydrate intake, and hepatic glucose production.
- Patients with DKA and hyperosmolar hyperglycemic syndrome (HHS) should be managed carefully in the Intensive Care Unit (ICU) with IV fluids, electrolytes, and an IV infusion of regular insulin based upon frequent BG measurements.

Hyperglycemia in the hospital

Hospitalized patients with diabetes mellitus (DM) commonly develop mild to moderate hyperglycemia (prevalence 90% in one survey) due to the IV infusion of glucose plus the metabolic stress response that occurs with acute illness and major surgery. An estimated 18% to 38% of DM patients have persistent hyperglycemia (3 consecutive days with BG >200 mg/dl) while in the hospital.[1] Many non-diabetic patients develop "stress hypergly-cemia" while in the hospital, a condition that completely resolves once the metabolic stress response has resolved.[2]

The prevalence of diagnosed DM is estimated to be 8.3% (25.8 million) of the US population; and the incidence may be increasing by 1.9 million cases per year. An additional 7.0 million Americans have DM that is currently undiagnosed and untreated. The preva-lence of pre-diabetes exceeds 26% of the US population (79 million) and is rapidly increasing, owing to the aging population and to obesity.[3]

Patients are diagnosed with diabetes if their fasting plasma glucose concentration consistently exceeds 126 mg/dl, if a random plasma glucose concentration exceeds 200 mg/dl, or the hemoglobin A1C (HbAIC) exceeds 6.5%. Diabetic patients with HbA1C >9% are considered in poor control, HbA1C 7–9% in below average control, and <7% in good control. Patients with below average and poor BG control are at increased risk for developing myocardial ischemia, myocardial infarction, congestive heart failure, stroke, deep vein thrombosis, pulmonary embolism, infection, chronic renal failure, blindness, limb amputation, and death.[4]

Patients with the diagnosis of DM can be divided into four categories:

1. **Type 1 diabetes mellitus** (T1DM) is an autoimmune disease that destroys all of the beta-cells within the pancreas. Patients with established T1DM do not make any insulin, and therefore require a continuous supply of exogenous insulin to avoid DKA and severe hyperglycemia. Many patients with T1DM inject long-acting insulin once or twice per day and inject rapid-acting insulin prior to each meal (multiple-dose injection therapy). Approximately 500 thousand of the 1.2 million people in the United States with T1DM deliver insulin with a pump and catheter inserted into the subcutaneous tissue that continuously infuses a small amount of rapid-acting insulin and a bolus dose of insulin prior to each meal (basal-bolus insulin therapy). Many patients with T1DM >5 years duration have hypoglycemia unawareness due to an attenuated release of epinephrine and glucagon, and are at increased risk for severe and prolonged hypoglycemia.

Frequent self-monitoring of blood glucose (SMBG) is the key to safe and effective insulin delivery with a low incidence of hypoglycemia.[3,4]

2. **Type 2 diabetes mellitus** (T2DM) is a chronic disease of cellular metabolism characterized by insulin resistance and progressive loss of beta-cell function. Patients with T2DM have abnormal carbohydrate, lipid, and protein metabolism, leading to diffuse atherosclerosis and microvascular disease at an early age. Treatment typically progresses from diet and exercise to one or more oral medications that increase endogenous insulin production and/or increase insulin sensitivity in hepatic and adipose tissue cells. Approximately 2.8 million of the 24 million people in the United States with T2DM are treated with SC injections of insulin each day. Some of these patients have severe loss of beta-cell function and are at risk for developing DKA and HHS.[3,4]

3. **Secondary diabetes** is caused by destruction of pancreas tissue secondary to infection, inflammation, surgical removal, cystic fibrosis, radiation therapy, tumors that secrete epinephrine, corticosteroid, or growth hormone, medications that increase hepatic glucose production (gluconeogenesis), and medications that increase insulin resistance. Many of the 100,000 patients in the United States with secondary diabetes require a continuous supply of exogenous insulin in the hospital to avoid hyperglycemia and ketoacidosis.[3,4]

4. **Gestational diabetes** occurs during the second and third trimesters of 80,000 pregnancies in the United States each year, and typically resolves after delivery of the baby. The mother's BG concentration should be maintained in the near-normal range with insulin to minimize the risk for birth defects, macrosomia, and neonatal hypoglycemia.[3,4]

Glycemic control and clinical outcome

Hyperglycemia, hypoglycemia, and glycemic variability have been independently associated with increased morbidity, mortality, length of stay, and cost in a variety of critical care and non-critical care patient populations in the hospital.[5–8] Observational trials in the hospital have revealed a moderate to strong association between hyperglycemia and an increased risk for nosocomial infection (surgical wound, ventilator-acquired pneumonia, CVS, urinary bladder catheter, bacteremia, and sepsis), deep vein thrombosis, pulmonary embolism, acute kidney injury, renal failure, neuropathy and worse clinical outcome after myocardial infarction, congestive heart failure, cerebral infarction, subarachnoid hemorrhage, burns, penetration trauma, and blunt trauma.[2,4–10]

The results from prospective randomized clinical trials (RCTs) designed to determine the risks and benefits of intensive insulin therapy and tight glycemic control have been confusing and conflicting.[11,12] Some prospective RCTs demonstrated a significant decrease in morbidity and mortality when the BG concentration was targeted to the near-normal BG range (80 to 110 mg/dl or 100 to 150 mg/dl) with IV insulin; while other RCTs in medical and surgical ICU patients did not show a clinical benefit from IV insulin therapy and tight glycemic control.[11–13] The RCT evidence supporting tight glycemic control with IV insulin is strongest in cardiac surgery patients and patients managed for >3 days in the surgical ICU.[12,13] Non-diabetic patients who develop stress hyperglycemia may actually benefit the most from intensive insulin therapy and tight glycemic control.[2,4,5]. Many of the RCTs were complicated by a high incidence of mild (70 to 61 mg/dl), moderate (60 to 41 mg/dl), and severe hypoglycemia (BG ≤40 mg/dl) and low percentage of time spent in the target range.[11–13]

Hospitalized patients are at increased risk for severe and prolonged hypoglycemia because sleep, sedatives, hypnotics, analgesics, and general anesthetics blunt the hypothalamus, autonomic nervous system, and adrenal gland response to hypoglycemia. In addition, the most sensitive signs of hypoglycemia (change in mentation, and tachycardia) may be lost in patients that are sedated or anesthetized. For these reasons, several of the major endocrinology and critical care societies recently changed their guidelines to a more conservative target BG range (140 to 180 mg/dl) to minimize the risk for hypoglycemia.[2, 14–16]

Of interest, none of the RCTs considered the effects of cardiac output or local tissue blood flow on the amount of glucose delivered to the tissues per minute. Future research is needed to determine the effects of glucose under-delivery or over-delivery to the tissues, and the effects on the incidence of adverse events and clinical outcome in hospitalized patients.

Recent research suggests that patients with poorly controlled BG prior to hospital admission (HbA1c >9%) may benefit from a higher BG target range (for example BG 140 to 180 mg/dl) while recovering from major surgery or illness. Patients with good pre-admission glucose control (HbA1c <7%) may benefit from a lower BG target range (for example 100 to 140 mg/dl) in the hospital. In general, the lower the target BG range the greater the risk for hypoglycemia.[2,7,15]

Summary: glycemic control and clinical outcome

Research and clinical evidence supports that: (1) prolonged hyperglycemia should be avoided because glycosuria leads to polyuria, dehydration, electrolyte imbalance, platelet activation, and decreased tissue blood flow; (2) glucose levels should be controlled in diabetic and non-diabetic patients that develop moderate to severe hyperglycemia; (3) the optimal target BG range for an individual patient depends upon their physiology at each stage of their illness or surgical care; (4) severe and prolonged hypoglycemia should be strictly avoided; and (5) perioperative nutrition and factors other than BG control greatly affect the incidence of adverse events and overall clinical outcome.

Treatment of hyperglycemia in the PACU

Type 1 diabetes

Surgical patients with T1DM require a continuous supply of insulin to control their carbohydrate, lipid, and protein metabolism. The very short pharmacokinetic half-life of an IV bolus of regular insulin injected into the bloodstream ($t_{1/2}$ = approximately 5 minutes) makes patients with T1DM highly susceptible to hyperglycemia, glycemic variability, dynamic fluid shifts, and variable tissue perfusion. The glucose-lowering effect (pharmacodynamic) of an IV bolus of regular insulin lasts from 2 hours (low dose) to 4 hours (high dose) (Table 17.1). Patients with T1DM will rapidly develop hyperlipidemia, ketosis, and DKA during a period of insulin deficiency. Therefore, surgical patients with T1DM must receive a continuous supply of insulin to minimize the risk for DKA, a life-threatening condition if not appropriately diagnosed and managed.[14–19]

Many clinicians use a variable rate IV infusion of regular insulin, based upon a validated insulin dosing algorithm, to manage their patients with T1DM. The IV insulin infusion dose (units/hr or mU/kg/min) should be adjusted every 30 minutes when the BG concentration is low or falling into the hypoglycemia range to every 2 hours when patient physiology and the BG concentration are stable. A small IV bolus dose of regular insulin

Table 17.1 PK and PD profiles for intravenous and subcutaneous tissue insulin formulations. Note the prolonged glucose-lowering effect (PD) following an IV bolus injection of regular insulin

Generic name	Brand name	Onset of action	Peak action	Duration of action
Rapid-acting insulin: subcutaneous tissue injection				
Insulin lispro	HumaLog	15 minutes	30–90 minutes	3–5 hours
Insulin aspart	NovoLog	15 minutes	30–90 minutes	3–5 hours
Insulin glulisine	Apidra	15 minutes	30–90 minutes	3–5 hours
Short-acting insulin: subcutaneous tissue injection				
Regular	Novolin R	30–60 minutes	2–4 hours	5–8 hours
Regular	Humulin R	30–60 minutes	2–4 hours	5–8 hours
Intermediate-acting insulin: subcutaneous tissue injection				
NPH	Novolin N	1–3 hours	8 hours	12–16 hours
NPH	Humulin N	1–3 hours	8 hours	12–16 hours
Long-acting insulin: subcutaneous tissue injection				
Insulin glargine	Lantus	1 hour	Peakless	20–26 hours
Insulin detemir	Levemir	1 hour	Peakless	20–26 hours
Intravenous infusion of regular insulin				
Regular	Novolin R	5 minutes	15 minutes	1–2 hours
Regular	Humulin R	5 minutes	15 minutes	1–2 hours

may be appropriate therapy, prior to starting the IV insulin infusion. Patients with T1DM undergoing major surgery have increased glycemic variability when managed with intermittent injections of IV regular insulin or intermittent injections of insulin injected into the subcutaneous tissue.[14,15]

Hyperglycemia should be controlled slowly to avoid intravascular dehydration and electrolyte imbalance due to the rapid movement of plasma fluid into the extracellular and intracellular fluid compartments. Patients with T1DM undergoing a minor or outpatient surgical procedure can be safely managed with their own insulin pump and a SC tissue infusion catheter. The infusion catheter and pump parameters should be carefully checked to minimize the risk for insulin delivery failure and DKA.[16]

Increased vigilance is required during an acute change in patient temperature, tissue blood flow, renal function, and nutrition therapy. Patients change from insulin-resistant during hypothermia to insulin-sensitive after returning to normal temperature. Ambulation increases muscle and adipose tissue blood flow, leading to greater insulin receptor binding and a rapid decrease in the BG concentration. An acute decrease in renal function can slow insulin excretion and prolong insulin's glucose-lowering effect.[14,15] Patients who develop DKA or HHS should be diagnosed early and managed aggressively in the ICU.[4] Clinicians are referred to their hospital's guidelines and methods for safely dosing insulin, with the goal being to avoid DKA and minimize the severity of hyperglycemia, hypoglycemia, and glycemic variability.

Type 2 diabetes

Surgical patients with T2DM should have their BG concentration monitored frequently in the OR and PACU to diagnose persistent hyperglycemia. T2DM patients with mild hyperglycemia in the PACU may not need treatment, while patients with moderate hyperglycemia (BG 180 to 240 mg/dl) and severe hyperglycemia (BG >240 mg/dl) should be treated with insulin. Surgical patients with prolonged hyperglycemia and dehydration should be evaluated for ketosis and/or lactic acidosis due to DKA or HHS.[4,14,15] Clinicians are referred to their hospital's guidelines and methods for safely dosing insulin to minimize the severity of hyperglycemia, hypoglycemia, and glycemic variability.

T2DM patients treated at home with insulin commonly require significantly more insulin in the hospital owing to the IV infusion of glucose and the metabolic stress response. Patients taking large doses of SC insulin at home may require very large doses of IV or SC tissue insulin while in the hospital. Many clinicians manage these patients with a continuous IV infusion of regular insulin and an IV infusion of dextrose, similar to the management of patients with T1DM.

Surgical patients with T2DM who use oral agents at home are commonly managed in the hospital with insulin. Clinicians in the PACU must consider the glucose-lowering effects of long-acting oral agents taken prior to hospital admission and the type, dose, and timing of insulin delivered prior to surgery and in the OR. It may be appropriate to withhold a scheduled dose of insulin in the PACU because of the residual effects of prior medication, the acute increase in insulin sensitivity that occurs with the return of normal temperature, and the increase in muscle glucose uptake that occurs with shivering. Additional insulin may be safely delivered as a SC injection, an IV bolus injection, or an IV infusion as long as the BG concentration is monitored frequently. Hyperglycemia should not be corrected too rapidly, to minimize the clinical consequences of rapidly shifting water, salt, glucose, and potassium from the extracellular fluid into the cells.

Postoperative patients are commonly transitioned from an IV infusion of regular insulin to intermittent SC injections of long-acting and rapid-acting insulin once they are stable and tolerating enteral nutrition. An IV insulin infusion should be discontinued 30 to 60 minutes after giving the first SC dose of insulin to minimize hyperglycemia. The concentration of BG should be monitored frequently and the dose of SC insulin adjusted frequently during the transition period.[14-19]

T2DM patients not previously managed with insulin at home may benefit from home insulin therapy after discharge from the hospital, following consultation with their primary care physician and/or endocrinologist. Many of these patients will not require home insulin therapy after the metabolic stress response resolves.

T2DM patients should be closely observed in the PACU for myocardial ischemia/infarction, congestive heart failure, deep vein thrombosis, and pulmonary embolism because hyperglycemia may cause hemoconcentration, platelet activation, and a hypercoagulable state. An accurate diagnosis may require serial electrocardiograms (ECGs), troponin levels, chest X-rays, CT scans, and/or a diagnostic catheterization because many T2DM surgical patients with myocardial ischemia will not develop angina or shortness of breath. Unstable PACU patients require timely and aggressive medical therapy to avoid a serious adverse event.

Blood glucose monitoring in the PACU

Safe and effective insulin therapy requires accurate and timely BG measurements.[2,17–19] The most accurate and precise BG measurements are obtained using blood sampled from a radial artery catheter that is assayed with a central laboratory glucose analyzer or an ICU blood gas analyzer. The measurement of BG is commonly complicated by pre-analytical and analytical error.[20] Whole blood samples obtained from a central venous catheter or a peripheral venous catheter may be contaminated or diluted by adjacent infusions. Of interest, the glucose concentration in peripheral arterial blood is higher than peripheral venous blood and central venous blood (atrioventricular [AV] difference 3 to 8 mg/dl). The concentration of glucose in the vena cava can be highly variable owing to hepatic/renal glucose production, and absorption of food from the intestines, in addition to contamination and dilution from adjacent infusions.[19]

The most timely but least accurate BG measurements are obtained using a fingerstick capillary blood sample and a POC glucose meter/test strip. Fingerstick capillary blood may produce an erroneous BG measurement due to poor tissue perfusion, dilution with edema fluid, or contamination from glucose on the skin surface. Accuracy of the POC meters can be adversely affected by anemia, polycythemia, hypoxemia, acidosis, drugs (acetaminophen, dopamine, mannitol, and maltose), and low sample volume.[14–16,20] BG measurements that are questionable should be repeated with a whole blood sample analyzed in the central laboratory as long as the time delay does not adversely affect clinical care.

A variety of continuous glucose monitoring (CGM) systems are being developed for the hospital that measure the concentration of glucose in the interstitial fluid of subcutaneous tissue or the bloodstream every 1 to 15 minutes (Figure 17.1). In the future, CGM systems and closed-loop computer control algorithms may be used to maintain the BG concentration in the desired target range, while eliminating the risk for hypoglycemia.

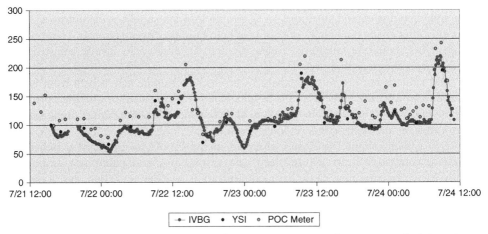

Figure 17.1 The concentration of BG was measured in a postoperative general surgery patient for 3 days using an IV continuous glucose monitoring system and peripheral venous blood (IVBG); a reference BG analyzer and radial artery blood (YSI); and a point-of-care BG meter/test strip and fingerstick capillary blood (POC meter).

References

1. D.J. Wexler, J.B. Meigs, E. Cagliero, D.M. Nathan, R.W. Grant. Prevalence of hyper- and hypoglycemia among inpatients with diabetes: a national survey of 44 U.S. hospitals. *Diabetes Care* 2007; 30:367–369.

2. G.E. Umpierrez, R. Hellman, M.T. Korytkowski, *et al.* Management of hyperglycemia in hospitalized patients in non-critical care setting: an Endocrine Society clinical practice guideline. *J Clin Endocrinol Metab* 2012; 97:16–38.

3. Available at: http://diabetes.niddk.nih.gov/dm/pubs/statistics/. Accessed 1 Dec 2014.

4. Standards of Medical Care in Diabetes – 2013. *Diabetes Care* 2013; 36:S1.

5. M. Egi, R. Bellomo, E. Stachowski, *et al.* Blood glucose concentration and outcome of critical illness: the impact of diabetes. *Crit Care Med* 2008; 36:2249–2255.

6. J.S. Krinsley. Glycemic variability: a strong independent predictor of mortality in critically ill patients. *Crit Care Med* 2008; 36:3008–3013.

7. M.H. Murad, J.A. Coburn, F. Coto-Yglesias, *et al.* Glycemic control in non-critically ill hospitalized patients: a systematic review and meta-analysis. *J Clin Endocrinol Metab* 2012; 97:49–58.

8. B. Mraovic, B.R. Hipszer, R.H. Epstein, *et al.* Preadmission hyperglycemia is an independent risk factor for in-hospital symptomatic pulmonary embolism after major orthopedic surgery. *J Arthroplasty* 2010; 25:64–70.

9. G.V. Bochicchio, J. Sung, J. Manjari, *et al.* Persistent hyperglycemia is predictive of outcome in critically ill trauma patients. *J Trauma* 2005; 58:921–924.

10. T.M. Vriesendorp, Q.J. Morelis, J.H. DeVries, D.A. Legemate, J.B.L. Hoekstra. Early postoperative glucose levels are an independent risk factor for infection after peripheral vascular surgery. A retrospective study. *Eur J Vasc Surg* 2004; 28:520–525.

11. S. Finfer, R. Bellomi, D. Blair, *et al.* Intensive versus conventional glucose control in critically ill patients. *N Engl J Med* 2009; 36:1283–1297.

12. E. Van den Berghe, P. Wouters, F. Weekers, *et al.* Intensive insulin therapy in critically ill patients. *N Engl J Med* 2001; 345:1359–1367.

13. G. Van den Berghe, A. Wilmer, G. Hermans, *et al.* Intensive insulin therapy in the medical ICU, *N Engl J Med* 2006; 354: 449–461.

14. E.S. Moghissi, M.T. Korytkowski, M. DiNardo, *et al.* American Association of Clinical Endocrinologists and American Diabetes Association consensus statement on inpatient glycemic control. *Diabetes Care* 2009; 32:1119–1131.

15. J. Jacobi, N. Bircher, J. Krinsley, *et al.* Guidelines for the use of an insulin infusion for the management of hyperglycemia in critically ill patients. *Crit Care Med* 2012; 40:3251–3276.

16. G.P. Joshi, F. Chung, M.A. Vann, *et al.* Society for Ambulatory Anesthesia consensus statement on perioperative blood glucose management in diabetic patients undergoing ambulatory surgery. *Anesth Analg* 2010; 111:1378–1387.

17. I. Hirsch, D.S. Paauw, J. Brunzell. Inpatient management of adults with diabetes. *Diabetes Care* 1995; 18:870–878.

18. P. Brian, M.B. Kavanagh, K.C. McCowen. Glycemic control in the ICU. *N Engl J Med* 2010; 363:2540–2546.

19. J.I. Joseph. Anesthesia and surgery in the diabetic patient. *Textbook of Type 2 Diabetes*, Chapter 31. Boca Raton: CRC Press 2008, pp. 475–500.

20. A. Desachy, A.C. Vuagnat, A.D. Ghazali, *et al.* Accuracy of bedside glucometry in critically ill patients: influence of clinical characteristics and perfusion index. *Mayo Clin Proc* 2008; 83:400–405.

Chapter 18

Electrolyte disorders

Michael Jon Williams

- Signs and symptoms of sodium abnormalities will often involve central nervous system (CNS) function.
- Potassium-level perturbations will threaten a patient because of the risk of cardiac arrhythmias.
- Other ionic abnormalities have far-reaching effects on both muscle tissue and neuron functions.

While the large majority of patients postoperatively can be treated with isotonic solutions such as normal saline or lactated Ringer's solution, there will be times when electrolyte abnormalities necessitate specialized solutions. In many cases these will be patients requiring intensive therapy, such as those with hypernatremia, or cases where iatrogenic causes may be the case, as in postoperative hypocalcemia after parathyroidectomy. This chapter describes various electrolyte abnormalities one may encounter in a Post-Anesthesia Care Unit (PACU) or Intensive Care Unit situation (see Table 18.1), their signs and symptoms, and treatments.

Sodium

Sodium is the most abundant cation in the extracellular fluid and is important in the generation of action potentials of neurological and cardiac tissue. In addition, it is important in the determination of plasma osmolality, along with glucose and urea. Hypothalamic osmoreceptors can detect small changes in serum osmolality and will secrete antidiuretic hormone (ADH) in response to an elevated serum osmolality. Control of sodium balance also occurs with atrial natriuretic peptide (ANP) and aldosterone through the renin–angiotensin system. The renin–angiotensin system serves to conserve sodium and can be activated by the sympathetic nervous system, by decreases of sodium delivery to the macula densa, or by decreases in blood pressure to the renal artery, all factors which can be seen in surgical stress.

Hypernatremia

Hypernatremia is defined as a serum sodium of 145 mEq/l or greater. The process is primarily thought of as an absolute or relative inadequate amount of free water for the amount of electrolyte content of plasma.[1] Normally, the osmolality of plasma is tightly regulated between 275 and 290 mOsm/kg by the renal effects of ADH and a normal physiological

Post-Anesthesia Care: Symptoms, Diagnosis, and Management, ed. James W. Heitz. Published by Cambridge University Press. © Cambridge University Press 2016.

Table 18.1 Postoperative electrolyte abnormalities

↑ Sodium	**Diuretics, hyperglycemia, acute tubular necrosis, vomiting, nasogastric suction, diarrhea, gastrointestinal drains, fistulas, diabetes insipidus, pituitary trauma (resections around sella turcica) or infarction (Sheehan's syndrome), or mineral corticoid administration**
↓ Sodium	**Hypovolemic:** emesis, diarrhea, burns, pancreatitis, small bowel obstruction, loop diuretics, osmotic diuretics (e.g. mannitol) **Euvolemic:** prostate resection, hysteroscopy [transurethral resection of prostate (TURP) and female TURP syndromes], syndrome of inappropriate antidiuretic hormone (SIADH) (pain, mechanical ventilation, oxytocin), cerebral salt wasting **Hypervolemic:** congestive heart failure, cirrhosis
↑ Potassium	Rhabdomyolysis, hemolysis, diabetic ketoacidosis acidosis, respiratory acidosis (opioid effect), crush injuries/massive tissue trauma Medications: angiotensin-converting enzyme inhibitor, angiotensin receptor blockers, potassium-sparing diuretics, non-steroidal anti-inflammatory drugs, selective cyclooxygenase-2 (COX-2) inhibitors, some immunosuppressants (cyclosporine and tacrolimus)
↓ Potassium	Diarrhea, hypomagnesemia (poor nutrition, alcohol abuse), hyperventilation, alkalosis, Cushing's syndrome, insulin, epinephrine, surgical stress
↑ Calcium	Malignancy, hyperparathyroidism, rebound after rhabdomyolysis, hyperthyroidism
↓ Calcium	Hypoparathyroidism after parathyroidectomy or thyroidectomy, hyperventilation, hungry bone syndrome, rhabdomyolysis
↑ Phosphate	Hypoparathyroidism after parathyroidectomy or thyroidectomy, acidosis, crush injury, rhabdomyolysis, hyperthermia, factitious (heparin-contaminated sample)
↓ Phosphate	Hyperventilation, poor nutrition, chronic alcohol abuse

thirst mechanism. With hypovolemia or an increase of plasma osmolality, increased ADH secretion and thirst come into play to restore the body's plasma volume and osmolality.

Hypernatremia can be seen with conditions where thirst is impaired, access to water is restricted, or in conditions where there is increased loss of hypotonic fluid such as gastrointestinal (GI) losses and burns. This could easily develop in the elderly, infants, or patients in intensive care units. Solute loading with continuing doses of sodium bicarbonate can lead to hypernatremia. Another cause of hypernatremia could be the lack of ADH secretion seen after pituitary surgery or head injury such as a basilar skull fracture. This condition is known as central diabetes insipidus or DI. Nephrogenic DI is caused by the kidney's inability to generate a hypertonic urinary output. This could be seen after ureteral obstruction is relieved, in medullary cyst disease, or after the use of various pharmacological agents such as lithium, glyburide, demeclocycline, or amphotericin B. Markedly increased levels of plasma vasopressin are seen with nephrogenic DI, owing to the kidney's inability to respond to this hormone.

Signs of hypernatremia depend on the rate of serum sodium increase. Acute hypernatremia can produce severe thirst, shock due to hypovolemia, coma, or convulsions. Most concerning is brain shrinkage that occurs when water follows the osmotic gradient and moves out of the intracellular volume; this could lead to tearing of meningeal vessels, producing intracranial or extracranial hemorrhage.

Determination of the cause of hypernatremia is by evaluation of the extracellular fluid volume, thereby separating patients into hypovolemic, euvolemic, or hypervolemic hypernatremia. Next, measurement of plasma and urine sodium concentration along with urine osmolality will determine non-renal or renal losses. A urine osmolality of greater than 400 mOsm/kg with low urine sodium concentration suggests non-renal causes of hypernatremia: that is, loss of water that is non-renal in cause. If a patient's urine output is greater than 1.5 cc/kg/hr along with the presence of hypernatremia, DI should be suspected. DI is likely with a urine mOsm of less than 300 and a serum sodium of greater than 150 mEq/l.

Management of hypernatremia consists of restoring the amount of free water loss by using hypotonic crystalloid solutions. One first measures the amount of free water deficit using the formula given below (TBW, total body water).

$$\text{TBW deficit} = 0.6 \times \text{body weight(kg)} \times [([\text{Na}^+] - 140)/140]$$

Once the amount of deficit is calculated, the serum sodium should be corrected at a rate of 10% of the offset from normal or about 0.7 mEq/l/hr.[1] This represents a replacement of water deficit over 24 to 48 hours. It is best to avoid rapid correction of this abnormality as it can cause possible brain edema and offers no real advantage in a patient with a chronic hypernatremia. If DI is the cause, additional use of DDAVP or vasopressin acetate is necessary for central DI. DDAVP is given subcutaneously in a dose of 1 to 2 mcg every 12 hours, or intranasally in a dose of 5 to 20 mcg, every 24 hours. In nephrogenic DI, the course is salt and water restriction, enhancing tubular water reabsorption, along with thiazide diuretics and treatment of the underlying cause of nephrogenic DI.

Hyponatremia

Hyponatremia is the most common electrolyte abnormality in hospitalized patients and exists when the level of serum sodium is less than 135 mEq/l. A mid-1980 study found that 4.4% of postoperative patients developed a serum sodium concentration of less than 130 mEq/l.[2]

In evaluating the cause of hyponatremia, one must first measure the serum osmolality. When osmolality is measured as normal or high, one should look for a cause of dilutional hyponatremia caused by another solute which brings water into the extracellular plasma, such as glucose or mannitol. For each 100 mg/dl rise in glucose, the serum sodium can decrease by approximately 2.4 mEq/l.[3] Another common cause of hyponatremia with a normal osmolality is in the TURP (transurethral resection of prostate) syndrome where amounts of sodium-free glycine or sorbitol irrigating solutions are used during resection of the prostate.[4]

If the serum osmolality is low, the total body sodium might still be high, as in various edematous states (congestive heart failure, cirrhosis, nephritis), which will be reflected in a urine sodium concentration of less than 15 mEq/l. Total body sodium is typically low in situations due to excess sodium loss with water replacement (GI losses, skin losses, peritonitis, renal failure, diuretic use). Finally, one of the most common causes of hyponatremia on the postoperative surgical arena is SIADH, which can be present with a normal total body sodium.

SIADH can occur after general surgery, opiate administration, CNS disorders, and various cancerous diseases. Urine osmolality in SIADH with normal renal function is greater than 300 to 400 mOsm/kg with a urinary sodium concentration of greater than 30 mEq/l in a euvolemic patient. Cardiac, renal, and hepatic functions should also be normal to avoid misdiagnosis of an edematous state as noted above.

Symptoms of hyponatremia are dependent on both the acuteness of sodium drop and on the absolute level of sodium concentration. Mostly this relates to brain swelling from water shifting into the brain owing to differences in extra and intracellular osmolality. Patients may initially complain of muscle weakness, but as the severity of hyponatremia progresses, seizures or coma may ensue once the serum sodium level drops to 120 mEq/l or less.

Management of hyponatremia with high serum osmolality consists of reducing the concentration of the responsible solute. Treatment of high glucose concentration requires insulin or dialysis with a high concentration of urea. With low serum osmolality, as in edematous states, restriction of sodium and water are required. SIADH management is restriction of free water administration and treatment of the inciting cause. Administration of furosemide will increase the amount of free water excretion. Severe hyponatremia with seizures may be treated with 3% saline to increase sodium concentration and furosemide to facilitate free water clearance. Aggressive treatment should only continue for one to two hours to avoid abrupt CNS dehydration with shrinkage or central pontine myelinolysis.[5] Ideally, sodium concentration should be increased at a rate of only 10 mEq/l/24 hours.

Potassium

Potassium is the body's most plentiful intracellular cation, with 98% of a person's potassium in cells. It is important in maintaining the resting membrane potential of cells and in generating action potentials in excitable cells. Daily balance of potassium consists of absorption through the GI tract of about 1 mEq/kg/day and excretion of some of the excess by the GI tract. Although potassium balance is managed predominantly by the kidney with some regulation by aldosterone.

Hypokalemia

Hypokalemia may be caused by a true deficiency in body potassium or by redistribution into intracellular volume. In perioperative cardiac surgical patients, a potassium level less than 3.5 mEq/l was associated with a higher incidence of arrhythmias, especially atrial.[6]

The most common causes of hypokalemia include reduced intake, excessive renal excretion, GI losses from diarrhea or nasogastric suctioning, or shifting of potassium from the extracellular space by alkalosis (hyperventilation), insulin, or β-adrenergic agonists. Particular concern is with patients who have diabetic ketoacidosis. Correction of the diabetes and acidosis will cause an abrupt decrease in serum potassium as the hyperglycemia and acidosis improve.

The signs and symptoms of hypokalemia usually present when plasma potassium reaches a level of 2 to 2.5 mEq/l. At this point muscle weakness, arrhythmias of atrial fibrillation and premature ventricular contractions, along with ECG changes including flat T waves, prominent U waves, and ST-segment depression may be seen. More severe abnormalities in the ECG may be seen in patients on digitalis therapy, since hypokalemia increases this drug's binding and toxicity.

Management of hypokalemia consists of replacement therapy, treatment of alkalemia, and removal of potassium-wasting drugs. As a general rule, 1 mEq/l decrease in the serum potassium concentration corresponds to a total body potassium deficit of 100 to 300 mEq. But because the potassium deficit is unpredictable, careful replacement must be at no more than 10 to 20 mEq/hr with ECG monitoring.

Hyperkalemia

Hyperkalemia is defined as a serum potassium greater than 5.0–5.3 mEq/l. Typically, the kidneys are able to maintain potassium homeostasis until the glomerular filtration rate drops below 15–20 ml/min.

Hyperkalemia is caused by two mechanisms: first, decreased excretion in renal failure as noted or use of potassium-sparing diuretics; and second, a shift of potassium to the extracellular space. This latter can be caused intraoperatively by tissue destruction (rhabdomyolysis, tumor lysis), reperfusion of a vascular bed after a period of ischemia, or use of succinylcholine. Elevations can also be caused by a shift of potassium from the intracellular space by acidosis.

Signs of hyperkalemia are mostly manifested in the cardiac system and rarely seen if the serum potassium is below 6.0 mEq/l. As potassium concentration increases, there is an increase in cardiac automaticity, tall peaked T waves, prolongation of the PR interval, a widening of the QRS wave, and finally, ventricular fibrillation or asystole. Although the cardiac effects necessitate the most rapid response, systemic muscle weakness will also occur, leading to the inability to talk or to respiratory paralysis.

Hyperkalemia management consists of removing the cause of the hyperkalemia, antagonizing the effects of potassium on the body, moving potassium from the extracellular space to the intracellular space, and removal of potassium from the body. Antagonism of high extracellular potassium consists of calcium chloride 1g over 3 minutes or two to three ampules of calcium gluconate over 5 minutes. Additional steps are necessary to transfer potassium into the intracellular space. This can be accomplished by giving insulin 5–10 units in an adult with 25–50 g of D50 glucose (1 to 2 ampules), treatment of acidosis with 1 mEq/kg sodium bicarbonate along with hyperventilation, and β-adrenergic agent administration. Action to rid the body of excess potassium involves diuretics that act on the distal tubule and collecting ducts, aldosterone agonists, and sodium polystyrene sulfonate resin (Kayexalate) can be given orally or as an enema. Finally, if time permits, emergent hemodialysis can remove 25 to 50 mEq of potassium per hour.

Calcium

While 99% of bodily calcium is present in bones, 1% of calcium exists as a divalent ion primarily found in the extracellular compartment. Normal values for ionized calcium are 4.5–5.1 mEq/l (9–10.2 mg/dl). It is important to remember that it exists in three forms in the extracellular volume (ECV): first as protein-bound calcium (40%), second as chelated calcium (10%), and finally as ionized calcium (50%). With changes in the pH of fluid, the amount of calcium bound to albumin can change, thereby increasing the amount of ionized calcium with acidemia and decreasing the amount of ionized calcium with alkalemia.

Hypocalcemia

Hypocalcemia in a perioperative setting is most commonly caused by hyperventilation with its resultant alkalosis or with the chelation of calcium by citrate by the rapid infusion of preserved blood products at a rate greater than 1.5 ml/kg/min. Parathyroid hormone (PTH) deficiency, a major regulator of calcium homeostasis, can be caused by surgical removal of the parathyroid glands or hypo or hypermagnesemia with resultant hypocalcemia. In addition, hyperphosphatemia from large cellular destruction (rhabdomyolysis) can cause precipitation of calcium phosphate complexes. Patients with nutritional deficiencies or illness can have low albumin levels and show low total plasma calcium levels with normal ionized calcium levels. Finally, large amounts of isotonic saline used during resuscitation can produce hypomagnesemia which can lead to impairment of vitamin D action and PTH suppression leading to hypocalcemia.

Signs and symptoms of hypocalcemia can include mental status changes, tingling of digits, and positive Chvostek's and Trousseau's signs. Muscle tetany can lead to bronchospasm, laryngospasm, abdominal cramping, or urinary frequency. Cardiovascular changes of hypotension, heart failure, heart block, and impairment of β-adrenergic therapy can also be seen.

Initial evaluation should concentrate on renal function and serum phosphate concentration, as well as duration and severity of the hypocalcemia. Impaired renal function with hyperphosphatemia suggests hypoparathyroidism, and management should be directed toward removal of phosphate rather than calcium supplementation which could lead to tissue calcification. Usually, mild asymptomatic hypocalcemia does not require treatment. If hypotension is present, treatment with calcium chloride or calcium gluconate can restore the calcium level back to normal. Given in equivalent doses (two to three ampules of calcium gluconate for every ampule of calcium chloride) both are equally effective but care must be used in giving calcium chloride as intravenous extravasation can cause tissue necrosis.

Hypercalcemia

Hypercalcemia is defined as a total serum calcium of 10.5 mg/dl or greater. Patients with mild to moderate hypercalcemia (11 to 14 mg/dl) may be asymptomatic or have symptoms of lethargy, anorexia, nausea, or polyuria, symptoms common in postoperative patients. Severe hypercalcemia (>15 mg/dl) can lead to stupor, coma, heart block, and cardiac arrest.

Causes of hypercalcemia can include malignancies (through bone destruction or malignant secretion of hypercalcemic hormones), hyperparathyroidism, thyrotoxicosis, immobilization, and granulomatous diseases (e.g. sarcoidosis). Sarcoidosis can produce calcitriol from granulomatous tissue, thus increasing gut absorption and bone resorption.

Management initially consists of general supportive therapy consisting of hydration with normal saline, which inhibits renal resorption of calcium, furosemide therapy to increase urine output and increase tubular sodium, correction of any electrolyte abnormalities, increased ambulation, and treatment of the underlying condition. Additional therapy includes the use of bisphosphonates to inhibit osteoclast function, mithramycin and calcitonin. In cases of impaired renal function, hemodialysis should be considered.

Magnesium

Another divalent cation found primarily in the intracellular space is magnesium. Most magnesium is located in bone with a smaller portion in muscle, and less than 1% of total body magnesium found in serum. In serum, it can be bound to protein, chelated, or (the majority, 55%) in ionized form. Magnesium is necessary for many enzymatic systems, maintenance of vascular tone, and regulation of PTH secretion as noted earlier. Magnesium is also used clinically to treat pre-eclampsia and premature labor, to prevent dysrhythmias after myocardial infarction or in congestive heart failure, and as treatment for torsades de pointes.

Hypomagnesemia

In most symptomatic patients the serum magnesium level is found to be <1.2 mg/dl (normal 1.5 to 1.9 mg/dl). Patients frequently have muscle weakness, paresthesias, and when severe, confusion and coma. Hypomagnesemia can also cause hypokalemia owing to renal potassium wasting, and an increased incidence of digitalis toxicity and congestive heart failure. Additionally, because end-organ response and secretion of PTH are dependent on magnesium, hypomagnesemia can be a cause of hypocalcemia. Finally, respiratory muscle function is impaired with hypomagnesemia, which could lead to impaired ventilator weaning after anesthesia.

Causes of hypomagnesemia commonly include inadequate gastrointestinal absorption due to prolonged nasogastric suctioning, gastrointestinal or biliary fistulas, or intestinal drainage. Thirty percent of alcoholic patients admitted to the hospital are hypomagnesemic.[7]

While mild hypomagnesemia can be treated with diet alone, severe magnesium depletion can be treated with 1 to 2 g (8 to 16 mEq) of magnesium sulfate over one hour followed by a slower infusion (2 to 4 mEq/h) dictated by the serum magnesium levels.

Hypermagnesemia

Hypermagnesemia (>2.5 mg/dl) is usually produced by iatrogenic administration (treatment of pre-eclampsia or parenteral nutrition), or the ingestion of magnesium antacids or laxatives, especially in patients with impaired renal function. In the treatment of pre-eclampsia the therapeutic level is 5 to 7 mg/dl. At this level it is a tocolytic and used to prevent seizures in pre-eclamptic patients. As levels reach 15 to 20 mg/dl, respiratory depression can become apparent. With levels above 20 mg/dl, sedation, decreased deep tendon reflexes, and muscle weakness appear, leading to areflexia and coma with higher levels. Because of these potential side effects, it is important to follow blood levels in patients receiving magnesium therapy.

Management of hypermagnesemia involves fluid loading and diuretic therapy, although in renal failure and emergency situations, dialysis may be necessary. Temporary reversal of magnesium effects can be achieved with calcium administration.

Phosphate

Phosphate is involved in cellular energy through high-energy bonds in ATP. It is also involved in cell membrane structure and 2,3-diphosphoglycerate, which is a necessary component of oxygen unloading from hemoglobin. In the body, 90% of phosphorus is in bone while 10% is intracellular and less than 1% is in the extracellular fluid. Absorption of phosphorus occurs in the small intestine, with excretion controlled by renal mechanisms. Normal serum levels of phosphate range from 2.7 to 4.5 mg/dl.

Hyperphosphatemia

Hyperphosphatemia can be caused by inadequate renal excretion due to renal failure, cellular necrosis and release of phosphate from cells, or excessive intestinal uptake. Renal failure is the most common cause of hyperphosphatemia. To determine the cause of hyperphosphatemia, measurement of renal function and urinary phosphate is necessary. Rapid increases in serum phosphate can lead to hypocalcemia due to decreased calcitriol production. If phosphate levels become high enough, frank precipitation of calcium and phosphate may occur in tissues.

Management of hyperphosphatemia includes treatment of the underlying cause of the increased phosphate load and increasing the urinary excretion of phosphate with fluid loading. Additionally, inhibiting phosphate absorption with phosphate-binding antacids is necessary. Dialysis may be necessary for patients with renal failure.

Hypophosphatemia

Severe hypophosphatemia can cause a wide range of organ dysfunction when the serum phosphate falls below 1 mg/dl. Neurological manifestations can be seen in parathesias, delirium, and coma. Muscle weakness with respiratory muscle failure and heart failure can be symptoms. Causes of hypophosphatemia come from an intracellular shift of phosphate, an increase in renal phosphate losses, or a decrease in GI absorption of phosphate. Common among hospitalized patients is hypophosphatemia caused by the refeeding syndrome, in which insulin mediates the uptake of carbohydrates and phosphate.[8]

Patients with severe hypophosphatemia should receive intravenous phosphate, 5 to 16 mg/kg over 12 hours, and additional therapy adjusted by the serum phosphate level. Phosphate should be given slowly to hypocalcemic patients to avoid possibly causing more severe hypocalcemia or causing soft tissue calcification in hypercalcemic patients. Also, phosphate should be given slowly to patients with renal failure, owing to the inability of renal phosphate excretion.

References

1. H.J. Adrogue, N.E. Madias. Primary care: hypernatremia. *N Engl J Med* 2000; 342:1493–1499.

2. H. Chung, R. Kluge, R.W. Schrier, R.J. Anderson. Postoperative hyponatremia. A prospective study. *Arch Intern Med* 1986; 146: 333–336.

3. A.S. Kashyap. Hyperglycemia-induced hyponatremia: is it time to correct the correction factor? *Arch Intern Med* 1999; 159: 2745–2746.

4. D. Gravenstein. Transurethral resection of the prostate (TURP) syndrome: a review of the pathophysiology and management. *Anesth Analg* 1997; 84:438–446.

5. W.D. Brown. Osmotic demyelination disorders: central pontine and extrapontine myelinolysis. *Curr Opin Neurol* 2000; 13:691–697.

6. J.A. Wahr, R. Parks, D. Boisvert *et al.* Preoperative serum potassium levels and perioperative outcomes in cardiac surgery patients. *JAMA* 1999; 281:2203–2210.

7. M. Elisaf, M. Merkouropoulos, E.V. Tsianos *et al.* Pathogenetic mechanisms of hypomagnesemia in alcoholic patients. *J Trace Elem Med Biol* 1995; 9:210–214.

8. M.J. Brooks, G. Melnik. The refeeding syndrome: an approach to understanding its complications and preventing its occurrence. *Pharmacotherapy* 1995; 15:713–726.

Chapter

19 Nausea and vomiting

James W. Heitz

- Postoperative nausea and vomiting is common.
- Rescue anti-emetic therapy is indicated when nausea or vomiting occurs after surgery and should be targeted towards receptors in the chemoreceptor trigger zone.
- Low-dose multimodal therapy with medications exhibiting different mechanisms of action maximizes efficacy and minimizes side effects.
- Dexamethasone and scopolamine patches are not indicated for rescue therapy.

Postoperative nausea and vomiting (PONV) was described over two decades ago as anesthesiology's "big 'little problem'."[1] Since that time, literally thousands of studies have been conducted, and multiple organizations have proposed guidelines, but PONV remains a frequent complication encountered after surgery.

The majority of the medical literature is focused upon prophylaxis of PONV. Rescue therapy of established PONV is less well studied.[2] Dozens of risk factors for PONV have been identified, but the predictive value of scoring systems is not improved by using more than four or five. Christian Apfel proposed a simplified scoring system examining four easily measured parameters: (1) female sex; (2) non-smoking; (3) previous PONV or motion sickness; and (4) postoperative opioids (see Figure 19.1).[3] The presence of each risk factor increases risk in linear fashion. This simple PONV risk assessment tool has been validated across diverse patient populations. While it fails to encompass all of the risk factors recognized in the most recent version of the Society for Ambulatory Anesthesiology Consensus Guidelines for the Management of Postoperative Nausea and Vomiting, the Apfel criteria remain one of the most clinically useful tools for predicting PONV risk (see Table 19.1).[4]

The accurate assessment of risk is important, since prophylaxis is only warranted for high-risk patients.[5] Prophylaxis of low-risk patients increases costs and the incidence of side effects without improving outcomes and is not recommended by most organizations offering guidelines. However, many patients who warrant prophylaxis do not receive therapy consistent with current recommendations.[6]

It is important that the above-mentioned factors be considered when treating PONV. The incidence of PONV may be affected by targeting a number of different receptors within

Post-Anesthesia Care: Symptoms, Diagnosis, and Management, ed. James W. Heitz. Published by Cambridge University Press. © Cambridge University Press 2016.

Table 19.1 PONV risk factors

Risk factors for PONV in adults	
Positive evidence	Female sex
	History of PONV or motion sickness
	Non-smoking
	Younger age
	Use of volatile agents
	Postoperative opioids
	Duration of anesthesia
	Type of surgery
Conflicting evidence	ASA physical status
	Menstrual cycle
	Level of anesthetist's experience
	Neuromuscular blockade antagonism

ASA, American Society of Anesthesiologists

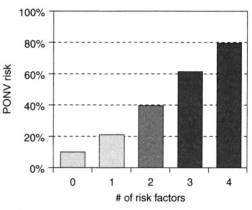

Risk factors	Points
Female sex	1
Non-smoker	1
History of PONV	1
Postoperative opioids	1
Sum =	0 ... 4

Figure 19.1 Apfel criteria for PONV risk. Adapted from ref. [3].

the central nervous system. High-risk patients may receive two or three anti-emetic therapies as prophylaxis prior to arrival in the Post-Anesthesia Care Unit (PACU). If prophylaxis has failed, it is important to establish which receptors have been already targeted so that therapy can be directed towards different receptors. Avoiding redundant therapy avoids unnecessary dose-related medication side effects.

Physiology

Emesis is a coordinated reflex in which gastric contents are forcibly expelled while the airway is protected and must be distinguished from the passive reflux of gastric contents in the presence of an unprotected airway. These separate processes are frequently

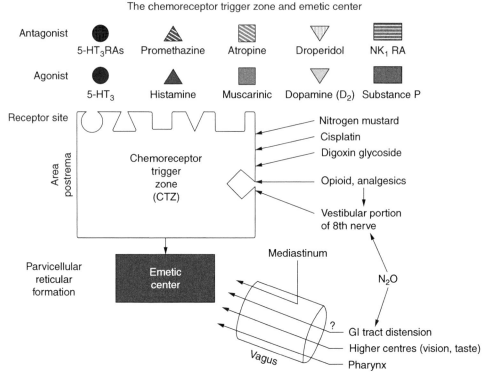

Figure 19.2 Chemoreceptor trigger zone receptors. From ref. [12].

confused, and the distinction between them has important implications for treatment. Whereas the treatment of passive reflux is aimed at limiting the sequela of pulmonary aspiration by increasing pH or decreasing volume, treatment of PONV is directed at preventing the initiation of the emesis reflex.

The chemoreceptor trigger zone (CTZ) is an area of the medulla which communicates with the emesis center in the area postrema via the nucleus tractus solitarius (NTS). The CTZ has an incomplete blood–brain barrier, so emetogenic chemicals in the blood may stimulate emesis. Additionally, the CTZ receives rich input from the middle ear, so the CTZ has a central role in emesis from motion sickness as well. A variety of neurotransmitters and receptors including acetylcholine, dopamine, histamine (H_1 receptor), substance P (NK_1 receptor), and serotonin (5-HT_3 receptor) are found in the CTZ, so an assortment of medications may reduce the incidence of PONV[12] (see Figure 19.2). Most pharmacological prophylaxis or treatment for PONV is directed at stabilizing the CTS, NTS, or both.

Although the emesis center is primarily involved in the motor function of emesis, it is important to note that emesis may be initiated by direct vagal afferents on the emesis center. A number of gastric or bowel irritants may directly initiate emesis without the involvement of the CTZ, and conventional therapy directed at CTZ receptor blockade will have limited efficacy in such cases. In the postoperative setting, this is primarily due to the irritating effect of swallowed blood on the stomach. Procedures in which blood is swallowed, including tonsillectomy, dental extractions, other surgeries within the mouth, and sinus surgery, may require unique therapy for PONV.

PONV management

Low-dose administration of medications from different classes is better than administration of higher doses of a single medication. Escalating the dose of a single agent often increases side effects significantly more than efficacy. Repeating a dose of a previously administered anti-emetic is rarely appropriate in the early postoperative period.[4]

In choosing an anti-emetic, consider mechanism of action, previously administered medications, patient allergies, and speed of onset. Some medications used for prophylaxis are inappropriate for rescue therapy owing to slow onset. Medications efficacious in the rescue therapy of PONV are presented in Table 19.2.

Failed prophylaxis

It is important to determine which anti-emetics may have already been administered when providing rescue therapy for PONV. Ondansetron targets the 5-HT$_3$ receptor and is highly efficacious. Ondansetron 1 mg IV is effective in the treatment of PONV with a number-needed-to-treat of 4.[8] Rescue therapy with ondansetron requires dosing of only 1 mg, which has a better side-effect profile than the 4 mg prophylactic dose. Ondansetron may cause headache at the 4 mg (number-needed-to-harm = 31), but not at the 1 mg dose.[9] However, its efficacy as rescue therapy is greatly diminished when it has already been administered for prophylaxis, with a 4 mg rescue dose being no more effective than placebo.[8]

No prophylaxis

In patients requiring treatment for PONV who have not received prophylaxis, administration of a single anti-emetic is indicated. Typically, these patients are low-risk patients for PONV and there are many anti-emetics which may be considered. 5-HT$_3$ antagonists are very effective for rescue treatment and carry a relatively benign side-effect profile, so are often appropriate for initial therapy, although some have been associated with QT-interval prolongation. Anticholinergics, antidopaminergics, or antihistaminics are appropriate for second-line therapy after rescue with an antiserotonergic medication has failed.

Swallowed blood

Procedures in which blood may be swallowed by the patient require special consideration, since gastric blood may induce emesis without excitation of the CTZ. Therefore, anti-emetic therapy targeting CTZ receptors may be ineffective. Antiserotonergic medications also exert a peripheral effect on gastric enterochromaffin cells, distinct from the central effect on the CTZ, and are efficacious in the therapy of PONV caused by blood in the stomach. Gastric prokinetics such as metoclopramide may also be beneficial, by removing the offending stimulus more quickly, keeping in mind it requires approximately 20 minutes for onset of action.

Non-pharmacological treatment

Some non-pharmacological interventions, including P6 acupressure and K-K9 Korean acupressure, have demonstrated efficacy in the treatment of PONV (see Figure 19.3).

Stimulation of these acupressure points, either by the application of direct pressure, electrical stimulation, or capsaicin ointment, have been validated in numerous trials for the

Table 19.2 PONV rescue therapy

Medication class	Examples	Comments
Corticosteroids	Dexamethasone 5–10 mg	Not indicated for rescue therapy
5-HT$_3$ receptor antagonists	Ondansetron 1 mg IV	Lower dose for rescue therapy than for prophylaxis
	Dolasetron 12.5, 25, 50, or 100 mg IV	No longer available in the USA, demonstrated efficacy for rescue therapy, little benefit from dose escalation
	Granisetron 2–20 mcg/kg	Less QT prolongation than ondansetron
	Tropisetron 0.5, 2 or 5 mg IV	Not available in the USA, demonstrated efficacy for rescue therapy, little benefit from dose escalation
	Ramosetron 0.3 mg IV	Not available in the USA
	Palonosetron 0.75 mg IV	Second generation, FDA approved for prophylaxis only
Antidopaminergics		
Butyrophenones	Droperidol 0.625–1.25 mg IV	FDA Black Box warning, ↑QT
	Haloperidol 0.5–1 mg IV	Not FDA approved for PONV, ↑QT
Benzamides	Metoclopramide 10 mg IV	Weak anti-emetic, gastric prokinetic
	Trimethobenzamide 200 mg IM	Very sedating, caution in renal insufficiency
Phenothiazines	Perphenazine 2.5 mg IV or IM	
	Promethazine 6.25 mg IV or IM	PO or PR if needed, avoid extravasation
	Prochlorperazine 5–10 mg IV/IM	Currently unavailable
	Chlorpromazine 25–50 mg IM/IV	Very sedating, extrapyramidal side effects, hypotension
Antihistamines	Dimenhydrinate 1 mg IV	
	Meclizine 25–50 mg PO	
	Diphenhydramine 25–50 mg IV/PO	Very sedating
Anticholinergics	Transdermal scopolamine	Not indicated for rescue therapy
	Scopolamine 0.3 mg sq or IM	Poor side-effect profile limits clinical usefulness: sedation, visual disturbances, confusion, dry mouth, hallucinations
NK-1 receptor antagonists	Aprepitant 40 mg PO	Efficacy as rescue not established
	Casopitant 50–150 mg PO	Investigational drug, not FDA approved
	Rolapitant 70–200 mg PO	Investigational drug, not FDA approved
Benzodiazepines	Midazolam 1 mg IV + 1 mg/hr IV	One small placebo-controlled trial in adults demonstrating efficacy in rescue therapy for emesis (nausea not measured)
Cannabinoids	Dronabinol 2.5–5 mg PO q 4–6 hr	Scant data for prophylaxis, not examined for PONV rescue therapy
Miscellaneous	Propofol 20 mg IV	May be administered in patient-controlled analgesia (PCA) form in PACU for rescue therapy
	Mirtazapine 30 mg PO	Effective for prophylaxis, unclear rescue efficacy
	Gabapentin 600 mg PO	Effective for prophylaxis, unclear rescue efficacy
	Isopropyl alcohol vapor inhalation	One small placebo-controlled trial in pediatrics demonstrating efficacy in rescue therapy for nausea and emesis

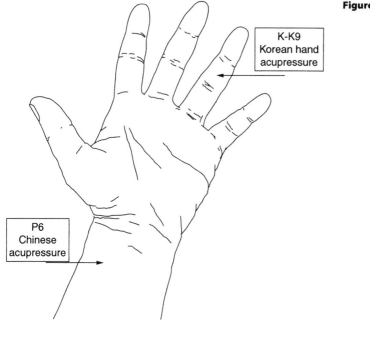

Figure 19.3 Acupressure points.

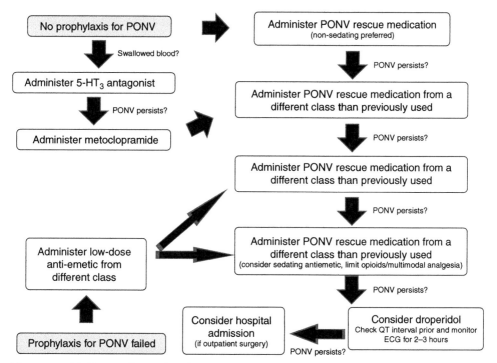

Figure 19.4 PONV rescue therapy algorithm.

prevention of PONV. In some studies, these modalities perform as well as ondansetron 4 mg IV for PONV prophylaxis.[10] Their efficacy for PONV rescue therapy is anecdotal and not yet validated by randomized placebo-controlled trials. The inhalation of isopropyl alcohol vapor from small disinfectant wipes was demonstrated to be effective as PONV rescue therapy for both nausea and emesis in a single small randomized placebo-controlled trial on pediatric patients.[11]

PONV rescue therapy will be most effective by selecting novel classes of medications in therapy rather than escalating doses, and minimizing postoperative opioids by utilizing multimodal pain therapy with non-opioid adjuvants when possible (see Figure 19.4).

References

1. P. Kapur. Editorial: The big "little problem." *Anesth Analg* 1991; 73:243–245.

2. F. Kazemi-Kjellberg, I. Henzi, M.R. Tramèr. Treatment of established postoperative nausea and vomiting: a quantitative systematic review. *BMC Anesthesiol* 2001; 1:2. doi:10.1186/1471-2253-1-2.

3. C.C. Apfel, E. Läärä, M. Koivuranta, C.A. Greim, N. Roewer. A simplified risk score for predicting postoperative nausea and vomiting: conclusions from cross-validations between two centers. *Anesthesiology* 1999; 91:693–700.

4. T.J. Gan, P. Diemunsch, A.S. Habib, *et al.* Consensus guidelines for the management of postoperative nausea and vomiting. *Anesth Analg* 2014; 118:85–113.

5. J.L. Apfelbaum, J.H. Silverstein, F.F. Chung, *et al.* American Society of Anesthesiologists Task Force on Postanesthetic Care. Practice guidelines for postanesthetic care. *Anesthesiology* 2013; 118:291–307.

6. P.F. White, J.F. O'Hara, C.R. Roberson, R.H. Wender, K.A. Candiotti and the POST-OP Study Group. The impact of current antiemetic practices on patient outcomes: a prospective study on high-risk patients. *Anesth Analg* 2008; 107:452–458.

7. M.R. Tramèr, R.A. Moore, D.J.M. Reynolds, H.J. McQuay. A quantitative systematic review of ondansetron in treatment of established postoperative nausea and vomiting. *Br Med J* 1997; 514:1088–1092.

8. M.R. Tramèr, D.J.M. Reynolds, R.A. Moore, H.J. McQuay. Efficacy, dose-response, and safety of ondansetron in prevention of postoperative nausea and vomiting: a quantitative systematic review of randomized placebo-controlled trials. *Anesthesiology* 1997; 87:1277–1289.

9. A.L. Kovac, T.A. O'Connor, M.H. Pearman, *et al.* Efficacy of repeat intravenous dosing of ondansetron in controlling postoperative nausea and vomiting: a randomized, double-blind, placebo-controlled multicenter trial. *J Clin Anesth* 1999; 11:153–159.

10. D.J. Rowbotham. Recent advances in the non-pharmacological management of postoperative nausea and vomiting. *Br J Anaesth* 2005; 95:77–81.

11. S.M. Wang, M.B. Hofstadter, Z.N. Kain. An alternative method to alleviate postoperative nausea and vomiting in children. *J Clin Anesth* 1999; 11:231–234.

12. M.F. Watch, P.F. White. Postoperative nausea and vomiting: its etiology, treatment, and prevention. *Anesthesiology* 1992; 77:162–184.

Pruritus

James W. Heitz

- Pruritus is common after surgery.
- Opioids account for most cases of postoperative pruritus.
- The therapeutic goal of patient comfort must be achieved without sacrificing analgesia.
- No single medication is universally effective in the treatment of postoperative pruritus.

Pruritus is virtually ubiquitous in the perioperative period. Everyone has the occasional itch. For patients, the severity of postoperative pruritus can range from inconsequential to extremely distressing. The etiology of postoperative pruritus may be divided into two broad categories: pharmacological and pathophysiological. Both etiology and severity need to be considered when selecting therapy. It is also essential to have an understanding of the physiology of pruritus.

Physiology: Pruritus shares anatomical and physiological similarity to pain. Both are unpleasant sensory experiences. Both elicit a specific behavioral response. Pruritus elicits scratch behavior. Pain elicits withdrawal behavior. Both are typically initiated by specialized receptors in the skin, transmitted via unmyelinated nerve fibers, conducted up the spinothalamic tracts, and may be modulated by inhibition from higher centers.

Although sharing similarities, pain and pruritus also appear to be mutually exclusive and do not normally co-exist. Non-noxious distracting stimuli reduce the intensity of pain and pruritus for only about 20 seconds, but noxious stimuli (pain) will suppress itch for up to 30 minutes, probably via spinal cord modulation.[1] Pain inhibits the perception of itch,[2] and, conversely, the inhibition of pain may enhance the perception of itch (Figure 20.1).[3] This creates the clinical dilemma that successful treatment of pain may exacerbate pruritus, and treatment of pruritus may reverse analgesia. Achieving a comfortable balance between analgesia and pruritus can be a daunting challenge for the clinician caring for the surgical patient.

Pruritus is mediated via dermal itch receptors, and knowledge of these receptors is rapidly evolving. Until recently believed to be a relatively undifferentiated receptor, it is now recognized that itch receptors are specialized similar to nociceptors. Itch receptors in primates are highly specialized to detect specific itch stimuli and send their input paired with nerve fibers carrying mechanical, thermal, or chemical nociception.[4]

Post-Anesthesia Care: Symptoms, Diagnosis, and Management, ed. James W. Heitz. Published by Cambridge University Press. © Cambridge University Press 2016.

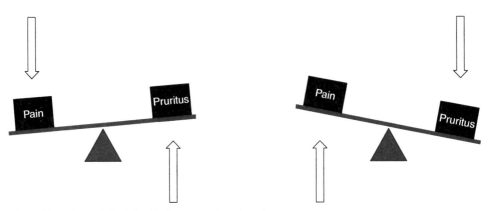

Figure 20.1 The clinical relationship between pain and pruritus.

Although the nerve fibers conducting itch sensation initially travel with fibers conveying nociceptive input, they synapse with second order neurons unique for itch in the dorsal horn of the spinal cord.[5] In rodent models, these second order neurons display a gastrin-releasing peptide receptor. The gene for this receptor has been identified, and mice bred without this gene do not display a scratch response to normally itchy stimuli.[6] Targeting this receptor could one day provide efficacious therapy for pruritus in humans. However, contemporary therapy is limited to targeting non-specific transmitters and inflammatory mediators either peripherally at the receptor level or centrally at the level of the spinothalamic tract.

The origin of pruritus may be dermal, neurogenic, psychogenic, neuropathic, or mixed.[7] As with pain, pruritus has the capacity to become neuropathic, causing a chronic pruritus which is difficult to treat. Effective perioperative pruritus therapy should be a clinical priority.

Management: Postoperative pruritus therapy currently utilizes a wide variety of pharmaceuticals with differing mechanisms of action and limited efficacy. No single agent is efficacious for all causes of pruritus or in all patients for a particular cause. Although the symptoms occur at the skin, postoperative pruritus is primarily neurogenic in etiology. Therapy should be directed at the neurogenic cause of pruritus. Topical creams and ointments are suitable for treatment of pruritus of dermal origin, but are generally not effective in the treatment of postoperative pruritus.

Pharmacological pruritus

Opioids: Opioids cause pruritus among 10% to 50% of patients with parenteral adminis-tration and between 20% and 100% with neuraxial administration.[8] Severe pruritic symptoms are experienced by only 1% of patients after neuraxial opioid administration, but therapy may be challenging for these patients.[9] Opioid-induced pruritus is neurogenic and occurs without rash or overt skin manifestations.

Opioids cause neurogenic pruritus primarily through action on the μ-receptor, although dopamine (D_2) receptors, serotonin (5-HT_3) receptors, γ-aminobutyric acid (GABA) receptors, glycine receptors, and prostaglandins have been identified as also being involved.[10] Complete μ-receptor antagonism may be achieved clinically with opioid antagonists and will effectively reverse both opioid-induced pruritus and opioid-induced analgesia, which is not tolerable for most surgical patients. Therefore, management of

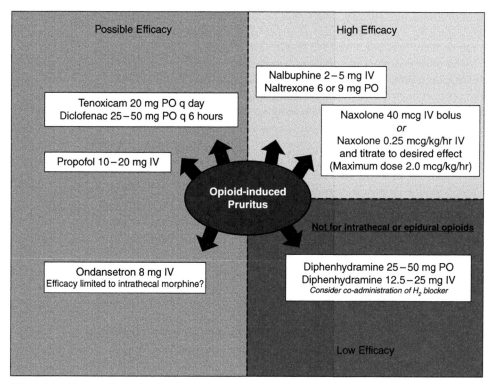

Figure 20.2 Therapy of opioid-induced pruritus.

opioid-induced pruritus either targets the μ-receptor with the aim of incomplete antagonism in order to treat pruritus without significant interference of analgesia or aims for blockade of one of the other involved receptors of lesser importance not crucial to analgesia (Figure 20.2). Management is further complicated by the fact that most studies have examined agents for prophylaxis of pruritus; there are too few studies examining the efficacy of rescue therapy for established postoperative pruritus to make evidence-based recommendations.[8]

Incomplete antagonism of the μ-receptor may be achieved either by ultralow-dose administration of an antagonist or by administration of a mixed opioid agonist–antagonist medication. Naloxone 40 mcg intravenous (IV) bolus may be administered for transient relief of opioid-induced pruritus. Continuous infusion of naloxone allows for dose titration and a longer duration of action. Naloxone infusions in the range of 0.17–2.0 mcg/kg/hr have reported efficacy with minimal reversal of analgesia. In most clinical situations, naloxone 0.25 mcg/kg/hr is an appropriate starting dose with slow upwards titration as needed to control symptoms.

Administration of a mixed agonist–antagonist such as nalbuphine or naltrexone may also successfully treat opioid-induced pruritus without reversal of analgesia by incomplete antagonism of the μ-receptor. Competitive binding at μ-receptors may reverse respiratory depression or pruritus (effectively functions as antagonist), but partial agonist effects at - kappa-receptors may maintain analgesia. Nalbuphine 2–5 mg IV has been demonstrated to provide effective rescue therapy for pruritus for adults after intrathecal administration of morphine, but efficacy could not be demonstrated in pediatric patients at a dose of 50 mcg/kg IV for treatment of pruritus from intravenous morphine.[10] Naltrexone 6 mg or 9 mg (but not 3 mg) PO is effective as well.[8]

The other receptors identified as involved in opioid-induced pruritus may be targeted, but these receptors appear to be less significant than the μ-receptor and clinically efficacy is also proportionately less. Good clinical results have been achieved by dopamine D_2 receptor antagonism. Droperidol 2.5 mg IV reduced the incidence of pruritus from 73% to 40% in one randomized control trial of women receiving morphine 2 mg via epidural catheter after cesarean section.[11] Interestingly, dose escalation to 5 mg IV negatively affects the efficacy of droperidol.[12] IV droperidol might offer some benefit in rescue therapy of pruritus, but the United States Food and Drug Administration's Black Box warning requires a pre-administration electrocardiogram (ECG) to confirm a normal QT interval followed by 2 to 3 hours of continuous ECG monitoring, which may not be clinically practical in all situations.

Ondansetron 8 mg IV has demonstrated ability to provide prophylaxis for intrathecal morphine, but not intrathecal sulfentanil administration.[5] Non-steroidal anti-inflammatory drugs might theoretically decrease pruritus via an anti-prostaglandin effect. Tenoxicam and diclofenac have some benefit in opioid-induced pruritus, but celecoxib has demonstrated conflicting results in clinical trials.[13] Studies of gabapentin are similarly conflicting with respect to efficacy of pruritus prophylaxis. While gabapentin has some efficacy in the treatment of chronic pruritus, it currently has no role as a rescue medication for pruritus in the perioperative period. Propofol may treat pruritus by inhibition of neuronal transmission at the level of the dorsal horn of the spinal cord. Subhypnotic doses of propofol 10 mg to 20 mg have been evaluated, also yielding conflicting results. Although a single study demonstrated sustained relief of pruritic symptoms (>1 hour) after a propofol 10 mg IV bolus,[14] subsequent studies found either less benefit or no benefit at all.

Although antihistamines have no role for neurogenic pruritus, they may effectively treat dermal pruritus. Morphine, codeine, and meperidine, with oral or parenteral administration, may release histamine and clinically present with a mixed pruritus of dermal and neurogenic origin. H_1 antihistamine therapy may benefit the dermal component. H_2 antihistamine therapy does not affect pruritus, but does improve the efficacy of H_1 antihistamines when administered in combination therapy. Response to antihistaminic therapy is predictably incomplete. Intrathecal or epidural administration of opioids do not release histamine, so this therapy is limited to oral or parenteral administration of certain opioids.[5]

Hetastarch: Hetastarch is a colloid that may be administered perioperatively in order to achieve intravascular volume expansion. Pruritus after administration of hetastarch appears to be common, but ascertaining the actual incidence of hetastarch-induced pruritus is complicated because symptoms may not appear for a month or longer after administration. The clinical association between the hetastarch and the delayed symptomatology may not be recognized in many cases. Hetastarch is most typically administered by anesthesiologists, surgeons, and intensivists, none of whom is likely to be involved in the care of the patient when symptoms develop. It has been estimated that over 12% of patients develop some pruritus after hetastarch administration.[15] The mechanism by which hetastarch causes pruritus is not fully understood, but tissue deposition in or in proximity to small peripheral nerves with direct irritant effect or indirect irritation from mediators released by affected cells appears to contribute.[16] Severe symptoms may be experienced by nearly one-half of affected patients, and symptoms may persist up to 2 years. Despite presentation late in the postoperative period, hetastarch-induced pruritus may occasionally be recognized in the first few postoperative days. Treatment is often ineffective, but there is anecdotal evidence of response to topical capsaicin ointment[17] or naltrexone.[18]

Vancomycin: Rapid administration of IV vancomycin may be accompanied by intense pruritus, cutaneous flush and hypotension ("red man syndrome" – see Chapter 30). Management is to discontinue the infusion and, after symptoms resolve, resume at a slower infusion rate.

Miscellaneous: Any medication causing a **Type I hypersensitivity reaction** (anaphylaxis) will cause pruritus that is usually associated with urticaria and other constitutional symptoms. Almost all medications may cause anaphylaxis, but the most commonly implicated causes of perioperative anaphylaxis are neuromuscular blocking agents, latex, and antibiotics.[19] Similarly, **acute transfusion reaction** may present with pruritus and urticaria and other constitutional symptoms. Many medications have some potential to cause pruritus, particularly during the polypharmacy of the perioperative period. Medications commonly initiated perioperatively implicated in pruritus include: angiotensin-converting enzyme inhibitors, angiotensin II antagonists, β-blockers, calcium entry blockers, fractionated heparins, antibiotics, tricyclic antidepressants, carbamazepine, non-steroidal anti-inflammatory drugs, and corticosteroids.[20] Evaluation of new-onset pruritus should include a search for these newly initiated medications.

Pathophysiological pruritus

Many underlying disease states are associated with pruritus, including renal failure, polycythemia vera, iron deficiency anemia, lymphoma, leukemia, hyper and hypothyroidism, diabetes, and carcinoid syndrome.[5] Few would be expected to present in the perioperative period, and most affected patients will already be treated. An important exception is cholestasis, a potent cause of pruritus. Cholestasis may develop acutely before or after surgery for a variety of reasons and may require therapy in the early postoperative period.

Cholestasis: Bilirubin is an irritant when deposited in the skin, and approximately 25% of jaundice patients will experience pruritus.[21] The pruritus of jaundice may be severe and refractory to pharmacological intervention, making it a difficult clinical problem in the surgical patient. Ondansetron has been reported to effectively treat jaundice-related pruritus when administered at higher doses (8 mg) than are needed for treatment of postoperative nausea and vomiting.[22,23] Serotonin-antagonists may treat pruritus by stabilizing the peripheral itch receptor.[24]

Koebner phenomenon: For patients with certain pre-existing dermatological conditions, minor trauma of unaffected skin may cause the appearance of new persistent skin lesions. This has been reported in patients with psoriasis, eczema, pityriasis rubra pilaris, lichen sclerosus, lichen nitidus, lichen planus, and vitiligo.[25] Postoperative pruritus when associated with vigorous scratching behavior may risk skin disease extension by Koebner phenomenon.[26] The relative risk is unknown, but patients with certain dermatological conditions may benefit from more aggressive treatment of postoperative pruritus when also associated with vigorous scratching behavior.

References

1. L. Ward, E. Wright, S.B. McMahon. A comparison of the effects of noxious and innocuous counterstimuli on experimentally induced itch and pain. *Pain* 1996; 64:129–138.

2. S.J. Brull, P.G. Atanassoff, D.G. Silverman, J. Zhang, L.H. Lamotte. Attenuation of experimental pruritus and mechanically evoked dysesthesiae in an area of cutaneous allodynia. *Somatosens Mot Res* 1999; 16:299–303.

3. P.G. Atanassoff, S.J. Brull, J. Zhang, et al. Enhancement of experimental pruritus and mechanically evoked dysesthesia with local anesthesia. *Somatosens Mot Res* 1999; 16:291–298.

4. S. Davidson, X. Zhang, C.H. Yoon, et al. The itch-producing agents histamine and cowhage activate separate populations of primate spinothalamic tract neurons. *J Neurosci* 2007; 27:10007–100014.

5. B. Waxler, Z.P. Dadabhoy, L. Stojiljkovic, S.F. Rabito. Primer of postoperative pruritus for anesthesiologists. *Anesthesiology* 2005; 103:168–178.

6. Y.G. Sun, A.F. Chen. A gastrin-releasing peptide receptor mediates the itch sensation in the spinal cord. *Nature* 2007; 448:700–703.

7. M. Schmelz. Itch: mediators and mechanisms. *J Dermatol Sci* 2002; 28:91–96.

8. F. Kjellberg, M.R. Tramer. Pharmacological control of opioid-induced pruritus: a quantitative systematic review of randomized trials. *Eur J Anaesthesiol* 2001; 18:346–357.

9. L. Krause, S. Shuster. Mechanism of action of antipruritic drugs. *Br Med J Clin Res Ed* 1983; 287:1199–1200.

10. A. Ganesh, L.G. Maxwell. Pathophysiology and management of opioid-induced pruritus. *Drugs* 2007; 67:2323–2333.

11. M.L. Horta, B.L. Horta. Inhibition of epidural morphine-induced pruritus by intravenous droperidol. *Reg Anesth* 1993; 18:118–120.

12. M. L. Horta, L. Ramos, Z.G. da Rocha, et al. Inhibition of epidural morphine-induced pruritus by intravenous droperidol: the effect of increasing the doses of morphine and of droperidol. *Reg Anesth* 1996: 21:312–317.

13. K. Kumar, S.I. Singh. Neuraxial opioid-induced pruritus: an update. *J Anaesthesiol Clin Pharmacol* 2013; 29:303–307.

14. A. Borgeat, O.H. Wilder-Smith, M. Saiah, K. Rifat. Subhypnotic doses of propofol relieve pruritus induced by epidural and intrathecal morphine. *Anesthesiology* 1992; 76:510–512.

15. M. Murphy, A.J. Carmichael, P.G. Lawler, M. White, N.H. Cox. The incidence of hydroxyethyl starch-associated pruritus. *Br J Dermatol* 2001; 144:973–976.

16. K. Bork. Pruritus precipitated by hydroxyethyl starch: a review. *Br J Dermatol* 2005; 152:3–12.

17. R.M. Szeimies, W. Stolz, U. Wlotzke, H.C. Korting, M. Landthaler. Successful treatment of hydroxyethyl starch-induced pruritus with topical capsaicin. *Br J Dermatol* 1994; 131:380–382.

18. D. Metze, S. Reimann, S. Beissert, T. Luger. Efficacy and safety of naltrexone, an oral opiate receptor antagonist, in the treatment of pruritus in internal and dermatological diseases. *J Am Acad Dermatol* 1999; 41:533–539.

19. D.L. Hepner, M.C. Castells. Anaphylaxis during the perioperative period. *Anesth Analg* 2003; 97:1381–1395.

20. A. Reich, S. Stander, J.C. Szepietowski. Drug-induced pruritus: a review. *Acta Derm Venereol* 2009; 89:236–244.

21. J. Crowe, E. Christensen, D. Doniach, et al. Early features of primary biliary cirrhosis: an analysis of 85 patients. *Am J Gastroenterol* 1985; 80:466–468.

22. M. Raderer, C. Muller, W. Sheithauer. Ondansetron for pruritus due to cholestasis. *N Engl J Med* 1994; 330:1540.

23. S. Dillon, J.D. Tobias. Ondansetron to treat pruritus due to cholestatic jaundice. *Pediatr Pharmacol Ther* 2013; 18:241–246.

24. S. Szarvas, D. Harmon, D. Murphy. Neuraxial opioid-induced pruritus: a review. *J Clin Anesth* 2003; 15:234–239.

25. G. Weiss, A. Shemer, H. Trau. The Koebner phenomenon: review of the literature. *J Eur Acad Dermatol Venereol* 2002; 16:241–248.

26. R. Mahajan, G.V. Kumar. Neuraxial opioids and Koebner phenomenon: implications for anesthesiologists. *Anesthesiology* 2003; 99:229–230.

Weakness

21

Donald Baumann

- Diffuse perioperative weakness may result from the residual effects of neuromuscular blockade.
- Weakness which interferes with breathing or the ability to protect the airway is an emergency.
- Weakness is occasionally associated with an underlying co-morbidity that may be undiagnosed at the time of surgery.

Postoperative weakness is an ongoing problem, still a major cause of perioperative morbidity and mortality despite recent advances in surgical technique, anesthesia, and pharmacotherapy.[1] Causes of postoperative weakness often involve the use of muscle relaxants given during general anesthesia, but there is evidence that weakness is still prevalent in anesthetized patients where muscle relaxants are not used.[2] Airway protection and ventilation is a primary concern in weak patients, which is an emergency and should be addressed immediately. However, non-airway-related weakness is still a potential emergency. When neuraxial anesthesia is used and block time exceeds the typical length, an evaluation for epidural hematoma should begin quickly with an urgent neurosurgical consult and computed tomography (CT) scan. The same is true for other regional anesthetic techniques such as peripheral nerve blocks, where hematoma or compartment syndrome can cause compression of nerves resulting in loss of function and potentially permanent injury. In these cases, physical exam can provide a quick diagnosis if compressing hematoma or compartment syndrome is present. If so, the surgical service should be contacted quickly to evaluate the patient and determine whether a return to the operating room is necessary. If there is no emergency present, the evaluation of a patient with postoperative weakness can still be done quickly and easily.

Evaluation

When evaluating a weak patient always consider the pre-procedural status. A patient having difficulty raising their leg off the bed may be a cause of great concern for a 20-year-old athlete who underwent a cholecystectomy, but may be the baseline strength for an inactive 80-year-old having the same operation. Always consider the operation and anesthetic choice as well. If the same 20-year-old athlete was given a femoral nerve block or epidural for an anterior cruciate ligament (ACL) repair, the level of concern would decrease since the

Post-Anesthesia Care: Symptoms, Diagnosis, and Management, ed. James W. Heitz. Published by Cambridge University Press. © Cambridge University Press 2016.

weakness is likely to be due to residual nerve block. Conversely, if he or she underwent a lumbar spinal fusion under general anesthesia, our level of concern would increase as we consider whether this is a surgical complication that needs immediate attention.

Other considerations for weak patients focus on pre-existing disease and home medications. If a patient has cerebrovascular disease with history of transient ischemic event or cerebrovascular accident, the differential diagnosis may consider a central rather than peripheral cause. Similarly, a patient who stopped taking warfarin 7 days prior to surgery but also, accidentally, stopped taking their thyroid hormone replacement may be profoundly hypothyroid with resulting muscle weakness.

When evaluating weak patients a good starting point is the neurological exam focusing on strength, motor function, and sensory. Adequate strength in the operating room (OR) can be assessed by firm handgrip or sustained head lift of at least 5 seconds, and the same can be done in the Post-Anesthesia Care Unit (PACU) if weakness is suspected. Depending on the operation performed, a baseline exam may be present in the patient's chart from either the surgeon or anesthesiologist. The type of operation performed, anesthetic type and medications given, and operative course is well documented in the anesthesia record available by the patient's bedside. Any questions not answered by the patient history and anesthesia record can be quickly obtained by a phone call to the OR where both the surgeon and anesthesiologist may still be present. It is generally good policy to notify the surgical and anesthesia services quickly if there are any deficits or neurological changes, since a return trip to the OR may be necessary depending on the underlying cause.

Neuromuscular blocking drugs

Neuromuscular blocking drugs are routinely given during general anesthesia to facilitate airway management, surgical exposure, and safety during operations where undesired movement could be detrimental. That being said, these drugs are also responsible for much of the postoperative morbidity and mortality associated with patient weakness. While new medications have been developed in recent years, our methods of monitoring the level of muscle relaxation are still underutilized and when used are lacking in sensitivity and subject to a wide range of interpretation among different providers. A basic understanding of how neuromuscular blocking drugs work and contribute to postoperative weakness is important when evaluating weak patients with or without neuromuscular disease.

Depolarizing muscle relaxants: Succinylcholine is the most common depolarizer currently used in clinical practice and is composed of two acetylcholine molecules linked through an ester bond.[3] The ester bond allows rapid hydrolysis by plasma enzymes, rendering succinylcholine breakdown largely independent of liver and kidney function. This makes a succinylcholine block very short-lived and predictable except in cases of inherited or acquired pseudocholinesterase deficiency.

Pseudocholinesterase deficiency: This condition, which is present in 1:3,200 individuals, may not be discovered until the patient is given succinylcholine in the OR and a prolonged recovery is seen. The inherited form is an autosomal dominant condition and affects the quality not the quantity of plasma pseudocholinesterase enzyme. Normal patients will demonstrate 90% recovery from succinylcholine block in 9 to 13 minutes, while heterozygous atypical patients will show prolonged recovery by 50 to 100%, and homozygous atypical patients may have a prolonged block lasting up to 4 to 6 hours.[3] The acquired form is secondary to drugs such as anticholinesterases, organophosphates, and oral contraceptives. Acquired deficiency can also be due to severe hepatic or renal disease, and even seen in normal physiological states such as pregnancy.[4] Management of pseudocholinesterase deficiency, whether inherited or acquired, is generally supportive with continued tracheal intubation and ventilation until the block wears off, although transfusion of plasma containing normal pseudocholinesterase may expedite recovery.[4]

Non-depolarizing muscle relaxants: The non-depolarizing neuromuscular blocking drugs are classified based on duration of action: short, intermediate, and long. They are metabolized and excreted by both hepatic and renal systems (with the exception of cisatracurium), so prolonged duration of action can be seen in patients with respective disease. The effects of non-depolarizers are measured by a train-of-four response using a twitch monitor attached to the overlying surface of various peripheral nerves, most commonly ulnar, posterior tibial, or facial. Four stimuli are given in rapid succession with response measured in number and intensity of twitch height. Misinterpretation of the train-of-four can cause both under- and over-assessment of relaxation and lead to problems with weakness postoperatively.

When non-depolarizers are used during surgery, they are generally reversed prior to extubation by acetylcholinesterase inhibitors, such as neostigmine. This increase in acetylcholine at the neuromuscular junction will compete with the non-depolarizing muscle relaxant at the receptor level and facilitate return of strength.

In weak patients without neuromuscular disease, residual block by non-depolarizing relaxants is often the cause. This can result from failure to administer reversal agent at the end of surgery, inadequate amount of reversal given, or reversal given too early with duration of block exceeding the half-life of reversal and subsequent recurarization. Management is dependent upon both the cause and severity of symptoms. For less severe causes, administration of additional pharmacological reversal agents is sufficient, but patients experiencing difficulties breathing may require intubation and mechanical ventilation.

Neuromuscular disease

Pre-existing neuromuscular disease leading to postoperative weakness can be classified into a few different broad categories: disorders of the neuromuscular junction, myopathies, and myotonia.[5] The major disorders of the neuromuscular junction are myasthenia gravis, Lambert–Eaton syndrome, and congenital myasthenic syndromes. These disorders render the patient extremely sensitive to neuromuscular blocking drugs, making their dosing and time to recovery very unpredictable. Additionally, drugs given during the perioperative period can exacerbate weakness in these patients. These drugs include: aminoglycosides, macrolides, beta-lactams, iodinated contrast dye, β-blockers, calcium channel blockers, lidocaine, bretylium, procainamide, quinidine, phenytoin, and phenothiazines.[6]

Myasthenia gravis: Myasthenia gravis is an autoimmune disease, which targets and decreases the number of acetylcholine receptors at the neuromuscular junction. Since reduced numbers of acetylcholine receptors are available, the patient will have an intensified and prolonged response to non-depolarizing muscle block. Often, greatly reduced dosages are required intraoperatively, and avoidance of muscle relaxation is preferable owing to the possibility of postoperative weakness. Even when muscle relaxation is not used, myasthenic patients may have postoperative weakness, which occurs in proportion to the severity of their disease.[3] Management is supportive with the primary concerns being respiratory insufficiency and airway protection. Inadequate oxygenation and decreased ability to remove carbon dioxide can necessitate reintubation and supportive ventilation until the patient returns to full strength.

Lambert–Eaton myasthenic syndrome (LEMS): LEMS is an autoimmune-mediated condition attacking the presynaptic neurons, resulting in decreased release of acetylcholine into the neuromuscular junction. This condition often manifests as a paraneoplastic syndrome, in approximately 60% of cases, and is most commonly seen with small cell lung cancer.[7] Patients with LEMS are sensitive to both depolarizing and non-depolarizing muscle block. Just as in myasthenia gravis, reduced dosages are required and postoperative weakness is frequently encountered. Management is supportive, as described above for myasthenia gravis.

Muscular dystrophy: There exists a large group of diseases that fall into the category of muscular dystrophy, the most common and serious being myotonic dystrophy and Duchenne or Becker muscular dystrophy. The clinical presentation of limb muscle weakness, respiratory weakness, and cardiac disease may not be diagnosed until early childhood or later. Anesthetic implications are similar and involve sensitivity to depolarizing muscle blockers, which are generally avoided in this population owing to the risk of cardiac arrest secondary to hyperkalemia, and sensitivity to non-depolarizing muscle blockers, which may be due to the pre-existing muscular weakness in these patients.[8]

Myotonic dystrophy: Myotonic dystrophy is the most common form of muscular dystrophy. The clinical presentation of weakness in limb and facial muscles is frequently not diagnosed until adulthood.[9] As in other muscular dystrophies, anesthetic complications arise from sensitivity to non-depolarizing muscular blocks, which can manifest as postoperative weakness. Succinylcholine and other depolarizing blockers are contraindicated owing to risk of hyperkalemia as well as sustained muscle contraction.

Hypokalemic periodic paralysis: Among the rare group of disorders categorized as periodic paralysis, hypokalemic periodic paralysis is the most common. The clinical presentation involves episodic weakness affecting the proximal more than distal limb muscles. Respiratory involvement is common. The triggers are generally ingestion of carbohydrate or sodium-rich foods or fluids. The diagnosis is generally one of exclusion, where measured serum potassium levels are low during an episode of paralysis.[8] Respiratory involvement may necessitate the need for supportive ventilation until the symptoms resolve. Treatment is to discontinue the triggers, such as stopping sodium or dextrose infusions, and to restore normal serum potassium levels.

In conclusion, assessment of weak PACU patients requires consideration of pre-procedural status, perioperative course, and co-morbidities. In most cases management is supportive; it may require reintubation and supportive ventilation in cases with airway compromise. Communication with surgical and anesthesia services should not be delayed, since correcting the underlying cause may require immediate surgery.

References

1. A. Marcus. Residual paralysis: the problem that won't go away. *Anesthesiol News* 2012; 38: 1–28.

2. W. Alkhazrajy, A.D. Khorasenee, W.J. Russell. Muscle weakness after muscle relaxants: an audit of clinical practice. *Anaesth Intensive Care* 2004; 32: 256–259.

3. M. Naguib, C.A. Lein. Pharmacology of muscle relaxants and their antagonists. In: R.D. Miller, ed. *Miller's Anesthesia* 6th Edition. Philadelphia, PA: Elsevier Churchill Livingstone; 2005; 481–572.

4. F.L. Soliday, Y.P. Conley, R. Henker. Pseudocholinesterase deficiency: a comprehensive review of genetic, acquired, and drug influences. *AANA J* 2010; 78: 313–320.

5. D. Quan, S.P. Ringel. Neuromuscular diseases. In: W.J. Weiner, C.G. Goetz, R.K. Shin, S.L. Lewis, eds. *Neurology for the Non-Neurologist* 6th Edition. Philadelphia, PA: Lippincott Williams & Wilkins; 2010; 344–374.

6. R.D. Stevens. Neuromuscular disorders and anesthesia. *Curr Opin Anaesthesiol* 2001; 14: 693–698.

7. T.B. Toothaker, M. Rubin. Paraneoplastic neurological syndromes: a review. *Neurologist* 2009; 15: 21–33.

8. G.N. O'Neill. Inherited disorders of the neuromuscular junction. *Int Anesthesiol Clin* 2006; 44: 91–106

9. J. Mathieu, P. Allard, G. Gobeil *et al.* Anesthetic and surgical complications in 219 cases of myotonic dystrophy. *Neurology* 1997; 49: 1646–1650.

Movement disorders

Nicole Renaldi

- Postoperative movement disorders are often secondary to the polypharmacy of the perioperative period.
- Extrapyramidal symptoms (e.g. dystonic reactions) are the most frequent movement disorders observed after surgery.
- Most postoperative movement disorders are transient and may be successfully managed with appropriate pharmacological intervention and reassurance to the affected patient and his or her family.

A variety of movement disorders may be encountered in the early postoperative setting. They range from benign to serious and from transient to long-term. Although most movement disorders seen in the Post-Anesthesia Care Unit (PACU) are more bothersome to the patient than they are life-threatening, some do place the airway at risk, and emergent airway management may be necessary. When evaluating patients with movement disorders, the focus should be on managing acute emergencies and uncovering the etiology, so that the disorder may be treated appropriately and future complications may be avoided. Many of the movement disorders encountered in the PACU often have an iatrogenic etiology from drugs given prior to, during, or after surgery. The movement disorders discussed in this chapter include: extrapyramidal symptoms (EPS), with a focus on dystonic reactions, myoclonus, and other drug-induced symptoms; restless legs syndrome (RLS); nystagmus; and shivering.

Extrapyramidal symptoms

Extrapyramidal symptoms include a wide range of signs and symptoms including acute dystonic reactions, akathisia, motor tics, myoclonus, and tardive dyskinesia. Patients may experience any one or a combination of these.

The type of reaction should be distinguished upon evaluation.

- *Acute dystonic reactions* display involuntary muscle contractions resulting in increased muscle tone, repetitive movements, or movements that result in twisting, pulling, or squeezing.[1]
- *Akathisia* is defined by both subjective and objective signs and symptoms; subjectively the patient may express feelings of restlessness, tension, or distress, and the patient may objectively display motor restlessness. It may be easily misdiagnosed as anxiety.[1]

Post-Anesthesia Care: Symptoms, Diagnosis, and Management, ed. James W. Heitz. Published by Cambridge University Press. © Cambridge University Press 2016.

- *Motor tics* are spastic muscle contractions, tonic or clonic, generally involving the face, neck, and/or shoulders.[1]
- *Myoclonus* can include involuntary muscle twitching, lightning-like jerks, or clonic spasm of a single muscle or group of muscles.[1,2]
- *Tardive dyskinesia* includes slow, rhythmic, stereotypical motor movements of the head, tongue, neck, arm, and/or upper trunk.[1]

Patients at risk for EPS include young women, pediatric patients, elderly patients, diabetics, patients with a history of neurological disorders, and patients receiving concurrent neuroleptics.[1] Case reports have also revealed EPS after uneventful anesthetics in healthy patients.

Dystonic reactions: Dystonic reactions following general anesthesia are rare. The differential diagnosis includes: adverse drug reaction, local anesthetic reaction, emergence delirium, hysterical response, and shivering. Case reports have demonstrated dystonic reactions following propofol and ondansetron. Most reported cases of abnormal movements following propofol occur following induction, emergence, or shortly thereafter with patients being fully awake and aware of the involuntary movements. Ondansetron has also been reported to result in EPS, with jerky movements of the head, neck, torso, and limbs, occurring in close proximity to drug administration.[3]

Rhythmic movement disorder (RMD) is classified as a sleep–wake transition disorder seen most commonly in infants and usually disappears by age 4 to 5, with a few cases presenting at a later age. Movements occur most frequently when falling asleep or between sleep stages. Movements most commonly seen with RMD include: head banging, head rolling, body rocking, and body rolling. The etiology is unknown, but the disorder has been shown to be benign, and usually resolves without intervention. A 2012 case report demonstrated RMD in a 10-year-old girl that developed in the PACU 30 minutes after a dose of IV ondansetron.[3]

Myoclonus: The differential diagnosis of the etiology of myoclonus is extensive, including drug reactions, essential myoclonus (idiopathic or hereditary), seizure, central nervous system (CNS) disease, infection, metabolic disorders, and nutritional deficiencies.[2] These should be considered upon evaluation of a patient demonstrating myoclonus in the PACU, with particular attention to drug reactions, as outlined below.

Postoperative myoclonic symptoms have been reported after the use of several inhalational anesthetic agents, induction drugs, and narcotics. Reviews reveal that postoperative myoclonic symptoms are frequently but not always associated with the use of central excitatory drugs, such as propofol and etomidate, and are associated with the use of potent narcotics.[4]

Myoclonus is a common side effect of induction with etomidate, thought to be due to subcortical disinhibition, with an incidence of 50–80% of patients who are not premedicated prior to induction with medications that inhibit subcortical activity, like benzodiazepines and fentanyl.[5] Both tonic and myoclonic muscle activity are well-known side effects of induction with opioids, including morphine, fentanyl, and fentanyl analogs. Cases report tonic rigidity and generalized myoclonus developing minutes to hours postoperatively, with successful naloxone termination of symptoms.[6]

Opisthotonus (spinal hyperextension and spasticity) has been reported to occur after anesthesia with propofol. One case even reported opisthotonus in association with torticollis, vertical nystagmus, obtundation, and periodic apnea, following an anesthetic that did not include propofol or drugs known to produce EPS symptoms. Symptomatic relief of the idiosyncratic reaction was achieved with administration of physostigmine, and the reaction was postulated to be due to central anticholinergic syndrome caused by fentanyl administration.[4]

Although rare, spinal myoclonus may be seen following intrathecal or epidural anesthesia. It is usually restricted to a limb or a few muscles of a limb, is not affected by peripheral stimuli, often persists in sleep, and is responsive to medical therapy with benzodiazepines, sodium valproate, and carbamazepine. Although symptoms may be demonstrated with conventional dosing, it is important to note that local anesthetic neurotoxicity has also been demonstrated as a possible etiology.[2]

Medication-induced EPS

As noted in the above discussion, in the PACU setting, EPS are often medication-induced. Medication-induced EPS are often recognized by the close proximity to administration of the offending medication. There are many medications known to induce EPS, including anti-emetics, drugs used for the treatment of vertigo, antidepressants, calcium channel antagonists, antiarrythmics, antiepileptics, cholinomimetics, and other drugs. Among those, dopamine receptor blocking agents are the most well-known culprits, including phenothiazines (e.g. prochlorperazine and chlorpromazine), butyrophenones (e.g. haloperidol and droperidol), and metoclopramide.

Metoclopramide-induced movement disorders are well documented. Tardive dyskinesia and Parkinsonism are seen after long-term use, while dystonia and akathisia, the two most common acute reactions, can occur after a single dose. The majority of reports of metoclopramide-induced movement disorders occur in conjunction with chronic therapy. If administering metoclopramide in the PACU, reduced doses should be considered in at-risk populations. It has also been shown that with slow metoclopramide administration over 15 minutes, severity and incidence of akathisia has been reduced compared with 2-minute administration; rapid injection has been shown to lead to anxiety, restlessness, and/or drowsiness.[1]

Treatment of drug-induced movement disorders/EPS involves prompt recognition. Discontinue the offending medication. Assess airway, breathing, and vital signs; severe acute dystonic reactions have been reported to result in airway obstruction. Be prepared to reintubate for airway protection if necessary. Treatment should begin with intravenous (IV) diphenhydramine 25–50 mg or 2 mg midazolam. If symptoms do not improve, akathisia has been treated with anticholinergics, benzodiazepines, β-blockers, α2-agonists, and opioids.[1] Continue to monitor vital signs and watch for resolution of EPS symptoms. Educate the patient about their reaction.

Restless legs syndrome

The prevalence of RLS is 7–10% of adults and 0.5–1% of children. RLS is most common among patients of European origin, with an increased prevalence among women, and ages 60–70 years.[7] RLS is defined by an irresistible urge to move the legs, which is often accompanied by unusual or unpleasant sensations in the legs that may be described as creeping, tugging, or pulling.[8]

Although evidence is conflicting, one study showed that spinal anesthesia caused postoperative RLS.[9,10] If a patient exhibits signs of new-onset or worsening RLS after anesthesia, opioids are a well-established and effective treatment.[7,11] Additionally, IV magnesium and physostigmine have provided symptomatic control anecdotally.

The use of compression stockings may also be beneficial.[7] Drugs that should be avoided for RLS patients, as they may exacerbate the condition, include: butyrophenones, sedative antihistamines, dopamine antagonist anti-emetics, and opioid antagonists.[7]

Nystagmus

Nystagmus, vertigo, and ataxia have been reported after injection of local anesthesia into the neck.[12] Case reports also describe vertical nystagmus after epidural administration of opioids, with both fentanyl and morphine. In these cases, resolution of the nystagmus was achieved with naloxone.[13] When a patient develops nystagmus after epidural opioid, it may be a benign side effect but could also be a sign of serious CNS lesions, especially in patients with underlying risk factors such as old age, diabetes, hypertension, and cerebrovascular disease.[13] Therefore, when evaluating a patient in the PACU, a thorough neurological exam should be performed, and pathological etiologies should be investigated if nystagmus does not improve with naloxone administration.

Shivering

Postoperative shivering is an acute complication of anesthesia frequently seen in the PACU setting. The incidence has been reported as 60% after general anesthesia with volatile agents[14] and 55% after neuraxial anesthesia.[15] Classic risk factors include: longer duration of surgery, male sex, anticholinergic premedication, spontaneous ventilation, higher American Association of Anesthesiologists (ASA) Physical Status, general versus orthopedic surgery, and administration of blood.[16] However, a more recent study reduced the number of risk factors to three: young age, endoprosthetic surgery, and hypothermia. While age was noted to be the most important, hypothermia was noted to be a weak risk factor for incidence, but greatly increased the duration of shivering when it occurred.[17]

Hypothermic shivering patients need rewarming and may require pharmacological intervention, while normothermic shivering patients need pharmacological intervention alone. For patients that remain ventilated, reversal should be held until the patient is rewarmed to near normal temperature and shivering attenuates.[18] Meperidine (12.5–25 mg IV) is an effective treatment, as it lowers the shivering threshold. It is often first-line therapy owing to the low side-effect profile; however, meperidine does lower the seizure threshold. Meperidine should therefore be avoided in patients with a history of seizure and/or renal failure, as its metabolites may accumulate and result in seizure. Many other pharmaceutical agents can lower the shivering threshold, including most anesthetic agents and opioids; fentanyl should be considered as an adjunct or when meperidine is contraindicated.

In the PACU, other causes of shivering, such as sepsis, drug allergy, and transfusion reaction, should be excluded.[18]

References

1. D.D. Moos, D.J. Hansen. Metoclopramide and extrapyramidal symptoms: a case report. *J Perianesth Nurs* 2008; 23: 292–9.

2. M.T. Sanjoaquín, J.V. Martinez-Quiñones, C. Teixeira *et al.* Spinal myoclonus following spinal anesthesia. *Internet J Anesthesiol* 2009; 19: 2.

3. A.O. Budde, M. Freestone-Bernd, S. Vaida. Rhythmic movement disorder after general anesthesia. *J Anaesthesiol Clin Pharmacol* 2012; 28: 371–3.

4. D. Dehring, B. Gupta, W.T. Peruzzi. Postoperative opisthotonus and toricollis after fentanyl, enflurane, and nitrous oxide. *Can J Anaesth* 1991; 38: 919–25.

5.   A.W. Doenicke, M.F. Roizen, J. Kugler
     et al. Reducing myoclonus after etomidate.
     Anesthesiology 1999; 90: 113–19.

6.   T.A. Bowdle, G.A. Rooke. Postoperative
     myoclonus and rigidity after anesthesia
     with opioids. *Anesth Analg* 1994; 78: 783–6.

7.   P. Smith, S. White. Anaesthesia and restless
     legs syndrome. *Eur J Anaesthesiol* 2009;
     26: 89–90.

8.   RLS foundation. About RLS: What is RLS?
     2007. http://www.rls.org/page.aspx?
     pid=477. (Accessed September 20, 2012.)

9.   T.A. Crozier, D. Karimdadian, S. Happe.
     Restless legs syndrome and spinal
     anesthesia. *N Engl J Med* 2008; 359: 2294–6.

10. B. Högl, B. Frauscher, K. Seppi *et al.*
     Transient restless legs syndrome after
     spinal anesthesia: a prospective study.
     Neurology 2002; 59: 1705–7.

11. B. Högl, C. Trenkwalder, W. Poewe.
     More on the restless legs syndrome and
     spinal anesthesia. *N Engl J Med* 2009;
     360: 1155–6.

12. P.T. de Jong, J.M. de Jong, B. Cohen,
     L.B. Jongkees. Ataxia and nystagmus
     induced by injection of local anesthetics in
     the neck. *Ann Neurol* 1977; 1: 240–6.

13. B.G. Lim, J.Y. Lee, H. Kim, D.K. Lee,
     M.K. Lee. Nystagmus caused by
     epidural fentanyl. *J Anesth* 2012;
     26: 94–6

14. P.K. Bhattacharya, L. Bhattacharya,
     R.K. Jain, R.C. Agarwal. Post anaesthesia
     shivering (PAS): a review. *Indian
     J Anaesthesiol* 2003; 47: 88–93.

15. L.J. Crowley, D.J. Buggy. Shivering and
     neuraxial anesthesia. *Reg Anesth Pain Med*
     2008; 33: 241–52.

16. A.W. Crossley. Six months of shivering
     in a district general hospital. *Anaesthesia*
     1992; 47: 845–8.

17. L.H.J. Eberhart, L. Doderlein, G. Eisenhardt
     et al. Independent risk factors for
     postoperative shivering. *Anesth Analg* 2005;
     101: 1849–57.

18. Postanesthesia care. Ch. 56 in: *Morgan &
     Mikhail's Clinical Anesthesiology*
     5th edition (ed JF Butterworth, DC
     Mackey, JD Wasnick) New York: McGraw-
     Hill, 2006; 1264–5.

Chapter

23

Limb paralysis

James W. Heitz

- Limb paralysis is a very rare event after surgery.
- Most cases of postoperative paralysis are traceable to surgical events.
- Compression neuropathy may occur as a complication of surgical positioning.
- Quadriplegia or paraplegia may be caused by exacerbation of pre-existing spine disease, spinal cord ischemia, or spinal hematoma.

Motor deficits caused by surgery

Direct trauma to the spinal cord or a peripheral nerve may occur with procedures of the spine or limbs. Surgical injury to nerves can be cause by transection, ischemia, compression, or stretching. Nerves in or near the operative field are at greatest risk of surgical injury. Total hip replacement produces an incidence of postoperative nerve palsy in the range of 0.6% to 3.7%.[1] Sciatic nerve injuries are most common and may impair leg flexion and dorsiflexion of the foot. Femoral nerve injuries occur with an incidence of 0.1% to 0.4%[1] and may impair leg extension and hip flexion. The vast majority of nerve palsies associated with hip replacement are noted in the early postoperative period. A small subset of nerve injury may present several weeks after surgery with new-onset leg weakness and pain. Some of these may be caused by a post-inflammatory neuropathy.[2] Abdominal hysterectomy may be associated with 10% incidence of postoperative femoral neuropathy, especially if self-retaining retractors are used for surgical exposure.[3] Brachial plexus injuries occur with a frequency of 0.1% to 4% during shoulder surgery depending upon the particular procedure.[4]

Management: New weakness after limb or spinal surgery needs to be brought to the attention of the surgeon. Post-inflammatory neuropathy may respond to intravenous (IV) methylprednisolone.[2]

Regional anesthesia

Regional anesthesia produces motor blockade in addition to anesthesia. While this is anticipated, motor blockade occasionally causes concern for patients, family, or healthcare providers. The duration of expected blockade is dependent upon several factors including whether it is a "single shot" or continuous infusion, the pharmacokinetics of the local anesthetic, the dose administered and the use of adjuvants in the block, such as epinephrine. Actual nerve injury from regional anesthesia is rare, but may occur from neural toxicity of local anesthetic solutions, mechanical trauma to the nerve from the needle, intraneural injection, and tourniquet-induced nerve compression or ischemia.[5] The incidence of nerve injury after brachial plexus blockade is very low and reported to be about 1.5 per 10,000 blocks,[6] but severe motor damage is occasionally reported.[7]

Management: Spontaneous recovery is typical, although the presence of a motor deficit is more ominous than is an isolated paresthesia. Concerns for either residual paresthesia or motor deficits in a patient receiving regional anesthesia should be referred to the anesthesiologist.

Compression neuropathy

Injury to peripheral nerves may occur because of stretch or compression. The most common nerve injury after surgery is ulnar neuropathy. Compression of the ulnar nerve in the olecranon fossa is the most commonly cited etiology, but the true etiology of ulnar neuropathy is probably multifactorial and more complex. The incidence of ulnar neuropathy after non-cardiac surgery is 1 in 2,729 procedures.[8] Half of these patients will be asymptomatic at one year. Cardiac procedures carry an increased risk of both ulnar and brachial plexus injury with an incidence range of 1.5% to 24% between studies.[9] The risk of brachial plexus injury is also increased for procedures in the lateral position including thoracotomy. Motor neuropathy is also seen after surgery in the lithotomy position with an incidence of 1 in 3,608 procedures.[10] The risk of motor neuropathy increases by two orders of magnitude for every hour in lithotomy position.

Management: Compression neuropathy limited purely to sensory deficits usually has a good prognosis with most patients achieving complete recovery after several weeks. Motor deficits are more ominous and although complete recovery is possible, consultation with a neurologist is prudent.

Compartment syndrome: Acute compartment syndrome may develop in a limb when elevated compartment pressure impairs perfusion. The compartmental pressure needed to cause cellular injury is therefore dependent upon systemic blood pressure, but compartmental pressure may become injurious when it approaches 20 mmHg[11] to 30 mmHg[12] of diastolic blood pressure. Compartment syndrome may develop in the perioperative period. Signs and symptoms of compartment syndrome may be remembered by the mnemonic of the 6 Ps: pain, paresthesia, paralysis, pallor, pulselessness, and poikilothermia (referring to cooling of the affected limb). While paralysis is a sign of compartment syndrome, it typically is a late finding. Paresthesia, severe pain exacerbated by passive movement of the limb, and pallor occur earlier and before pulselessness or paralysis develop.

Table 23.1 Motor deficits associated with common compression neuropathy

Symptom	Injury
Weakness of arm	Brachial plexus
Weak hand grip, unable to pinch between thumb and 5th digit	Ulnar nerve
Weak lower extremity extension	Femoral nerve
Weak lower extremity flexion	Sciatic nerve
Foot drop	Common peroneal nerve

6 Ps of compartment syndrome
Paralysis
Pain
Pallor
Paresthesia
Pulselessness
Poikilothermia

Acute compartment syndrome is most frequently observed in trauma patients with either long bone fractures or crush injuries, or may occur after reperfusion of an ischemic limb.[13] Vascular puncture causing bleeding into the limb may cause acute compartment syndrome, especially in patients with pre-existing coagulopathy. Acute compartment syndrome may occur as a complication of intraoperative positioning, particularly for procedures performed in lithotomy syndrome.[14–17] Mean arterial pressure decreases 2 mmHg for each inch above the level of the heart,[18] so higher positioning of the legs when combined with intraoperative reduction in blood pressure may place the legs at risk. Longer surgeries (>4–6 hours) and higher patient body mass index also appear to carry increased perioperative risk. Although some clinicians have expressed concern that calf compression devices may cause compartment syndrome in conjunction with lithotomy positioning,[14,16] these devices have been found to reduce compartment pressures in non-anesthetized healthy volunteers in lithotomy position.[19]

Compartment syndrome may develop after infiltration of an IV catheter, particularly if the infusion is administered under pressure,[20,21] or mannitol[22] or IV contrast dye[23] has been administered. Intraosseous fluid administration has rarely been associated with the subsequent development of compartment syndrome. This infrequent complication has been reported primarily among pediatric patients,[24–29] who typically receive intraosseous administration more frequently than do adult patients. However, intraosseous administration of fluids and medications for the resuscitation of the unstable adult patient without IV access has been recommended by the American Heart Association since 2010.[30] More recently, compartment syndrome has been reported in an adult patient in the intraosseous line.[31] The development of compartment syndrome with intraosseous fluid administration has been associated with greater volumes and rates of fluid infusion, the use of hypertonic crystalloids, needle malposition, bone fracture, or recent (<48 hours) prior intraosseous infusion in the same bone.[32] It should be emphasized that although fluid extravasation occurs in as many as 22% of pediatric patients with intraosseous fluid infusions,[33] development of compartment syndrome is a rarely observed complication. Compartment syndrome has been very rarely reported with IV regional anesthesia (Bier block) of the upper[34] or lower extremity.[35] Compartment syndrome may occur at any point during the postoperative period, but is most typically recognized within 24 hours of surgery.[36,37]

Management: The management of acute compartment syndrome is surgical. Best outcomes for limb function are achieved when fasciotomy is performed within 12 hours. Delayed diagnosis is limb-threatening, and compartment syndrome lasting more than

4 hours may result in acute kidney injury from rhabdomyolysis. Intravenous hydration and alkalization of the urine may be renal protective.

Quadriplegia

New-onset quadriplegia after surgery is rare and terrifying. If surgery involved the cervical spine, neurological deficits may be secondary to direct cord trauma, cord ischemia, or epidural hematoma. However, quadriplegia has been reported after procedures remote from the cervical spine including procedures of the lumbar spine, ophthalmological, cardiac, thoracic, and general surgical procedures. The diagnosis of the etiology of quadriplegia after procedures distant from the spinal cord is clinically challenging. Postoperative quadriplegia has been reported in patients with known cervical spine pathology, subclinical pathology, and in patients without pre-existing pathology.

Quadriplegia related to pre-existing spine pathology: Atlanto-axial instability is a feature of numerous diseases and syndromes, most notably rheumatoid arthritis and Down's syndrome. While there is anecdotal evidence of injury to the cervical spinal cord from airway management in patients with unstable cervical spines either due to trauma or medical co-morbidity, these reports are rare, and causality is uncertain.[38–43]

Pre-existing cervical spondylosis or spinal stenosis may create increase risk for cord injury during laryngoscopy or surgical positioning. Transient quadriplegia has been reported after endotracheal intubation in two patients with stable cervical spines who had

Atlanto-axial instability
Ankylosing spondylitis
Chondrodysplasia punctata
Congenital scoliosis
Down's syndrome
Grisel syndrome
Kniest syndrome
Larsen syndrome
Metatropic dysplasia
Morquio syndrome
Neurofibromatosis
Os odontoideum
Osteogenesis imperfecta
Psoriatic arthritis
Reiter syndrome
Rheumatoid arthritis
Spondyloepiphyseal dysplasia congenita
Systemic lupus erythematosus
Trauma

cervical spondylosis.[44] The mechanism of injury was presumably neck extension during laryngoscopy, although causality was not proven, and unrecognized disturbances of spinal cord perfusion during surgery could also have been contributory. Fortunately, outcome for both these patients was excellent and symptoms resolved within 24 hours. Undiagnosed cervical spondylosis and spinal stenosis contributed to permanent quadriplegia after lengthy neck extension for dental extractions under general anesthesia.[45]

Central cord syndrome may also be triggered by neck hyperextension in the presence of spondylosis or spinal stenosis. Central cord syndrome presents as incomplete quadriplegia, usually with greater motor impairment of the upper extremities and spasticity of the lower extremities. It may be seen as a complication of neck extension of laryngoscopy.[46,47] It may also occur as a consequence of the surgical procedure and has also been reported after cervical decompression.[48] Spinal cord injury with the edematous changes to spinal cord gray matter has been implicated in central cord syndrome, so it may present in the early postoperative period or in some cases be a delayed finding. Prognosis is variable, but recovery is common.

Prolonged neck flexion has been associated with midcervical quadriplegia secondary to stretch of the cervical spinal cord. This rare injury has been most frequently reported from intracranial surgery in the sitting position with neck flexion.[49,50] Prolonged neck flexion during any surgery imparts some risk, and midcervical quadriplegia has been reported from tracheal resection in a young woman maintained with neck flexion after surgery.[51] Phrenic nerve function may be spared, but overall prognosis for neurological recovery is generally poor. Extreme neck extension in a crime victim who was bound with his head between his ankles for 12 hours resulted in an incomplete cervical injury with recovery at 8 weeks.[52] This suggests this is a positioning injury and not attributable solely to other variables during surgery.

Management: Management is determined by the underlying etiology. High-dose IV steroid protocols used in other forms of spinal cord injury have been utilized with good results in some patients.

Quadriplegia unrelated to pre-existing spine pathology: Disruption of the anterior spinal artery may cause anterior spinal cord ischemia and subsequent damage to the corticospinal and spinothalamic tracts, with impairment of motor function and pain/temperature sensation and relative sparing of proprioception and vibratory sense. The majority of reported cases have resulted in paraplegia, but quadriplegia may result from more cephalad disruptions of the vasculature.[53–55]

Cervical spinal hematoma is a feared complication that may rapidly cause spinal cord ischemia in the confined space of the vertebral column. Most perioperative cases can be attributed to surgical complications. Spinal hematoma very rarely develops after injections of the cervical spine. Spontaneous spinal hematoma is possible, and most reported cases have been associated with coagulopathy.[56] Although coincidental cervical spinal hematoma would seem very unlikely in the postoperative period, coincidental lumbar hematoma related to perioperative dilutional thrombocytopenia has been reported.[57]

An interesting cause of transient postoperative quadriplegia is hypokalemic periodic paralysis. This typically presents as episodic subjective muscle weakness. However, transient quadriplegia has been reported among individuals with periodic paralysis due to Addison's disease[58] and hyperthyroidism.[59] A single report of postoperative hypokalemic periodic paralysis presented as transient quadriplegia.[60] In distinction to high cervical cord injury, patients with periodic paralysis have intact phrenic nerve function and are able to breathe normally and phonate. Periodic paralysis results from a number of different channelopathies and may also be associated with eukalemia or hyperkalemia, so acute electrolyte testing during an episode of paralysis may or may not aid in diagnosis.

Management: Cervical epidural hematomas require immediate surgical decompression. Episodes of periodic paralysis are self-limited, and management is supportive. General medical management includes treatment of a causative co-morbidity (e.g. thyrotoxicosis) and avoidance of triggers such as carbohydrate loading, stress, or sudden changes in temperature.[61] Surgery has not been implicated as a trigger to date.

Paraplegia

New-onset paraplegia after surgery is more common than quadriplegia and usually related to direct surgical injury to the spine. Major vascular and orthopedic procedures have been associated with a low incidence of postoperative paraplegia.

Anterior spinal cord syndrome is an important cause of postoperative paraplegia. Thoracic aortic and thoracoabdominal surgery are the most common causes of postoperative spinal cord ischemia resulting in paralysis. In most people, the artery of Adamkiewicz arises from the aorta between the T_8 and L_1 vertebral bodies, but significant variation in normal anatomy exists.[62] This vessel is at risk during abdominal aortic aneurysm repair, and subsequent paraplegia has been observed.[63–67] Aortic dissection may sometimes cause anterior spinal cord syndrome, whether it occurs spontaneously or is caused by the presence of an intra-aortic balloon pump.[68,69] Anterior spinal cord syndrome has been infrequently reported after other non-vascular procedures including procedures of the thorax.[70]

Spinal hematoma may be caused by either surgery or neuraxial anesthesia and results in postoperative paraplegia. Spinal hematoma occurs after 1 in 150,000 epidural anesthetics and 1 in 222,000 spinal anesthetics.[71] More than half of the cases of neuraxial anesthesia in the American Society of Anesthesiologists (ASA) Closed Claims Database arise from vascular procedures with the second most common procedure being orthopedic.[72] Back pain is the cardinal symptom of spinal hematoma and has been reported in approximately 80% of the more than 600 case reports in the literature.[73] Interestingly, back pain was present in only 25% of the cases in the ASA Closed Claims Database. This may reflect a decreased incidence of back pain in perioperative hematomas (secondary to opioids, sedation, or distracting pain) or bias for abnormal presentations of spinal hematoma having delayed diagnosis and worse clinical outcomes.[74] Bowel or bladder incontinence with motor impairment were the most common clinical presentations.

The accumulation of air in the epidural space from the injection of air during epidural catheter placement has been implicated in a variety of neurological deficits including, in very rare cases, transient paraplegia.[75,76] Inadvertent injection directly into the spinal cord during spinal or epidural anesthesia can cause paraplegia. These injections are typically performed in awake patients who should be able to report pain during injection, but intracord injection with permanent paraplegia has been reported despite this precaution.[77]

Transverse myelitis has been reported after both spinal and epidural injections.[78–83] The etiology is unknown and causality unproven. In most of these reports, symptoms appeared between 6 hours and 2 days after injection, but may be delayed for 1 to 2 weeks. Adhesive arachnoiditis has been reported after injection with tainted pharmaceuticals. In most cases the symptoms are after an interval of weeks to months,[84] but in a single report developed within six hours of injection.[85]

Management: Acute-onset paraplegia needs rapid imaging (CAT scan or MRI). Management of paraplegia is dependent upon etiology, but radiographic imaging should be obtained without delay to make the diagnosis of spinal hematomas. Hematomas need prompt surgical decompression, with the best results usually obtained if performed within 8 to 12 hours from the onset of symptoms.

Stroke

Acute ischemic or hemorrhagic cerebrovascular events may occur after procedures that do not involve intracranial trespass or manipulation of cerebral vasculature. Cardiac procedures are at increased risk because of embolic events related to cardiopulmonary bypass. While the clinical presentation of stroke is varied, it may include limb weakness or hemiplegia. The incidence of stroke within 30 days of non-cardiac, non-neurological surgery is between 0.05% and 7.4%.[86] Since these incidences are derived from retrospective review of databases of postoperative complications, they may underestimate the actual incidence of neurological events, owing to underreporting of transient events such as transient ischemic attacks or reversible ischemic neurological defects. The proinflammatory effects of surgery are implicated in the etiology of postoperative ischemic stroke after general surgery, with interleukin-6 appearing to be a significant mediator.[87] While perioperative hypotension could cause cerebral ischemia, patient co-morbidities including chronic obstructive pulmonary disease, prior cerebrovascular accident, and peripheral vascular disease appear to be more important than hypotensive episodes.[88] Advanced age, atrial fibrillation, and renal disease have also been identified as important predictors of perioperative stroke.[86]

Management: A head computed tomography scan or diffusion-weighted MRI (if available) should be obtained without delay if stroke is suspected. Management in consultation with the neurologist is based upon the etiology of the event and on institutional resources and protocols for stroke management.

Conversion disorder

Conversion disorder is characterized by functional symptoms without organic cause precipitated by emotional stress. Affected patients may display "La belle indifférence," being relatively unconcerned about significant symptoms. Conversion disorder is rarely observed after surgery, but single limb paralysis,[89,90] paraplegia,[91,92] quadriplegia,[93] and unilateral hemiplegia[94] have all been observed after surgery owing to conversion disorder. Conversion disorder is a diagnosis of exclusion, and organic causes must be ruled out.

Management: The prognosis for conversion disorder is good. Treatment requires psychiatric consultation and may include psychotherapy in combination with psychiatric medications as needed on a case by case basis.

References

1. T.P. Schmalzried, S. Noordin, H.C. Amstutz. Update on nerve palsy associated with total hip replacement. Clin Orthop Relat Res 1997; 344:188–206.

2. R.S. Laughlin, P.J.B. Dyck, J.C. Watson, et al. Ipsilateral inflammatory neuropathy after hip surgery. Mayo Clin Proc 2014; 89:454–461.

3. J.K. Chan, A. Manetta. Prevention of femoral nerve injuries in gynecologic surgery. Am J Obstet Gynecol 2002; 186:1–7.

4. A.W. Kam, P.H. Lam, G.A.C. Murrell. Brachial plexus injuries during shoulder

athroplasty: what causes them and how to prevent them. *Tech Should Surg* 2014; 15:109–114.

5. Q.H. Hogan. Pathophysiology of peripheral nerve injury during regional anesthesia. *Reg Anesth Pain Med* 2008; 33:435–441.

6. C.L. Jeng, T.M. Torrillo, M.A. Rosenblatt. Complications of peripheral nerve blocks. *Br J Anaesth* 2010; 105(Suppl 1):i97–i107.

7. J.M. Royer, M. Freysz, P.J. Regnard, A. Ahouanbevi, M. Wilkening. Severe paralysis of the upper limb after axillary brachial plexus block. *Ann Fr Anesth Reanim* 1991; 10:168–170.

8. M.A. Warner, M.E. Warner, J.T. Martin. Ulnar neuropathy: incidence, outcome, and risk factors in sedated or anesthetized patients. *Anesthesiology* 1994; 81:1332–1340.

9. R.C. Prielipp, R.C. Morell, J. Butterworth. Ulnar nerve injury and perioperative arm positioning. *Anesthesiol Clin North Am* 2002; 20:589–603.

10. M.A. Warner, J.T. Martin, D.R. Schroeder, K.P. Offord, C.G. Chute. Lower extremity motor neuropathy associated with surgery performed on patients in a lithotomy position. *Anesthesiology* 1994; 81:6–12.

11. T.E. Whitesides, T.C. Haney, K. Morimoto, H. Harada. Tissue pressure measurements as a determinant for the need of fasciotomy. *Clin Orthop Relat Res* 1975; 113:43–45.

12. M.M. McQueen, C.M. Court-Brown. Compartment monitoring in tibial fractures. The pressure threshold for decompression. *J Bone Joint Surg Br* 1996; 78:99–104.

13. S. Gourgiotis, C. Villas, S. Germanos, A. Foukas, M.P. Ridolfini. Acute limb compartment syndrome: a review. *J Surg Educ* 2007; 64:178–186.

14. M.S. Simms, J.R. Terry. Well leg compartment syndrome after pelvic and perineal surgery in lithotomy position. *Postgrad Med J* 2005; 81:534–536.

15. C. Prakash, A.A. Bonajmah, A. Ahmed. A case of acute compartment syndrome following prolonged lithotomy positioning for urological syndrome. *IJCRI* 2011; 2:19–22.

16. M.H. Verdolin, A.S. Toth, R. Schroeder. Bilateral lower extremity compartment syndromes following prolonged surgery in the low lithotomy position with serial compression stockings. *Anesthesiology* 2000; 92:1189–1191.

17. J. Tuckey. Bilateral compartment syndrome complicating prolonged lithotomy. *Br J Anaesth* 1996; 77:546–549.

18. G.E.H. Enderby. Postural ischaemia and blood pressure. *Lancet* 1954; 266:185–187.

19. S.D. Pfeffer, J.R. Halliwill, M.A. Warner. Effects of lithotomy position and external compression on lower leg muscle compartment pressure. *Anesthesiology* 2001; 95:632–636.

20. S.G. Talbot, G.F. Rogers. Pediatric compartment syndrome caused by intravenous infiltration. *Ann Plast Surg* 2011; 67:531–533.

21. D. Willsey, R. Peterfreund. Compartment syndrome of the upper arm after pressurized infiltration of intravenous fluids. *J Clin Anesth* 1997; 9:428–430.

22. J.J. Edwards, D. Samuels, E.S. Fu. Forearm compartment syndrome from intravenous mannitol extravasation during general anesthesia. *Anesth Analg* 2003; 96:245–246.

23. A. Grand, B. Yeager, R. Wollstein. Compartment syndrome presenting as ischemia following extravasation of contrast material. *Can J Plast Surg* 2008; 16:173–174.

24. S. Rimer, J.A. Wentry, R.L. Rodriguez. Compartment syndrome in an infant following emergency intraosseous infusion. *Clin Pediatr* 1988; 27:259–260.

25. R. Moscati, G.P. Moore. Compartment syndrome with resultant amputation following intraosseous infusion. *Am J Emerg Med* 1990; 8:470–471.

26. R.D. Galpin, J.B. Kronick, R.B. Willis, T.C. Frewen. Bilateral lower extremity compartment syndromes secondary to

intraosseous fluid resuscitation. *J Pediatr Orthop* 1991; 11:773–776.

27 R. Vidal, N. Kissoon, M. Gayle. Compartment syndrome following intraosseous infusion. *Pediatrics* 1993; 91:1201–1202.

28. M. Gayle, N. Kissoon. A case of compartment syndrome following intraosseous infusions. *Pediatr Emerg Care* 1994; 10:378.

29. R. Wright, S.L. Reynolds, B. Nachtsheim. Compartment syndrome secondary to prolonged intraosseous infusion. *Pediatr Emerg Care* 1994; 10:157–159.

30. R.W. Neumar, C.W. Otto, M.S. Link, *et al.* Part 8: Adult advanced cardiovascular life support: 2010 American Heart Association guidelines for cardiopulmonary resuscitation and emergency cardiovascular care. *Circulation* 2010; 122(18 Suppl 3): S729–S767.

31. A. d'Heurle, M.T. Archdeacon. Compartment syndrome after intraosseous infusion associated with a fracture of the tibia. A case report. *JBJS Case Connect* 2013; 3:e20. http://dx.doi.org/10.2106/JBJS.CC.L.00231.

32. J.A. Anson. Vascular access in resuscitation. Is there a role for the intraosseous route? *Anesthesiology* 2014; 120:1015–1031.

33. J.H. Paxton. Intraosseous vascular access. A review. *J Trauma* 2012; 14:195–232.

34. C. Ananthanarayan, C. Castro, N. McKee, G. Sakotic. Compartment syndrome following intravenous regional anesthesia. *Can J Anaesth* 2000; 47:1094–1098.

35. G.B. Maletis, R.C. Watson, S. Scott. Compartment syndrome following intravenous regional anesthesia in the reduction of lower leg shaft fractures. *Injury* 2008; 39:1204–1209.

36. G. Bocca, J.A. van Moorselaar, W.F. Feltz, F.H. van der Staak, L.A. Monnens. Compartment syndrome, rhabdomyolysis and risk of acute renal failure as complications of lithotomy position. *J Nephrol* 2002; 15:183–185.

37. N. Kikuno, S. Urakami, K. Shigeno, *et al.* Traumatic rhabdomyolysis resulting from continuous compression in the exaggerated lithotomy position for radical prostatectomy. *Int J Urol* 2002; 9:521–524.

38. D.J.J. Muckart, S. Bhagwanjee, R. van der Merwe. Spinal cord injury as a result of endotracheal intubation in patients with undiagnosed cervical fractures. *Anesthesiology* 1997; 87:418–420.

39. G. Redl. Massive pyramidal tract signs after endotracheal intubation: a case report of spondyloepiphyseal dysplasia congenita. *Anesthesiology* 1998; 89:1262–1264.

40. K. Yan, M.F. Diggan. A case of central cord syndrome caused by intubation: a case report. *J Spinal Cord Med* 1997; 20:230–232.

41. J. Farmer, A. Vaccaro, T.J. Albert, *et al.* Neurologic deterioration after cervical spinal cord injury. *J Spinal Disord* 1998; 11:192–196.

42. R.H. Hastings, S.D. Kelley. Neurologic deterioration associated with airway management in a cervical spine-injured patient. *Anesthesiology* 1993; 78:380–383.

43. M.J. Yaszemski, T.R. Shepler. Sudden death from cord compression associated with atlanto-axial instability in rheumatoid arthritis. *Spine* 1990; 15:580–583.

44. T. Kudo, Y. Sato, K. Kowatari, T. Nitobe, K. Hirota. Postoperative transient tetraplegia in two patients caused by cervical spondylotic myelopathy. *Anaesthesia* 2011; 66:213–216.

45. J.H. Whiteson, N. Panaro, J.H. Ahn, H. Firooznia. Tetraparesis following dental extraction: case report and discussion of preventive measures for cervical spinal hyperextension injury. *J Spinal Cord Med* 1997; 20:422–425.

46. J.M. Buchowski, K.M. Kebaish, K.S. Suk, J.P. Kostuik. Central cord syndrome after total hip arthroplasty: a patient report. *Spine* 2005; 30:E103–E105.

47. T. Wantanabe, D. Takizawa, T. Sato, *et al.* A case of central cord syndrome following thyroidectomy. *J Clin Anesth* 2010; 22:307–309.

48. W.J. Levy, D.F. Dohn, R.W. Hardy. Central cord syndrome as a delayed complication of decompressive

laminectomy. *Neurosurgery* 1982; 11:491–495.

49. M. Standefer, J.W. Bay, R. Trusso. The sitting position in neurosurgery: a retrospective analysis of 488 cases. *Neurosurgery* 1984; 14:649–658.

50. B.L. Wilder. Hypothesis. The etiology of midcervical quadriplegia after operation with the patient in the sitting position. *Neurosurgery* 1982; 11:530–531.

51. J. Dominguez, J.J. Rivas, R.D. Lobato, V. Díaz, E. Larrú. Irreversible tetraplegia after tracheal resection. *Ann Thorac Surg* 1996; 62:278–280.

52. L.M. Levy. An unusual case of flexion injury of the cervical spine. *Surg Neurol* 1982; 11:255–259.

53. K.R. Chin, J. Seale, V. Cumming. "White cord syndrome" of acute tetraplegia after anterior cervical decompression and fusion for chronic spinal cord compression: a case report. *Case Rep Orthop* 2013; 2013: 697918; doi.org/10.1155/2013/697918.

54. M.H. Lee, Y.D. Cha, J.H. Song, *et al.* Transient quadriplegia after fluoroscopic-guided selective cervical nerve root block in a patient who received cervical interbody fusion. A case report. *Korean J Anesthesiol* 2010; 59(Suppl):S95–S98.

55. A.F.K. Moore. Tetraplegia after elective abdominal aortic aneurysm repair. *J Vasc Surg* 2006; 44:401–403.

56. R.M. Beatty, K.R. Winston. Spontaneous cervical epidural hematoma. A consideration of etiology *Neurosurgery* 1984; 61:143–148.

57. G. Metzger, G. Singbartl. Spinal epidural hematomas following epidural anesthesia versus spontaneous spinal subdural hematoma. Two case reports. *Acta Anaesthesiol Scand* 1991; 35:105–107.

58. J.M. Sowden, D.Q. Borsey. Hyperkalemic periodic paralysis: a rare presentation of Addison's disease. *Postgrad Med J* 1989; 65:238–240.

59. F. Kokenge, H. Moenig. Thyrotoxic periodic paralysis. A peculiar case with weekend-related quadriplegia. *Endocrinologist* 2005; 15:297–299.

60. H. Abbas, N. Kothart, J. Bogra. Hypokalemic periodic paralysis. *Nat J Maxillofacial Surg* 2012; 3:220–221.

61. J.O. Leavitt. Practical aspects in the management of hypokalemic periodic paralysis. *J Transl Med* 2008; 6:18; doi: 10.1186/1479-5876-6-18.

62. I.O. Mehrez, D.C. Nabseth, E.L. Hogan, R.A. Deterling. Paraplegia following resection of abdominal aortic aneurysm. *Ann Surg* 1962; 156:501–503.

63. G. Lazorthes, A. Gouaze, J.O. Zadeh, *et al.* Arterial vascularization of the spinal cord. *Neurosurgery* 1971; 35:253–262.

64. W.F. Zuber, M.R. Gaspar, P.D. Rothschild. The anterior spinal artery syndrome – a complication of abdominal aortic surgery: report of five cases and review of the literature. *Ann Surg* 1970; 172:909–915.

65. J.A. Reid, D.J. Mole, L.C. Johnston. Delayed paraplegia after endovascular repair of abdominal aortic aneurysm. *J Vasc Surg* 2003; 37:1322–1323.

66. I.H. Mallick, S. Kumar, A. Samy. Paraplegia after elective repair of an infrarenal aortic aneurysm. *J R Soc Med* 2003; 96:501–503.

67. Y. Takahashi, Y. Tsutsumi, O. Monta, *et al.* Acute onset of paraplegia after repair of abdominal aortic aneurysm in a patient with acute type B aortic dissection. *Interact Cardiovasc Thorac Surg* 2009; 8:240–242.

68. B.M. Singh, A.E. Fass, R.W. Pooley. Paraplegia associated with intraaortic balloon pump counterpulsation. *Stroke* 1983; 14:983–985.

69. P. Trabattoni, S. Zoli, L. Dainese, *et al.* Aortic dissection complicating intraaortic balloon pumping: percutaneous management of delayed spinal cord ischemia. *Ann Thorac Surg* 2009; 88:e60–e62.

70. K. Popat, T. Ngyugen, A. Kowalski, *et al.* Postoperative paraplegia after nonvascular thoracic surgery. *Internet J Anesthesiol* 2003; 8; https://ispub.com/IJA/8/1/5155

71. T.T. Horlocker, D.J. Wedel. Anticoagulation and neuraxial block: historical perspective, anesthetic implications and risk management.

Reg Anesth Pain Med 1998; 23(Suppl 2): 129–134.

72. L.A. Lee, K.L. Posner, K.B. Domino, *et al.* Injuries associated with regional anesthesia in the 1980s and 1990s: a closed claims analysis. *Anesthesiology* 2004; 101:143–152.

73. D. Kreppel, G. Antoniadis, W. Seeling. Spinal hematoma: a literature survey with meta-analysis of 613 patients. *Neurosurg Rev* 2003; 26:1–49.

74. J.W. Heitz, E.R. Viscusi. Neuraxial anesthesia and anticoagulants. *Tech Orthop* 2008; 23:259–272.

75. P.G. Nay, R. Milaszkiewicz, S. Jothiligam. Extradural air as a cause of paraplegia following lumbar analgesia. *Anaesthesia* 1993; 48:402–404.

76. J. Dalmau-Carolà. An old complication of a new technique: pneumorrhachis from caudal epidural pulsed radiofrequency. *Pain Physician* 2014; 17:E790–E793.

77. M. Tripathi, S.S. Nath, R.K. Gupta. Paraplegia after intracord injection during attempted epidural steroid injection in an awake-patient. *Anesth Analg* 2005; 101:1209–1211.

78. K.K. Girdha, N. Banerjee. Transverse myelitis following spinal anesthesia-a case report. *Indian J Anaesth* 2002; 46:476–477.

79. E. Martinez-Garcia, E. Pelaez, J.C. Roman, A. Perez-Gallardo. Transverse myelitis following general and epidural anaesthesia in a paediatric patient. *Anaesthesia* 2005; 60:921–923.

80. S. Jha, R. Kumar. Transverse myelitis following spinal anesthesia. *Neurol India* 2006; 54:425–427.

81. M.D. Globokar, V.P. Erzen, V.N. Jankovic. Transverse myelitis following general and thoracic epidural anaesthesia. *Signa Vitae* 2010; 5:29–31.

82. J.H. Seok, Y.H. Lim, S.H. Woo, J.H. Yon. Transverse myelitis following combined spinal-epidural anesthesia. *Korean J Anesthesiol* 2012; 63:473–474.

83. O.F. Dueñas-Garcia, M. Diaz-Sotomayor. Postpartum complicated by transverse myelitis *West Indian Med J* 2012; 61:643–645.

84. T. Killeen, A. Kamat, D. Walsh, A. Parker, A. Aliashkevich. Severe adhesive arachnoiditis resulting in progressive paraplegia following obstetric spinal anaesthesia: a case report and review. *Anaesthesia* 2012; 67:1386–1394.

85. P. Petty, P. Hudgson, W. Hare. Symptomatic lumbar spinal arachnoiditis: fact or fallacy? *J Clin Neurosci* 2000; 7:395–399.

86. J.L. Ng, M.T. Chan, A.W. Geth. Perioperative stroke in noncardiac, nonneurosurgical surgery. *Anesthesiology* 2011; 155:879–890.

87. T.T. Dong, A.W. Gelb. Perioperative stroke remains an underappreciated cause of morbidity and mortality. *J Anesth Periop Med* 2014; 1:57–59.

88. M. Limburg, E.F. Wijdicks, H. Li. Ischemic stroke after surgical procedures: clinical features, neuroimaging, and risk factors. *Neurology* 1998; 50:895–901.

89. K. Yokoyama, Y. Okutsu, H. Fujita. A case of monoplegia from conversion disorder after spinal anesthesia. *Masui* 2002; 51:1363–1367.

90. R. Gihyeong, S.H. Song, K.H. Lee. Monolimb paralysis after laparoscopic appendectomy due to conversion disorder. *Korean J Fam Med* 2014; 35:321–324.

91. L. Berhane, R. Kurman, S. Smith. Lower extremity paralysis after operative laparoscopy from conversion disorder. A case report. *J Reprod Med* 1998; 43:831–835.

92. D. Hirjak, P.A. Thomann, R.C. Wolf, N. Weidner, E.P. Wilder-Smith. Dissociative paraplegia after epidural anesthesia: a case report. *Int Med Case Rep J* 2013; 7:56; doi:10.1186/1752-1947-7-56.

93. D. Han, N.R. Connelly, A. Weintraub, P. Kanev, E. Solis. Conversion locked-in syndrome after implantation of a spinal cord stimulator. *Anesth Analg* 2007; 104:163–165.

94. A. Judge, F. Spielman. Postoperative conversion disorder in a pediatric patient. *Paediatr Anaesth* 2010; 20:1052–1054.

Rigidity

Ashley Caplan and James W. Heitz

- Muscular rigidity after surgery often occurs as a side effect of perioperative medications.
- Although muscular rigidity often raises concern for malignant hyperthermia, it is usually attributable to other causes.
- Muscular rigidity and hyperthermia are an ominous combination of signs which require immediate evaluation and treatment.

Muscular rigidity is a state of involuntary muscle tension with resistance to passive movement. The perioperative causes range from incidental to catastrophic. When muscular rigidity is encountered after surgery, it is typically iatrogenic and secondary to medications administered, but may also be related to metabolic derangement. Malignant hyperthermia (MH), neuroleptic malignant syndrome (NMS), and serotonin syndrome are the most ominous causes of postoperative rigidity. Other drug-induced and metabolic causes include opioid-induced rigidity, propofol-related dystonia, extrapyramidal reactions, and hypocalcemia (see Figure 24.1).

Malignant hyperthermia

The incidence of MH is 1 per 100,000 general anesthetics delivered in hospitals and 0.31 per 100,000 anesthetics delivered in ambulatory care centers.[1] Although observed so infrequently that many career anesthesiologists never encounter a single case, MH accounted for 1% of all anesthesia-related mortality in the United States between the years 1999 and 2005.[2] The incidence of cardiac arrest during an episode of MH is 2.7%.[3] While most episodes of MH present in the operating room during the anesthetic, MH can rarely be initially recognized in the postoperative setting either as the initial episode or a recrudescence of previously treated crisis.[4–12] A recent observational study suggests that delayed presentation of MH to the second or third hour of the anesthetic is becoming more frequent.[13] Modern anesthetics might not be as strongly triggering for MH, and contemporary presentations of the syndrome are more indolent, increasing the likelihood of late recognition. Prompt diagnosis and therapy greatly reduces mortality, so it is important that clinicians caring for surgical patients recognize the syndrome (Table 24.1).

MH susceptibility is inherited in an autosomal dominant fashion and is thought to be caused by a mutation in the type 1 ryanodine receptor. This abnormality results in

---

Post-Anesthesia Care: Symptoms, Diagnosis, and Management, ed. James W. Heitz. Published by Cambridge University Press. © Cambridge University Press 2016.

Table 24.1 Malignant hyperthermia diagnostic criteria

Points	Diagnostic criteria
1	Respiratory acidosis (end-tidal CO_2 >55 mmHg/7.32 kPa or arterial pCO_2 >60 mmHg/7.98 kPa)
1	Cardiac involvement (sinus tachycardia, ventricular tachycardia, or ventricular fibrillation)
1	Metabolic acidosis (base excess lower than −8, pH <7.25)
1	Muscle rigidity (generalized rigidity including severe masseter muscle rigidity)
1	Muscle breakdown creatine kinase (CK) >20,000 U/l, cola-colored urine, myoglobinuria, plasma K^+ >6 mmol/l)
1	Temperature increase (rapidly increasing temperature, T >38.8 °C)
1	Other (rapid reversal of MH signs with dantrolene, elevated resting serum CK levels)
1	Family history (autosomal dominant pattern)

abnormal calcium transport and sustained muscle contraction with resultant rigidity and hyperthermia. Several genetic mutations have been identified that increase sensitivity to "triggering agents" including all volatile anesthetics and the depolarizing muscle relaxant succinylcholine.

The earliest clinical signs include elevated end-tidal CO_2, tachycardia, and muscle rigidity. Untreated, the syndrome progresses to acidosis, renal failure, rhabdomyolysis, hyperkalemia, and cardiac arrhythmias. Metabolic acidosis and respiratory acidosis occur simultaneously. A 1994 consensus conference led to the formulation of a set of diagnostic criteria.[14] The higher the score (greater than 6 following), the more likely a reaction constituted MH.

If recognized in the postoperative setting, treatment must be instituted rapidly with an intravenous (IV) loading dose of dantrolene 2.5 mg/kg. Each 20 mg vial of dantrolene must be dissolved in 60 ml of sterile water for injection. Preparation of dantrolene may take 20 minutes or more. In July 2014, the US Food and Drug Administration approved a new formulation of dantrolene (*Ryanodex®*, Eagle Pharmaceuticals, Woodcliff Lake, NJ), which is packaged in a 250 mg vial that requires reconstitution in only 5 ml sterile water and can be prepared in under 1 minute. Although clinical experience is limited, this formulation may improve outcomes by allowing faster treatment. Periodic readministration of dantrolene may be needed for several days to prevent recurrence. Cooling measures should be instituted to decrease core body temperature. Frequent monitoring of arterial blood gas, serum electrolytes, and coagulation studies should be performed. Sodium bicarbonate should be administered to treat hyperkalemia and metabolic acidosis as needed. An arterial line for frequent blood sampling and close monitoring of blood pressure would be beneficial. End-tidal CO_2 monitoring is helpful in monitoring response to therapy if available, but $PaCO_2$ may be monitored by frequent arterial blood gas sampling instead. Urine output should be maintained to prevent acute renal failure from rhabdomyolysis.

Neuroleptic malignant syndrome

NMS may occur after administration of medications that block the dopaminergic system. Haloperidol and chlorpromazine carry the highest risk, but metoclopramide, lithium, desipramine, phenelzine, reserpine, tetrabenazine, and abrupt discontinuation

Table 24.2 Neuroleptic malignant syndrome

Major criteria:	Fever
	Rigidity
	Elevated CK
Minor criteria:	Tachycardia
	Tachypnea
	Altered mental status
	Hypotension or hypertension
	Diaphoresis
	Leukocytosis

of levodopa have all been implicated in NMS.[15] The pathogenesis is thought to possibly be a result of neuroleptic-induced alteration of central neuroregulatory mechanisms versus an abnormal reaction of predisposed skeletal muscle. Diagnosis is made by confirming the presence of three major criteria, or two major and four minor criteria (see Table 24.2).

Management should include discontinuation of the offending agent, supportive care (i.e. mechanical ventilation, antiarrhythmic medication, pacing), and dantrolene 1 to 2.5 mg/kg IV repeated to a maximum of 10 mg/kg daily, slowly tapered over 10 days. Bromocriptine 2.5 mg by mouth every 6 to 8 hours and amantadine 100 mg by mouth every 12 hours are alternative pharmacological therapies.

Serotonin syndrome

Monoamine oxidase inhibitors (MAOIs), tricyclic antidepressants (TCAs), selective serotonin reuptake inhibitors (SSRIs), and serotonin-norepinephrine reuptake inhibitors (SNRIs) may trigger serotonin syndrome through excessive stimulation of central and peripheral postsynaptic $5\text{-}HT_{2A}$ receptors. The risk is increased when multiple medications modulating serotonin pathways are used in combination. Many surgical patients are on chronic SSRI or TCA therapy and are at increased risk for developing perioperative serotonin syndrome during the polypharmacy of the postoperative period. Serotonin syndrome may be triggered by cocaine, amphetamine, the street drug ecstasy, L-tryptophan, and buspirone among outpatients.[16] The surgical patient taking SSRIs, TCAs, or MAOIs is placed at risk from the many serotonergic medications commonly administered in the perioperative period, including opioids. Serotonergic opioids including fentanyl, tramadol, oxycodone, methadone, dextromethorphan, meperidine, codeine, and buprenorphine have been reported to contribute to the development of serotonin syndrome.[17] These medications are only weakly serotonergic, and the syndrome is rare after anesthesia and surgery. The combination of SSRI and intraoperative methylene blue was reported to cause serotonin syndrome in a susceptible individual.[18]

Excessive serotonin activity has cognitive, autonomic, and somatic effects. Patients may exhibit peripheral or ocular clonus, agitation, diaphoresis, tremor, tachycardia, hyperreflexia, hypertonism, shivering, diarrhea, and body temperature $>38\,°C$. A diagnosis of serotonin syndrome by Hunter criteria may be made by a history of serotonergic agents and at least one of the following signs: clonus (spontaneous, inducible, ocular), agitation, autonomic dysfunction (hyperthermia), tremor, or hyperreflexia.[18]

Management involves cessation of serotonergic medications and supportive care. Severely affected patients may require mechanical ventilation and/or dialysis, anticonvulsants if seizures develop, and propranolol to treat tachycardia. Severe cases may be treated with cyproheptadine 2 mg PO in incremental doses until symptoms resolve (max dose 12 to 32 mg/day) or chlorpromazine 50 to 100 mg IV if unable to take oral medications.[16]

Opioid-induced rigidity

Opioid-induced rigidity is sometimes observed following induction of general anesthesia. This often occurs within 60 to 90 seconds of IV administration of sufentanil, fentanyl, alfentanil, or remifentanil.[19–21] It can lead to difficulty with bag mask ventilation. Characteristics include chest wall rigidity, wrist flexion, closure of vocal cords, hoarseness, reduced pulmonary compliance and decreased functional residual capacity, and occasionally tonic-clonic movements. It has been linked to elevated central venous pressures and increased pulmonary vascular resistance.

Occurrence is dependent on dose, anatomical patient considerations, concomitant muscle relaxant use, and patient age. The mechanism of opioid-induced rigidity is poorly understood, but may be related to activation of GABAergic interneurons in the striatum and nucleus pontis raphe of the brain. It is common practice for anesthesiologists to administer a priming dose of non-depolarizing paralytic agent or succinylcholine to facilitate ventilation after large IV doses of opioids.

Rarely, rigidity is present on emergence from general anesthesia,[22] and in exceptionally rare circumstances this has been reported to occur more than 3 hours after the last dose of opioid.[23] Awareness of this syndrome is therefore important for clinicians caring for the surgical patient. When rigidity interferes with breathing, naloxone 4 mg IV should be administered.

Antidopaminergic medication effects

Dopamine antagonists or drugs with antidopaminergic side effects can cause extrapyramidal side effects, which can manifest as a number of related movement disorders, including Parkinsonism which includes rigidity, bradykinesia, and tremor. Many perioperative medications may cause extrapyramidal side effects, including droperidol,[24] ondansetron,[25] and metoclopramide.[26] Additionally, abrupt discontinuation of anti-Parkinsonian medications, especially levodopa, can lead to spastic rigidity in the perioperative period if the patient is unable to take oral medications for a prolonged period of time. Management of acute extrapyramidal symptoms is administration of diphenhydramine 50 mg IV.

Other medication effects

Propofol has been associated with excitatory neurological reactions, including seizure-like activity and dystonia.[27] The mechanism of this is poorly understood, but may be related to an imbalance in basal ganglia transmission. Since propofol is thought to act through GABA receptors, patients taking medications that affect this system, such as gabapentin, may be more susceptible to this side effect. Dystonic reactions with propofol have been described most commonly at induction of general anesthesia; however, several case reports of longer-term dystonia exist.

Hypocalcemia

Acute hypocalcemia due to post-surgical hypoparathyroidism must be considered post-operatively after total thyroidectomy or parathyroidectomy. This condition may be manifested by tetany, rigidity, laryngospasm, papilledema, prolonged QT interval, and, in severe cases, heart failure. Hypocalcemia is affected by acid–base status, hypomagnesemia, and potassium balance, and symptoms rarely occur unless ionized calcium is <4.3 mg/dl.[28] This condition is treated with IV calcium chloride or calcium glutamate.

Parkinsonism

Parkinsonism-like symptoms are occasionally observed in the perioperative period, and in the few published reports symptoms have been transient.[29] More recently, a case series of four patients displaying permanent symptoms with abrupt onset after general or spinal anesthesia has been reported.[30] The mechanism of this phenomenon is not yet identified.

Baclofen withdrawal

Baclofen is a $GABA_B$ receptor agonist efficacious in the treatment of spasticity due to spinal cord trauma, cerebral palsy, and multiple sclerosis. In severe cases of spasticity, baclofen may be administered by intrathecal pump. Acute interruption of intrathecal baclofen due to pump failure may be associated with rigidity, hyperthermia, disseminated intravascular

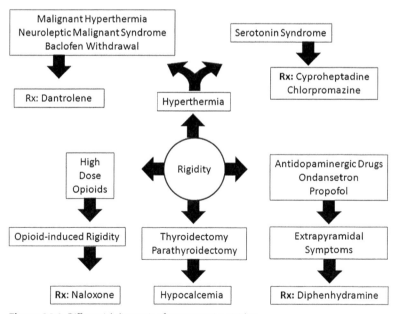

Figure 24.1 Differential diagnosis of postoperative rigidity.

coagulation, rhabdomyolysis, and acute renal failure.[31,32] In severe form, baclofen withdrawal may resemble MH or NMS, and mortality may exceed 20%.[33] Oral baclofen appears to be ineffective in the treatment of intrathecal baclofen withdrawal.[34] Successful management has been reported by intrathecal baclofen infusion by spinal catheter,[35] IV dantrolene,[36] IV propofol,[37] and IV benzodiazepines.[32]

References

1. T. Aderibigbe, B.H. Lang, H. Rosenberg, Q. Chen, G. Li. Cost-effectiveness analysis of stocking dantrolene in ambulatory surgery centers for the treatment of malignant hyperthermia. Anesthesiology 2014; 120(6):1333–1338.

2. G. Li, M. Warner, L. Huang, L.S. Sun. Epidemiology of anesthesia-related mortality in the United States, 1999–2005. Anesthesiology 2009; 110(4):759–765.

3. M.G. Larach, B.W. Brandorn, G.C. Allen, G.A. Gronert, E.B. Lehman. Malignant hyperthermia deaths related to inadequate temperature monitoring, 2007–2012: a report from the North American Malignant Hyperthermia Registry of the Malignant Hyperthermia Association of the United States. Anesth Analg 2014; 119(6):1359–1366.

4. B.J. Kripke, T.J.J. Blanck, D.A. Sizemore, et al. Association of post-anaesthetic hyperthermia with abnormal muscle characteristics: a case report. Can Anaesth Soc J 1983; 30(3):290–294.

5. J. Schulte-Sasse, W. Hess, J. Eberlein. Postoperative malignant hyperthermia and dantrolene therapy. Can Anaesth Soc J 1983; 30(6):635–640.

6. J. Grinberg, G. Edelist, J. Gordon. Postoperative malignant hyperthermia episodes in patients who received "safe" anesthetics. Can Anaesth Soc J 1983; 30(3):273–276.

7. A. Mathieu, A.J. Bogosian, J.F. Ryan, R.K. Crone, D. Crocker. Recrudescence after survival of initial episode of malignant hyperthermia. Anesthesiology 1979; 51(5):454–455.

8. R. Fletcher, G. Blennow, A.-K. Olsson, E. Ranklev, K. Törnebrandt. Malignant hyperthermia in a myopathic child.

Prolonged postoperative course requiring dantrolene. Acta Anaesthesiol Scand 1982; 26(5):435–438.

9. H. Rutenberg, E. Håkanson. Malignant hyperthermia: clinical course and metabolic changes in two patients. Acta Anaesthesiol Scand 1986; 30(3):211–214.

10. C. R. Souliere, S.J. Weintraub, C. Kirchner. Markedly delayed postoperative malignant hyperthermia. Arch Otolaryngol Head Neck Surg 1986; 112(5):564–566.

11. J.A. Short, C.M.S. Cooper. Suspected recurrence of malignant hyperthermia after post-extubation shivering in the intensive care unit, 18 h after tonsillectomy. Br J Anaesth 1999; 82(6):945–947.

12. C.W. Hoenemann, T.B. Halene-Holtgraeve, M. Booke, et al. Delayed onset of malignant hyperthermia in desflurane anesthesia. Anesth Analg 2003; 96(1):165–167.

13. M. Visoiu, M.C. Youn, K. Wieland, B.W. Brandom. Anesthetic drugs and onset of malignant hyperthermia. Anesth Analg 2014; 118(2):388–396.

14. M.G. Larach, A.R. Localio, G.C. Allen, et al. A clinical grading scale to predict malignant hyperthermia susceptibility. Anesthesiology 1994; 80(4):771–779.

15. P. Adnet, P. Lestavel, R. Krisvosic-Horber. Neuroleptic malignant syndrome. Br J Anaesth 2000; 85(1):129–135.

16. R.P. Muhnoz. Serotonin syndrome induced by a combination of bupropion and SSRIs. Clin Neuropharmacol 2004; 27(5):219–222.

17. R. Rastogi, R.A. Swarm, T.A. Patel. Case scenario: opioid association with serotonin syndrome: implications to the practitioners. Anesthesiology 2011; 115(6):1291–1298.

18. S. Izdes, N.D. Altintas, C. Soykut. Serotonin syndrome caused by administration of methylene blue

to a patient receiving selective serotonin reuptake inhibitors. *Anesth Analg* 2014; 2(9):111–112.

19. J.L. Benthuysen, N.T. Smith, T.J. Sanford, N. Head, H. Dec-Silver. Physiology of alfentanil-induced rigidity. *Anesthesiology* 1986; 64(4):440–446.

20. T.A. Bowdle, A. Rooke. Postoperative myoclonus and rigidity after anesthesia with opioids. *Anesth Analg* 1994; 78(4):783–786.

21. C.M. Christian, J.L. Waller, C.C. Moldenhauer. Postoperative rigidity following fentanyl anesthesia. *Anesthesiology* 1983; 58(3):275–277.

22. S. Roy, L.P. Fortier. Fentanyl-induced rigidity during emergence from general anesthesia potentiated by venlafaxine. *Can J Anaesth* 2003; 50(1):32–35.

23. J.M. Klausner, J. Caspi, S. Leluek, *et al.* Delayed muscular rigidity and respiratory depression following fentanyl anesthesia. *Arch Surg* 1988; 123(1):66–67.

24. B.M. Melnick. Extrapyramidal reactions to low-dose droperidol. *Anesthesiology* 1988; 69(3):424–425.

25. M.M. Tolan, T.M. Fuhrman, K. Tsueda. S.B. Lippmann. Perioperative extrapyramidal reactions associated with ondansetron. *Anesthesiology* 1999; 90(1):340–341.

26. Y.Y. Jo, Y.B. Kim, M.R. Yang, Y.J. Chang. Extrapyramidal side effects after metoclopramide administration in a post-anesthesia care unit: a case report. *Korean J Anesthesiol* 2012; 63(3):274–276.

27. C. Constantino, L. Torres. Propofol-induced paroxysmal dystonia. *Parkinsonism Relat Disord* 2012; 18(2):115–116.

28. J.F. Tohme, J.P. Bilezikian. Hypocalcemic emergencies. *Endocrinol Metab Clin North Am* 1993; 22(2):363–375.

29. S. Muravchick, D.S. Smith. Parkinsonian symptoms during emergence from general anesthesia. *Anesthesiology* 1995; 82(1):305–307.

30. M.B. Ramani, M.L. Rabin, R. Kurlan. Postoperative and postpartum onset of chronic parkinsonism: four case reports. *Int J Med Students* 2014; 2(1):22–23.

31. L.W. Kao, Y. Amin, M.A. Kirk, *et al.* Intrathecal baclofen withdrawal mimicking sepsis. *J Emerg Med* 2003; 24(4):423–427.

32. R.J. Coffey, T.S. Edgar, G.E. Francisco, *et al.* Abrupt withdrawal from intrathecal baclofen: recognition and management of a potentially life-threatening syndrome. *Arch Phys Med Rehabil* 2002; 83(10):735–741.

33. U.S. Food and Drug Administration. MedWatch. The FDA Safety Information and Adverse Event Reporting Program. Lioresal Intrathecal (baclofen injection) [cited April 2002]. Available from: http://www.fda.gov/Safety/MedWatch/SafetyInformation/SafetyAlertsforHuman MedicalProducts/ucm154505.htm.

34. I. Mohammed, A. Hussain. Intrathecal baclofen withdrawal syndrome-a life-threatening complication of baclofen pump: a case report. *BMC Clin Pharmacol* 2004; 4:6; doi:10.1186/1472-6904-4-6.

35. B.S. Duhon, J.D. MacDonald. Infusion of intrathecal baclofen for acute withdrawal. *J Neurosurg* 2007; 107(4):878–880.

36. A. Khorasani, W.T. Peruzzi. Dantrolene treatment for abrupt intrathecal baclofen withdrawal. *Anesth Analg* 1995; 80(5):1054–1056.

37. G.L. Ackland, R. Fox. Low-dose propofol infusion for controlling acute hyperspasticity after withdrawal of intrathecal baclofen therapy. *Anesthesiology* 2005; 103(3):663–665.

Chapter

Seizure

25

James W. Heitz and Michelle Beam

- Most postoperative seizures may be pharmacologically aborted with benzodiazepines or barbiturates in small doses.
- The clinical differentiation between true seizure and seizure-like movements may be difficult.
- A high degree of clinical suspicion is necessary to recognize and treat local anesthetic systemic toxicity in the postoperative patient.

Seizure may be observed in the postoperative setting both in patients with pre-existing epilepsy and among patients without a prior history of seizures. The introduction of a new medication may provoke seizures in some patients and, for others, the absence of a chronic medication may lead to withdrawal seizures. Some surgical patients may experience seizure as a result of co-morbidities, while other seizures result from the underlying procedure. The differential diagnosis of postoperative seizure is robust and complicated by the fact that not all seizure activity results in abnormal movements and not all abnormal rhythmic movements represent true seizure activity (see Figure 25.1).

Myoclonus is common in surgical patients and in extreme form can appear like convulsions. Perioperative medications, such as metoclopramide, can trigger extrapyramidal symptoms and include oculogyric crisis (involuntary upward rotation of the eyes), dystonia (muscle spasms), torticollis (involuntary lateral neck flexion), and rarely tardive dyskinesia (involuntary repetitive movements).[1] Vigorous shivering or rigors may resemble convulsions. Possible seizure activity is usually observed in the perioperative setting without electroencephalographic (EEG) confirmation, further hindering the certainty of diagnosis.

Management

Although heterogeneous in presentation and etiology, postoperative seizures may be effectively managed in similar fashion (see Figure 25.2). The first step is symptom-guided therapy to treat the seizure. Once acutely managed, the second step is to determine the cause of the seizure. Etiologies requiring immediate intervention (hypoxia, hypoglycemia, local anesthetic toxicity [LAST]) need to be excluded first, then the broad differential can be systematically explored. Laboratory studies or radiographic imaging may aid the diagnosis. When the etiology is determined, the third step is to provide diagnosis-guided therapy.

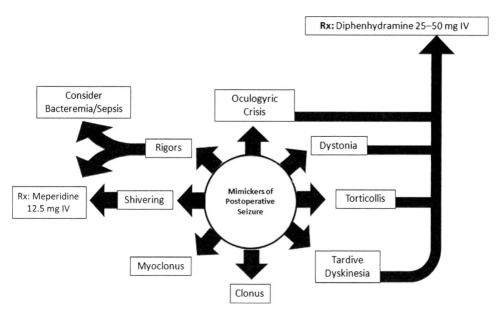

Figure 25.1 Mimickers of postoperative seizure.

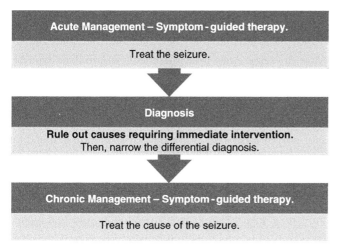

Figure 25.2 Clinical algorithm for postoperative seizures.

The acute management of all postoperative seizures is initially supportive (Figure 25.3). Ensure ventilation, provide supplemental oxygen, and protect the patient from self-injury during the event. With the absence of a structural lesion of the central nervous system (CNS), the majority of postoperative seizures are brief and self-limited. However, if needed, benzodiazepines or barbiturates will usually terminate a seizure with

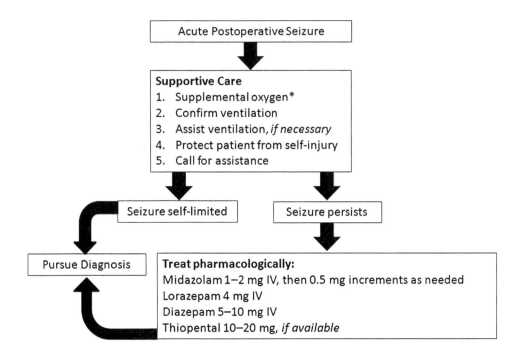

*If hypoxia or cyanosis, endotracheal intubation, mechanical ventilation, 100% oxygen.

Figure 25.3 Acute management of postoperative seizures.

administration of low doses. After the seizure has been successfully controlled, hypoxia, LAST, and hypoglycemia need to be considered and immediately addressed if present (Figure 25.4).

Hypoxia needs to be immediately excluded as a cause for postoperative seizure. In the early postoperative period, any CNS symptom (confusion, agitation, delirium, seizure) should be treated as hypoxia until proven otherwise. If low oxygen saturation is noted by pulse oximetry or central cyanosis is observed, endotracheal intubation and mechanical ventilation with 100% oxygen should be initiated.

LAST needs to be considered for any perioperative patient, especially if a nerve block or regional anesthesia has been performed. Local anesthetics cause neurological and cardiac toxicity, but the plasma levels for cardiac toxicity are generally two fold to four fold higher than needed for seizure. Most patients with LAST presenting with convulsions require only supportive care. Bupivacaine is an important exception and the plasma level of bupivacaine needed to provoke asystole is similar to the level to provoke seizure. If a seizure is caused by bupivacaine, cardiac arrest may be impending. Respiratory acidosis and hypoxia worsens LAST, so ventilation should be supported if necessary. If bupivacaine has been administered or cardiac symptoms (bradycardia, hypotension) are present with LAST from any type, lipid rescue should be implemented without delay.[2] Multiple case reports and reviews have been published showing survival of patients after lipid therapy for LAST.[3–9] Cardiovascular collapse may be the FIRST sign of bupivacaine toxicity in 40% of cases and may be delayed up to an hour after injection.[10]

Emergency treatment for local anesthetic toxicity
1. Airway management with 100% O_2 and cardiovascular support.
2. Seizure suppression. Administer midazolam 1–2 mg IV or another benzodiazepine.
3. Bolus 1.5 ml/kg lean body mass 20% lipid emulsion over 1 minute.
4. Start infusion 0.25 ml/kg/min.
5. Repeat bolus 1–2× for continued cardiovascular collapse.
6. Double the infusion rate to 0.5 ml/kg/min if patient remains hypotensive.
   Additional information may be found at http://www.lipidrescue.org/
7. Continue infusion for 10 minutes beyond establishing normal circulation.
8. Upper limit = 10 ml/kg in first 30 minutes.

A blood glucose measurement should be rapidly obtained for any patient with a new-onset postoperative seizure, but is of particular importance for patients with diabetes mellitus, chronic ethanol abuse, or malnutrition. Hypoglycemia and seizure is a medical emergency and if present should be treated with $D_{50}W$ 50 g IV.

If the etiology of the seizure has not been identified, an arterial blood gas and electrolytes including sodium, magnesium, calcium, and phosphate should be obtained. Abnormalities detected should be appropriately treated. If the patient is on anticonvulsant medications for epilepsy, blood should also be obtained for therapeutic level monitoring, if applicable. Serum levels of anticonvulsants are not always obtained preoperatively,

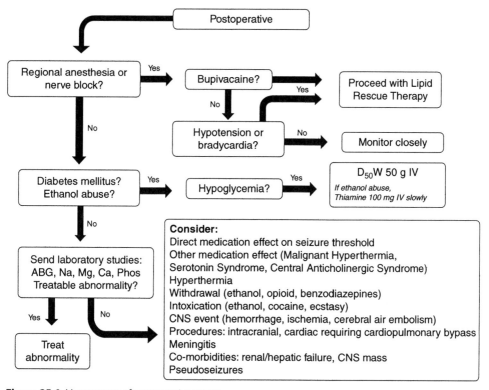

Figure 25.4 Management of postoperative seizure.

since many patients may have seizures controlled with "sub-therapeutic" plasma levels. However, a sub-therapeutic level of an antiepileptic medication should be increased if seizures occur.

The etiology of postoperative seizure is broad. Seizures are common after intracranial procedures and cardiopulmonary bypass. Seizures after neurological surgery are often persistent and require anticonvulsant therapy. The perioperative period is a time of poly-pharmacy, and if LAST has been eliminated as the cause of the convulsion, other medication effects need to be considered.

Medication effects

Many anesthetic medications may display both proconvulsive and anticonvulsive activity (Table 25.1).[11,12] This seemingly paradoxical clinical observation is attributable to the crucial importance of context and dosing. In low doses, some medications may cause CNS excitation and seizure, but at higher doses cause CNS depression and abort seizures. This phenomenon explains the clinical adage, "Wrong drug and not enough of it!" In some instances, administering more of the medication that provoked the seizure will also terminate it.

Induction agents: Intravenous agents for the induction of general anesthesia are a pharmacologically diverse group of medications with differing seizure effects. Many medications may be utilized to induce general anesthesia, but only five are in common clinical use for this purpose: thiopental, methohexital, etomidate, ketamine, and propofol. Barbiturates typically display strong anticonvulsant activity at clinical doses. Thiopental is a barbiturate that has strong anticonvulsive properties, but is not commercially available in the United States at this time. Methohexital is a unique barbiturate since it possesses proconvulsive properties. Methohexital administration has been associated with seizures in patients with prior epilepsy and among patients without prior seizure activity.[13]

Etomidate is an imidazole derivative with marked proconvulsive properties. Seizures from etomidate administration have been reported in epileptics and non-epileptic patients.[14,15] Ketamine is an N-methyl-D-aspartate (NMDA) receptor antagonist. While ketamine is frequently cited in anesthesia texts as being proconvulsant, scant evidence supports this assertion. Ketamine administered in combination with IV aminophylline, both bronchodilators once co-administered during anesthesia to asthmatic patients, was reported to cause seizure activity. Ketamine as a single agent is rarely implicated in provoking seizures even among epileptic patients. Moreover, ketamine administration may successfully terminate status epilepticus[16] and has been used by intramuscular administration to abort seizures in pediatric patients without IV access.[17,18]

Propofol (2,6-diisopropylphenol) is a non-barbiturate induction agent in widespread clinical use. The effect of propofol administration on seizure threshold is controversial. Propofol was introduced into clinical usage with the assumption that it had no significant pro- or anticonvulsant properties.[19] However, its anticonvulsant effects soon became apparent. Propofol reduces the seizure duration during electroconvulsive therapy by 63% compared with the strongly anticonvulsant thiopental[20] and appears to reduce duration without raising the seizure threshold.[21] There are numerous reports of propofol terminating seizures of status epilepticus. Conversely, there are also numerous reports of propofol inducing seizure activity in patients with and without prior epilepsy. Most of these

Table 25.1 Medications associated with seizures[26,36,37]

Amoxapine

Chlorpromazine

Clozapine

Maprotiline

Clomipramine

Bupropion

Venlafaxine

Meperidine

Flumazenil

Theophylline

Isoniazid

Alkylating antineoplastic agents (etoposide, ifosfamide, cisplatin)

Cyclosporine

Penicillin

Cephalosporins

Imipenem

Fluoroquinolones

Cocaine

Amphetamines

Hallucinogens

Local anesthetics

Withdrawal from:

Barbiturates

Benzodiazepines

Baclofen

Meprobamate

Chloral hydrate

Zolpidem

Narcotics

Anticonvulsants

Alcohol

have been observed during emergence from anesthesia, but some have occurred in the postoperative period.[22] There is some controversy over whether these are observations of myoclonus or true seizure. Although propofol is commonly administered to epileptic patients in the United States, the Committee on Safety of Medications in the United Kingdom and the Australian Adverse Drug Reactions Advisory Committee have both issued warnings about the use of propofol in epileptic patients.[23,24] In one small study of slowly titrated (0.5 mg/kg increments) propofol induction with EEG monitoring, spike wave activity was increased at levels below 2 mg/kg, then decreased at levels surpassing this dose.[25] One patient with a history of epileptic seizure experienced a seizure at 1 mg/kg of propofol which was terminated by administration of another 0.5 mg/kg. This suggests the propofol may display both pro- and anticonvulsant properties depending upon the dose administered.

Opioids: Mu-receptor agonists may induce seizures,[26] but few do so at clinically relevant doses. Alfentanil, sulfentanil, fentanyl, remifentanil, morphine, and hydromorphone have all been rarely reported in causing seizure activity. Meperidine is metabolized to normeperidine, which has renal elimination and has been often observed to cause seizure when plasma levels accumulate in patients with renal insufficiency. With adequate renal function, meperidine is not associated with seizures at therapeutic dosing even among individuals with established epilepsy.[27]

Nitrous oxide: Nitrous oxide has been associated with seizures in mice, but has not been reported to cause seizures in humans when used in modern anesthetic practice. The historical practice of 100% nitrous oxide inductions was reported to cause seizure-like activity associated with cyanosis, and these were almost certainly hypoxia-induced seizures. Similarly, nitrous oxide can also induce seizure activity when administered under hyperbaric conditions.[28]

Volatile agents: Enflurane was frequently observed to cause seizures when administered in high concentrations, but this agent is no longer in clinical use in the United States. Sevoflurane has been reported to cause seizures at clinical doses[29-31] and there is some EEG evidence that these are true seizures.[32,33]

Neuromuscular blockers (NMB): NMB are administered during most general anesthetics and will block the motor activity associated with tonic-clonic seizure, but not the seizure. Atracurium is metabolized to laudanosine, which has been associated with seizures in animal models. Prolonged continuous infusion of atracurium during postoperative mechanical ventilation has been associated with serum levels sufficient to cause seizures in animal models, but seizures in humans have not been reported.[27]

Other significant medication effects would include syndromes that include seizures, including malignant hyperthermia, serotonin syndrome, and central anticholinergic syndrome, but seizure would seldom be the first sign of any of these.

Alcohol withdrawal syndrome (delirium tremens) should be considered for any patient presenting with postoperative seizure. Alcohol withdrawal syndrome presents with fever, sweating, tachycardia, tremor, CNS manifestations (confusion, hallucinations), agitation, and seizures. General anesthesia may mask the early signs, and seizure may be the first recognized sign in the early postoperative period. Unhealthy alcohol use is common, but patients presenting for surgeries for head and neck cancers are at increased risk. Treatment is with benzodiazepines. Oxazepam or lorazepam may be preferred in patients with concurrent liver disease.

Pseudoseizures may occasionally be observed in the early postoperative period.[34,35]

References

1. S. Tesche, C. Henckell, F.U. Metternich. Therapy of postoperative nausea and vomiting in ENT–tardive dyskinesia as an adverse effect of metoclopramide – a case report. *Laryngorhinootologie* 2006; 85:824–826.

2. G.L. Weinberg. Treatment of local anesthetic toxicity (LAST). *Reg Anesth Pain Med* 2010; 35:188–193.

3. M.A. Rosenblatt, M. Abel, G.W. Fischer, C.J. Itzkovich, J.B. Eisenkraft. Successful use of 20% lipid emulsion to resuscitate a patient after a presumed bupivacaine-induced cardiac arrest. *Anesthesiology* 2006; 105:217–218.

4. G. Foxall, R. McCahon, L. Lamb, J.G. Hardman, N.M. Bedforth. Levobupivacaine-induced seizures and cardiovascular collapse treated with Intralipid. *Anaesthesia* 2007; 62:516–518.

5. A.G. Spence. Lipid reversal of central nervous system symptoms of bupivacaine toxicity. *Anesthesiology* 2007; 107:516–517.

6. T. McCutchen, J.C. Gerancher. Early intralipid therapy may have prevented bupivacaine-associated cardiac arrest. *Reg Anesth Pain Med* 2008; 22:178–180.

7. G. Di Gregorio, J.M. Neal, R.W. Rosenquist, G.L. Weinberg. Clinical presentation of local anesthetic systemic toxicity: a review of published cases, 1979–2009. *Reg Anesth Pain Med* 2010; 35:181–187.

8. G.L. Weinberg. Treatment of local anesthetic toxicity (LAST). *Reg Anesth Pain Med* 2010; 35:188–193.

9. G.L. Weinberg. Lipid emulsion infusion – resuscitation for local anesthetic and other drug overdoses. *Anesthesiology* 2012; 117:180–187.

10. C. Gevirtz. Local anesthetic systemic toxicity – prevention and treatment. *Top Pain Management* 2012; 27:1–6.

11. P. Modica, R. Tempelhoff, P.F. White. Pro- and anticonvulsant effects of anesthetics. Part I. *Anesth Analg* 1990; 70:303–315.

12. P. Modica, R. Tempelhoff, P.F. White. Pro- and anticonvulsant effects of anesthetics. Part II. *Anesth Analg* 1990; 70:433–444.

13. H. Folkerts. Spontaneous seizure after concurrent use of methohexital anesthesia for electroconvulsive therapy and paroxetine: a case report. *J Nerv Ment Dis* 1995; 183:115–116.

14. W. Krieger, J. Copperman, K.D. Laxer. Seizures with etomidate anesthesia. *Anesth Analg* 1985; 64:1226–1227.

15. H.C. Hansen, N.E. Drenck. Generalized seizures after etomidate anaesthesia. *Anaesthesia* 1988; 43:805–806.

16. D.J. Borris, E.H. Bertram, J. Kapur. Ketamine controls prolonged status epilepticus. *Epilepsy Res* 2000; 42:117–122.

17. M.M. Fisher. Use of ketamine hydrochloride in the treatment of convulsions *Anaesth Intensive Care* 1974; 2:266–268.

18. R.W. Davis, G.C. Tolstoshev. Ketamine use in severe febrile convulsions. *Med J Aust* 1976; 2:465–466.

19. J.C. Bevan. Propofol-related convulsions. *Can J Anaesth* 1993; 40:805–809.

20. B.A. Martin, R.M. Cooper, S.V. Parikh. Propofol anesthesia, seizure duration, and ECT: a case report and literature review. *J ECT* 1998; 14:99–108.

21. G. Gábor, T. Judit, I. Zsolt. Comparison of propofol and etomidate regarding impact on seizure threshold during electroconvulsive therapy in patients with schizophrenia *Neuropsychopharmacol Hung* 2007; 9:125–130.

22. B. Walder, M.R. Tramer, M. Seeck. Seizure-like phenomena and propofol: a systemic review. *Neurology* 2002; 58:1327–1332.

23. Committee on Safety of Medicines, Medicine Control Agency M, UK: UK Summary of product of characteristics (SPC) for Diprivan 2%, 1992.

24. Australian Adverse Drug Reactions Advisory Committee A: Propofol,

Convulsions. *Australian Adverse Drug Reactions Publications* 1993;12:7.

25. B. Wang, Q. Bai, X. Jiao, E. Wang, P.F. White. Effect of sedative and hypnotic doses of propofol on the EEG activity of patients with or without a history of seizure disorders. *J Neurosurg Anesthesiol* 1997; 9:335–340.

26. L.J. Voss, J.W. Sleigh, J.P.M. Barnard, H.E. Kirsch. The howling cortex: seizures and general anesthetic drugs. *Anesth Analg* 2008; 107:1689–1703.

27. K.S. Schlick, T.M. Hemmen, P.D. Lyden. Seizures and Meperidine: overstated and underutilized. *Ther. Hypothermia Temp. Manag.* 2015; 5:223–227.

28. T.F. Hornbein, E.I. Eger, P.M. Winter, *et al.* The minimum alveolar concentration of nitrous oxide in man. *Anesth Analg* 1982; 61:553–556.

29. M. Zacharias. Convulsive movements with sevoflurane in children. *Anaesth Intensive Care* 1997; 25:727.

30. D. Baines. Convulsive movements with sevoflurane. *Anaesth Intensive Care* 1998; 26:329.

31. C.A. Hilty, J.C. Drummond. Seizure-like activity on emergence from sevoflurane anesthesia. *Anesthesiology* 2000; 93:1357–1359.

32. T. Iijima, Z. Nakamura, Y. Iwao, H. Sankawa. The epileptogenic properties of the volatile anesthetics sevoflurane and isoflurane in patients with epilepsy. *Anesth Analg* 2000; 91:989–995.

33. K. Hisada, T. Morioka, K. Fukui, *et al.* Effects of sevoflurane and isoflurane on electrocorticographic activities in patients with temporal lobe epilepsy. *J Neurosurg Anesthesiol* 2001; 13:333–337.

34. L. Ng, N. Chambers. Postoperative pseudoepileptic seizures in a known epileptic: complications in recovery. *Br J Anaesth* 2000; 91:598–600.

35. J.A. Ramos, S.J. Brull. Psychogenic non-epileptic seizures in the post-anesthesia recovery unit. *Rev Bras Anestesiol* 2014 (in press); doi:10.1016/j.bjane.2013.10.005 accessed December 5, 2014.

36. N. Delanty, C.J. Vaughan, J.A. French. Medical causes of seizures. *Lancet* 1998; 352:383–390.

37. P. Beleza. Acute symptomatic seizures: a clinically oriented review. *Neurologist* 2012; 18:109–119.

Delirium

James W. Heitz

- Management of postoperative delirium is usually based upon principles for management of delirium in the medical patient.
- Unlike medical patients, surgical patients are less likely to display acid–base or electrolyte disturbances when presenting with delirium.
- Non-pharmacological interventions have demonstrated efficacy in the treatment of delirium and should be attempted before pharmacological interventions.

Delirium is an acute disturbance of cognitive functioning characterized by an abrupt onset and a fluctuating course of confusion, disorganized thinking, and inattention.[1] Psycho-motor components including agitation or lethargy, hallucinations, and emotional disturbances may also be present. Delirium may be differentiated on the basis of its motor manifestations and may be described as hyperactive, hypoactive, or mixed (alternating lethargy and agitation). Each motor subtype is observed after surgery. Different motor manifestations of delirium predict dissimilar clinical behavior (such as hyperactivity and pulling out of intravenous[IV] lines and surgical drains). More recent evidence suggests that patients with varying motor subtypes also display unique disturbances in cognitive processing.[2]

Postoperative delirium typically will present 1 to 3 days after surgery. However, delirium may be recognized earlier in the postoperative course and may complicate the admission to the Post-Anesthesia Care Unit (PACU). The incidence of delirium in the PACU has been reported to be between 3%[3] and 4.7%.[4] Hypoactive delirium may be more common among surgical patients than medical patients,[5,6] and the patient with "quiet delirium" may be recognized in the PACU less frequently than is the agitated or combative patient. Delirium is only recognized by healthcare providers in 31% of affected ward patients,[7] and a similar proportion of delirious surgical patients may go undiagnosed in the PACU. When all patients arriving to the PACU are actively screened for confused thinking, the incidence of delirium is as high as 17% to 45%.[8,9]

Early postoperative delirium as recognized in the PACU is inadequately studied and may be referred to by various terminology including: postoperative delirium, PACU delirium, recovery room delirium, emergence excitement, emergence agitation, emergence confusion, or emergence delirium.[4] There is a lack of standardized nomenclature, and some may use these terms synonymously, while others attempt to draw nuanced distinctions between them based upon where in the hospital the delirium is first detected. For clarity, delirium presenting after surgery will be referred to as "postoperative delirium," and delirium detected on the day of surgery will be referred to as "early postoperative delirium."

The development of delirium during the hospitalization increases costs, length of stay, and short-term and long-term mortality.[10-16] Although delirium is rarely the direct cause of mortality, delirium is a marker for diminished cognitive reserve and a poor prognostic sign when it develops during the hospitalization. The development of delirium in the surgical patient may predict future cognitive decline.[17,18]

Delirium during hospitalization is multifactorial and has been best characterized among medical patient populations. Nearly a dozen mnemonic devices have been developed and published to aid in the differential diagnosis of delirium, the two most complete of which are the ominous IWATCHDEATH[19] and DELIRIUMS[20] (Table 26.1). While clinically useful in remembering the diverse etiologies of delirium, mnemonics derived from medical patient populations serve less well for surgical patient populations and fail to include the more common etiologies of this cohort, including pain.

Postoperative delirium is very different than medical delirium. In medical delirium, organ dysfunction and acid–base disturbances are common. Postoperative delirium typically occurs without laboratory abnormalities. An imbalance of cortical and

Table 26.1 Delirium differential diagnosis mnemonic devices

I	Infectious (encephalitis, meningitis, UTI, pneumonia)	D	Drugs
W	Withdrawal (alcohol, barbiturates, benzodiazepines)	E	Emotional
A	Acute metabolic disorder (electrolyte, hepatic or renal failure)	L	Low PaO_2 (anemia, PE, MI, CVA)
T	Trauma (head injury, postoperative)	I	Infection
C	CNS pathology (CVA, hemorrhage, tumor, seizure, Parkinson's)	R	Retention (urine or fecal)
H	Hypoxia (anemia, cardiac failure, pulmonary embolism)	I	Ictal states
D	Deficiencies (vitamin B12, folic acid, thiamine)	U	Undernutrition/underhydration
E	Endocrinopathies (thyroid, glucose, parathyroid, adrenal)	M	Metabolic disorders (organ failure)
A	Acute vascular (shock, vasculitis, hypertensive encephalopathy)	S	Subdural hematoma
T	Toxins (alcohol, anesthetics, anticholinergics, narcotics)		
H	Heavy metals (arsenic, lead, mercury)		

UTI = urinary tract infection, CNS = central nervous system, CVA = cerebrovascular accident, PE = pulmonary embolism, MI = myocardial infarction

Table 26.2 Common etiologies of early postoperative delirium in the PACU

P	Pain and Pain medications (opioids)
A	Anxiolytics, Analgesia deficit (Pain)
C	Cytokines, C-reactive protein and other inflammatory mediators
U	Unease (full bladder, hypoxia, hypercapnia) and Under-resuscitation (hypovolemia, hypotension)

subcortical neurotransmitters, particularly too little cholinergic and too much dopaminergic, appears to predominate. Increases in GABAergic, serotonergic, and noradrenergic neurotransmission have also been implicated. Surgical stress, with the release of inflammatory mediators including interleukin-6, C-reactive protein, and cortisol may also be involved.[21] Different surgical procedures have disparate rates of postoperative delirium, perhaps in part due to differing release of inflammatory mediators. Postoperative delirium occurs in 3 of 4 lung transplant recipients, but only 1 in 50 patients after laparoscopic general surgery.[22]

Early postoperative delirium: Delirium is frequently observed in pediatric surgical patients and is self-limited with a benign prognosis. Delirium in adults observed in the PACU may have a less worrisome prognosis than delirium presenting later after surgery.[23] Early postoperative delirium has been considered a response to anesthetic agents and not a sign of limited cognitive reserve. While this appears to be true for younger patients with early postoperative delirium, recent evidence suggests early postoperative adult delirium may be distinct. Early postoperative delirium may predict both delirium later in the hospitalization[24] and later cognitive decline.[9] Limited study into the risk factors for early postoperative delirium in the adult patient has identified non-modifiable procedural risk factors including breast or abdominal surgery and long surgical duration. The one modifiable risk factor for early postoperative delirium in adults is preoperative sedation with benzodiazepines.[4] Whereas sedation with benzodiazepines has been demonstrated to be protective against early postoperative delirium for pediatric surgical patients, the administration of benzodiazepines increases early postoperative delirium in adults. Recently published data in abstract form implicated increased opioid doses as a risk factor as well,[8] but it is currently unclear whether this is an independent risk factor or associated with longer and more extensive surgical procedures.

Management of early postoperative delirium: See Figure 26.1. Any confusion or mental status change experienced by a surgical patient in the PACU should be treated as hypoxia until proven otherwise. Although the risk for hypoxia would seem to diminish linearly as time out-of-anesthesia increases, recent data suggest the majority of hypoxic events in the PACU occur more than 30 minutes after patient arrival.[25] The recognition of delirium should immediately elicit a clinical assessment for hypoxia, hypercarbia, or hypotension for any patient in the PACU regardless of how long they have been monitored there. These signs should be appropriately treated if identified. Hypoglycemia also needs to be rapidly identified and remedied in the confused patient. Postoperative urinary retention is a common and a readily treatable delirium trigger in the adult patient. Bladder over-distension may be very uncomfortable, and adults are very strongly

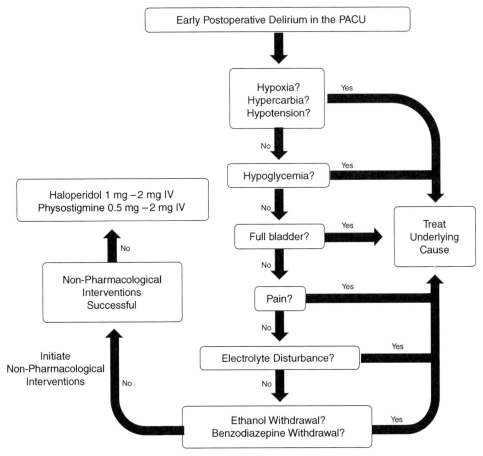

Figure 26.1 Algorithm for treatment of early postoperative delirium.

socialized not to wet the bed. The agitated patient may struggle to get off the stretcher without being able to vocalize the source of their discomfort. A bladder scan, if readily available, or percussion of the bladder will reveal postoperative urinary retention. Bladder palpation is discouraged in adults as it may cause bradycardia. Paradoxically, both pain and opioid administration may trigger delirium in the surgical patient. Multimodal analgesia utilizing non-opioid analgesics is clinically prudent for the patient with early postoperative delirium and has been validated in the prevention of delirium.[26–28] Alcohol withdrawal syndrome needs to be considered in the differential diagnosis of the adult with hyperactive delirium. Hallucinations and tremor are commonly present, and fever, tachycardia, or seizures may also occur. Treatment with benzodiazepines is indicated for delirium caused by alcohol or benzodiazepine withdrawal. The routine administration of benzodiazepines in the hyperactive delirious patient is discouraged, since it may worsen the underlying confusion. Routine laboratory work may occasionally reveal electrolyte disturbances requiring correction.

If a treatable underlying cause for early postoperative delirium is not identified, non-pharmacological interventions are indicated. Calm reassurance and orientation may be helpful for the surgical patient. Reassurance to the patient that they are safe is often beneficial. Reorientation to time, place, and situation should be repeated as needed. Limiting unnecessary stimulation including noise from loud talking and monitor alarms may also help. Restoration of sensory input by returning glasses or hearing aids, if applicable, should also be attempted. Although not formally studied in the early postoperative setting, simple non-pharmacological interventions shortened both the duration and severity of delirium in hospitalized medical patients.[28] The risk–benefit ratio favors these benign interventions for delirium in the PACU not caused by a reversible underlying cause in a patient who is not so agitated as to pose a danger to self or staff.

If pharmacological treatment of early postoperative delirium is needed, physostigmine 0.5 mg to 2 mg IV (not faster than 1 mg per minute) is efficacious in reversing CNS anticholinergic effects. Physostigmine can cause bradycardia and asystole, particularly with too rapid injection. Caution is needed in patients with reactive airway disease because of the risk of bronchospasm. Rigidity and tremors can be exacerbated in patients with Parkinson's disease. Haloperidol 1–2 mg IV may be considered. Side effects include sedation, tardive dyskinesia, priapism, malignant neuroleptic syndrome, dry mouth, and QT prolongation. Haloperidol is also contraindicated in Parkinson's disease. The pharmacological treatment of early postoperative delirium should be reserved for only the most severe cases.

Postoperative delirium management: Delirium in the surgical patient that presents after the early postoperative period requires special management. Therapeutic goals are to decrease the duration and/or severity of the delirium while ensuring patient safety. Non-pharmacological interventions in medical patients with delirium including reorientation, reassurance, cognitive stimulation, sleep hygiene, improvement of hearing or visual impairment, and correction of dehydration have been demonstrated to be both efficacious and cost-effective.[29] Guidelines for the treatment of delirium in medical patients include sleep promotion by noise and lighting regulation, avoidance of unnecessary polypharmacy, hydration with associated electrolyte correction, and prophylaxis for alcohol withdrawal for at-risk patients.[30]

Towards this aim, the American Geriatrics Society issued Clinical Practice Guidelines for Postoperative Delirium in November 2014.[31] While limited to the older adult patient, this represents the first attempt by a medical organization to offer guidelines for postoperative delirium specifically. Although the aim was to construct evidence-based recommendations, the quality of evidence underlying nearly all the recommendations was low. The recommendation for institutions to establish interdisciplinary (physician, nurses, ancillary staff) teams to deliver multicomponent non-pharmacological interventions was deemed to be supported by moderate evidence. Despite a paucity of evidence, the panel did agree upon several strong recommendations. These included formal education for staff to recognize and treat delirium in the postoperative patient, medical evaluation of the delirious patient, opioid-sparing multimodal analgesia, and the avoidance of the routine use of cholinesterase inhibitors to treat or prevent delirium. The routine use of benzodiazepines was strongly discouraged, except to treat benzodiazipine or alcohol withdrawal syndrome.[31]

References

1. J. Mantz, H.C. Hemmings, J. Boddaert. Case scenario: postoperative delirium in elderly surgical patients. *Anesthesiology* 2010; 112:189–195.

2. S. Grover, A. Sharma, M. Aggarwal, et al. Comparison of symptoms of delirium across various motoric subtypes. *Psychiatry Clin Neurosci* 2014; 68:283–291.

3. D.K. Rose. Recovery room problems or problems in the PACU. *Can J Anaesth* 1996; 43:R116–R128.

4. C. Lepousé, C.A. Lautner, L. Liu, P. Gomis, A. Leon. Emergence delirium in adults in the post-anesthesia care unit. *Br J Anaesth* 2006; 96:747–752.

5. J.F. Peteron, B.T. Pun, R.S. Dittus, et al. Delirium and its motor subtypes: a study of 614 critically ill patients. *J Am Geriatr Soc* 2006; 54:479–484.

6. T.N. Robinson, C.D. Raeburn, Z.V. Tran, L.A. Brenner, M. Moss. The motor subtypes of postoperative delirium in the elderly. *Arch Surg* 2011; 146:295–300.

7. S.K. Inouye, M.D. Foreman, L.C. Mion, K.H. Katz, L.M. Cooney. Nurses' recognition of delirium and symptoms: comparison of nurse and researcher ratings. *Arch Intern Med* 2001; 161:2467–2473.

8. E. Card, C. Hughes, C. Tomes, et al. Incidence and risk factors for emergence and PACU delirium. *J Perianesth Nurs* 2014; 29:e35–e36.

9. K.J. Neufeld, J.M.S. Leoutsakos, F.E. Sieber, et al. Outcomes of early delirium diagnosis after general anesthesia in the elderly. *Anesth Analg* 2013; 117:471–478.

10. K. Franco, D. Litaker, J. Locala, et al. The cost of delirium in the surgical patient. *Psychosomatics* 2001; 43:68–73.

11. J. McCusker, M.G. Cole, N. Dendukuri, E. Belzile. Does delirium increase hospital stay? *J Am Geriatr Soc* 2003; 51:1539–1546.

12. M. Cole, J. McCusker, N. Dendukuri, L. Han. The prognostic significance of subsyndromal delirium in elderly medical inpatients. *J Am Geriatr Soc* 2003; 51:754–760.

13. M.M. Dolan, W.G. Hawkes, S.I. Zimmerman, et al. Delirium on hospital admission in aged hip fracture patients: prediction of mortality and 2-year functional outcomes. *J Gerontol A Biol Sci Med Sci* 2000; 55A:M527–M534.

14. K. Rockwood, S. Cosway, D. Carver, et al. The risk of dementia and death after delirium. *Age Ageing* 1999; 28:551–556.

15. E.W Ely, S. Gautam, R. Margolin, et al. The impact of delirium in the intensive care unit on hospital length of stay. *Intensive Care Med* 2001; 27:1892–1900.

16. J. McCusker, M. Cole, M. Abrahamowicz, F. Primeau, E. Belzile. Delirium predicts 12-month mortality. *Arch Intern Med* 2002; 162:457–463.

17. A.L. Gruber-Baldini, S. Zimmerman, R.S. Morrison, et al. Cognitive impairment in hip fracture patients: Timing of detection and longitudinal follow-up. *J Am Geriatr Soc* 2003; 51:1227–1236.

18. M. Lundström, A. Edlund, G. Bucht, S. Karlsson, Y. Gustafson. Dementia after delirium in patients with femoral neck fractures. *J Am Geriatr Soc* 2003; 51:1002–1006.

19. J. Smith, J. Seirafi. Delirium and dementia. In: Marx JA III, Hockberger RS, Walls RM, editors. *Rosen's Emergency Medicine Concepts and Clinical Practices.* 7th edn. Philadelphia, PA: Elsevier; 2010. pp. 1367–1373.

20. J.H. Flaherty, J.E. Morley. Delirium: a call to improve current standards of care. *J Gerontol A Biol Sci Med Sci* 2004; 59A:341–343.

21. J. Mantz, H.C. Hemmings, J. Boddaert. Case scenario: postoperative delirium in elderly surgical patients. *Anesthesiology* 2010; 112:189–195.

22. F.E. Sieber. Postoperative delirium and the elderly surgical patient. *Anesthesiol Clin* 2009; 27:451–464.

23. S. Deiner, J.H. Silverstein. Postoperative delirium and cognitive dysfunction. *Br J Anaesth* 2009; 103:141–146.

24. P.T. Sharma, F.E. Sieber, J. Khwaja, et al. Recovery room delirium predicts

postoperative delirium after hip-fracture repair. *Anesth Analg* 2005; 105:1215–1220.

25. R.H. Epstein, F. Dexter, M.G. Lopez, J.M. Ehrenfeld. Anesthesiologist staffing considerations consequent to the temporal distribution of hypoxemic episodes in the postanesthesia care unit. *Anesth Analg* 2014; 119:1322–1333.

26. T.M. Halaszynski. Pain management in the elderly and cognitively impaired patient: the role of regional anesthesia and analgesia. *Curr Opin Anaesthesiol* 2009; 22:594–599.

27. L. Krenk, L.S. Rasmussen, T.B. Hansen, et al. Delirium after fast-track hip and knee arthroplasty. *Br J Anaesth* 2012; 108:607–611.

28. H. Li, Y. Qing, F-S. Yang, et al. The study of multimodal analgesia on postoperative delirium in elder patients with hip fracture. *Chin J Orthop* 2013; 33:736–740.

29. S.K. Inouye, S.T. Bogardus, P.A. Charpentier, et al. A multicomponent intervention to prevent delirium in hospitalized older patients. *N Engl J Med* 1999; 340:669–676.

30. L. Michaud, C. Büla, A. Berney, et al. Delirium: guidelines for general hospitals. *J Psychosom Res* 2007; 62:371–383.

31. American Geriatrics Society. Postoperative delirium in older adults: best practice statement from the American Geriatrics Society. *J Am Coll Surg* 2015; 220:136–148.

Headache

James W. Heitz

- Caffeine withdrawal is the most common cause of headache in the surgical patient.
- 5-HT$_3$ antagonists may cause severe headache.
- Postdural puncture headache should be suspected after spinal anesthesia for headaches with a strong postural component.

Postoperative headache is a common phenomenon affecting 13% to 80% of surgical patients at some point during the postoperative period. For the majority of patients, history is crucial to identifying the etiology. Physical examination and laboratory studies have a secondary role in the evaluation of most postoperative headaches.

Headaches may be classified into two broad categories: primary and secondary headache (Table 27.1).[1] Primary headaches are not associated with structural abnormalities or systemic disease. Tension, migraine, and cluster headaches account for most headaches experienced in medical patient populations. Secondary headaches are caused by underlying disease. Infection, mass, hemorrhage, or vasculitis are the most serious causes of secondary headaches experienced in medical patient populations. Primary headache disorders account for 90% of headaches experienced by medical patients.[2]

The surgical patient may experience either primary or secondary headache (see Table 27.1). Secondary headaches occur with greater frequency after surgery. Many of the causes of secondary headache among surgical patients are unique to the perioperative period. The first step in the evaluation of any headache is to search for a secondary cause.

Postoperative secondary headache

Four Hs: Clinical consideration must be given to the four "Hs" of postoperative headache: hypoxia, hypercarbia, hypoglycemia, and hypovolemia (Figure 27.1). Hypoxia, hypercarbia, or hypoglycemia may contribute to headache by causing cerebral vasodilation. Intravascular hypovolemia may cause headache by creating traction upon dural sinuses. While not the most common etiology of postoperative headache, these are frequent problems in surgical patients and should be considered in the differential diagnosis of every postoperative headache. Assessment of ventilation and risk of hypoglycemia is prudent for any patient with new-onset headache after surgery. Arterial blood gas analysis or blood glucose

Table 27.1 Postoperative headache differential diagnosis

	Suspect if…
Minor secondary causes	
Hypoxia, hypercarbia, hypoglycemia, hypovolemia	In all postoperative patients until excluded
Caffeine withdrawal syndrome	Habitual caffeine ingested, coffee drinker, throbbing headache
Nicotine withdrawal syndrome	Smokers
Opioid withdrawal syndrome	Chronic opioids
Medication overuse headache	Chronic primary headache, most common in middle-age women with co-morbidity of depression
$5-HT_3$ antagonist medication	Onset temporally related to anti-emetic administration
Opioids	Opioid-naïve patient
Postdural puncture headache	Younger patient, spinal anesthesia, headache relieved by lying flat, may have cranial nerve involvement
Intrathecal/epidural air	Neuraxial anesthesia, headache exacerbated by lying flat
Eclampsia	Pregnancy
Post-traumatic headache	Closed head injury/concussion
Serious secondary causes	
Increased intracranial pressure	Hypertension, bradycardia, altered mental status, papilledema, intracranial process, procedure, or trauma
Subarachnoid hemorrhage	Focal neurological findings, altered mental status, thunderclap headache, hypertension
Subdural hematoma	Chronic alcohol, anticoagulants
Cerebral ischemia	Focal neurological signs, headache is usual symptom
Acute narrow-angle glaucoma	Anisocoria, conjunctival erythema, photophobia
Meningitis	Fever, nuchal rigidity, photophobia, several days to several weeks after otorhinolaryngology, neurosurgical, or maxillofacial procedure
Primary headaches	
Tension	Band-like discomfort, headache not affected by activity
Migraines	With or without aura, history of prior migraine, women, headache exacerbated by activity
Cluster headache	Abrupt onset of periocular pain, male over 50 years with smoking history

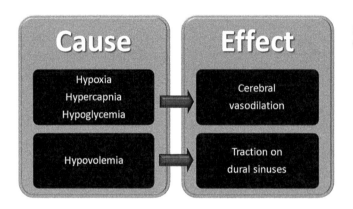

Figure 27.1 The 4 Hs of perioperative headache.

measurement is not indicated routinely in the evaluation of all postoperative headaches, but should be employed when justified by clinical suspicion. Intravascular hypovolemia is common in surgical patients and may cause headache which is exacerbated by upright posture or movements of the head.[3] Hypovolemia has also been implicated in the exacerbation of migraine headaches.[4]

Management: While these headaches will respond to analgesics including non-steroidal anti-inflammatory drugs (NSAIDs) or acetaminophen, correction of the underlying abnormality is indicated.

Withdrawal headache

Perioperative fasting may produce headache of withdrawal. The most common perioperative headache in adult patients is caused by caffeine withdrawal.

Caffeine withdrawal headache: Over 85% of Americans consume at least one beverage containing caffeine every day, with a US average daily caffeine intake of 165 mg per person.[5] Symptomatic caffeine withdrawal may occur in as few as 8 hours in individuals consuming as little as 100 mg caffeine per day.[6] Most adult surgical patients are at risk for caffeine withdrawal headache. The symptoms of caffeine withdrawal are protean and may also include fatigue, drowsiness, irritability, anxiety, cognitive impairment, muscular aches, or nausea. Headache is the most commonly reported symptom of caffeine withdrawal, presenting in 47% of affected individuals.[7] Mean daily caffeine consumption is a strong predictor of postoperative headache, with a 12% increase in incidence per 100 mg of daily consumption.[8] Among outpatient surgical patients, mean daily caffeine consumption greater than 400 mg and surgery starting after 12 pm predict postoperative headache.[9] The headache of caffeine withdrawal is typically moderate to severe, diffuse, and may be described as "pounding."

Management: Preoperative ingestion of caffeine will offer prophylaxis against postoperative headache. In one small randomized, placebo-controlled study, replacement of the daily caffeine intake in pill form (50% preoperative, 50% postoperative) reduced the incidence of headache from 50% to 0%.[10] Intravenous (IV) caffeine is also efficacious,[11] but IV caffeine benzoate was withdrawn from the US market in 2011. Recent relaxation in the fasting requirements prior to anesthesia to allow for the ingestion of clear liquids (including coffee or tea *without* milk or cream)[12] may prevent withdrawal for some patients. NSAIDs or acetaminophen may offer benefit for some patients, but best results will be obtained by allowing patients who are able to take liquids to ingest caffeine. Small quantities of caffeine may relieve withdrawal symptoms even in heavy users. A benefit of caffeine pills over caffeinated beverages in the surgical patient able to tolerate liquids has not been demonstrated.

Medication overuse headache (MOH): Also known as "rebound headache," headache may be caused by the withdrawal of many chronic analgesics including acetaminophen, aspirin, NSAIDs, ergotamine, triptans, barbiturates, codeine, hydrocodone, oxycodone, meperidine, morphine, butorphanol, and nalbuphine.[13] This typically occurs in patients with long-standing primary headaches and may present as the typical primary headache or as a less severe, bilateral headache. MOH may occur after a few hours of abstinence, and severely affected individuals may routinely experience nocturnal awakening due to MOH. MOH is infrequently recognized in the perioperative period, but can be produced by fasting and an inability to take pills. There is no test for MOH, and the diagnosis is clinical. A history of heavy medication use suggests a diagnosis of MOH, but affected individuals often attempt to conceal their analgesic usage from healthcare providers.[13]

Management: The definitive treatment of MOH is difficult, but in the acute setting, return of the withdrawn agent will provide benefit. For the surgical patient unable to take pills, each of these medications (or similar medication in the same class) is clinically available in injectable, sublingual, or suppository form.

Recreational substance withdrawal: Headache may present as part of the withdrawal symptoms of nicotine, alcohol, or opioids. Headache is a consistent symptom of withdrawal from acute intoxication of alcohol ("hangover"), but less frequently observed in withdrawal from chronic abuse. Headache is a frequent symptom of nicotine withdrawal. Hospitalized smokers may experience headache as may former smokers who are habitual nicotine gum chewers.[14]

Management: The surgical patient with opioid dependence should receive their daily maintenance dose of opioid in addition to the postoperative analgesic needs. Acute withdrawal from alcohol intoxication is treated with benzodiazepines, the associated headache may be treated with NSAIDs, acetaminophen, and IV hydration. Perioperative nicotine replacement therapy for smokers remains controversial. Smoking impairs wound healing, and although nicotine replacement therapy does not appear to inhibit healing, some evidence suggests nicotine replacement therapy may have some impact on post-surgical inflammatory tissue response.[15] The effectiveness of nicotine replacement therapy in the perioperative period has not been established. In one randomized placebo-controlled trial, nicotine replacement therapy did not diminish perioperative stress or withdrawal symptoms in surgical patients.[16] Moreover, nicotine replacement therapy may contribute to excess mortality among cardiac patients after coronary artery bypass.[17] NSAIDs or acetaminophen would be alternative treatments for smokers with headache for whom nicotine replacement therapy is not deemed appropriate.

Anti-emetic medication-induced headache

5-HT$_3$ receptor antagonists administered as anti-emetics, including ondansetron, granisetron, dolasetron, and palonosetron, may cause headache. Ondansetron administration is associated with headache in 1 of every 36 administrations.[18] The headache is most often mild, but may be abrupt and severe in some individuals. Early clinical experience indicated that surgical patients with primary headache syndromes were not at increased risk for ondansetron-induced headache,[19] but a higher incidence among migraine patients has more recently been reported.[20] Although the clinical association between primary headache and an increased risk of headache with 5-HT$_3$ antagonists is unproven, the weak 5-HT$_1$ receptor antagonism these medications possess could increase the risk of headache for surgical patients with a history of migraine or experiencing caffeine withdrawal.[21]

Management: The headache is mild and can usually be treated with NSAIDs or acetaminophen as needed. Reducing the dose of ondansetron from 4 mg to 1 mg eliminates the risk of headache without compromising efficacy when administered for rescue therapy of established postoperative nausea or vomiting.[22]

Opioids: Opioid withdrawal is the most commonly implicated medication in MOH,[23] but conversely opioids may also cause headache from acute administration. In the largest published comparison of two opioids ($n = 1,941$), the incidence of postoperative headache was higher in patients receiving postoperative analgesia with fentanyl iontophoretic transdermal system (11.1%) compared with morphin IV patient-controlled analgesia (7.3%).[24] Only 2 (headache and pruritus) of the 17 side effects monitored were significantly different. The mechanism of opioid-induced headache is not known, but hypercapnia has been postulated as contributing.

Management: Minimizing opioids in the perioperative setting and utilizing non-opioid adjuvants may be beneficial. Establishing the adequacy of ventilation for all patients receiving opioids and complaining of headache is important. Supportive care and NSAIDs or acetaminophen may be helpful.

Other medications

Headache is reported in low incidence from most medications and may occur in the postoperative setting owing to polypharmacy. The most commonly implicated perioperative medications in causing headache include nitrates, calcium channel blockers, and phosphodiesterase inhibitors.

Management: Discontinuation of the offending medication may be beneficial, but only after a clinical evaluation of risk and benefit. In instances where benefit outweighs risk (e.g. medication is potentially life-saving) attenuation of the side effect is often observed over time.

Anesthesia-related causes

Postdural puncture headache (PDPHA): A PDPHA ("spinal headache") may occur after puncture of the dura and arachnoid mater. Clinically, PDPHA is observed after spinal anesthesia, failed epidural catheter placement with inadvertent dural puncture, myelography, and diagnostic lumbar puncture. Modifiable risk factors for spinal headache include needle size and design, and technique. Non-modifiable risk factors include younger patient age and pregnancy. Female sex is a frequently cited but controversial risk factor.[25] PDPHA occurs in low frequency after spinal anesthesia despite strict adherence to techniques to reduce modifiable risk factors. In one retrospective study of 4,767 spinal anesthetics, the incidence of PDPHA was 1.3%.[26]

PDPHA is typically bilateral, fronto-occipital, with a strong postural component. Nausea, emesis, and visual and auditory disturbances are frequently reported. The International Headache Society has defined PDPHA as a headache that develops within 7 days of lumbar puncture, resolves within 14 days, worsens within 15 minutes of becoming upright, and improves within 30 minutes of recumbency.[27] This definition may not be completely adequate, since PDPHA persisting weeks, months, or even years are infrequently reported.

Headache after spinal anesthesia should raise clinical suspicion for PDPHA, but is not diagnostic. It is clinically important to remember that other diagnostic possibilities exist. In one study of parturients after spinal anesthesia (very high-risk patient population) only 16% of headaches were PDPHA.[28] Tension headaches and eclampsia were more frequently observed etiologies. Other etiologies require different therapy, so PDPHA should *not* be assumed for all patients receiving spinal anesthesia and experiencing headache.

Management: IV hydration and epidural blood patch are the major treatment for PDPHA. Abdominal binding is a historical practice no longer recommended. Recumbency provides symptomatic relief, but is neither curative nor preventative.[25] IV caffeine benzoate has some efficacy, but is no longer available in the United States. IV aminophylline, a methylxanthine with structural similarity to caffeine, has some reported efficacy. In retrospective analysis, slightly more than 1/3 of affected patients required epidural blood patch.[26]

Epidural or intrathecal air: Small quantities of air may be injected to identify the epidural space during neuraxial anesthesia administration (loss-of-resistance technique). Large quantities of epidural air or small quantities of intrathecal air may cause sudden and profound headache. Like PDPHA, epidural or intrathecal air may occur after neuraxial anesthesia, but the headache is generally *exacerbated* by recumbency.

Management: Computed tomography may aid in diagnosis and exclude other etiologies such as hemorrhage. This headache is typically self-limited, but may persist for days and be relatively refractory to treatment. Analgesics may provide partial, if incomplete, relief.

Monday morning headache: A headache observed in the Post-Anesthesia Care Unit (PACU) early Monday morning should raise consideration of carbon monoxide poisoning. Carbon monoxide may rarely be produced from an interaction of volatile agents with desiccated carbon dioxide absorbent. This very rare phenomenon has been infrequently reported and typically occurs after a weekend or holiday when oxygen flow through an anesthesia machine causes desiccation of the absorbent.[29]

Management: Carbon monoxide poisoning may be confirmed by arterial blood gas analysis for carboxyhemoglobin level. Treatment is with 100% oxygen. Hyperbaric oxygen and endotracheal intubation are reserved for the most severe cases. If carbon monoxide is identified in the PACU, identification of the offending anesthesia equipment and replacement of the carbon dioxide absorbent is mandatory.

Procedure-related headaches: Neurovascular procedures including intracranial stent or carotid stenting may be associated with postoperative headache, perhaps owing to perfusion changes within the brain. Intracranial procedures are commonly associated with postoperative headache. Sinus surgery is frequently associated with headache lasting for several weeks. Postoperative edema formation and the development of pressure are implicated in the etiology.

Management: Although certain procedures may cause headache requiring complex treatment regimens (e.g. acoustic neuroma resection), most ambulatory procedures cause mild headaches responsive to mild analgesics.

Miscellaneous postoperative causes: Headache in the gravid patient should cause suspicion for eclampsia. Postoperative hypertension may cause headache and requires immediate treatment of blood pressure. The incidence of post-traumatic headache after closed head injury without demonstrable lesion may occur in up to 60% of individuals.[30] Treatment is supportive, but imaging to exclude structural lesion is usually necessary to confirm the diagnosis. Sepsis may cause headache, but this is rarely the presenting symptom. Hypotension, fever, hypothermia, or rigors would be more common. Acute narrow-angle glaucoma can present in the early perioperative period with photophobia and anisocoria (unequal pupils), conjunctival hyperemia, nausea and vomiting. Although eye pain is the cardinal symptom, in some individuals this pain is generalized and perceived as headache.

Recognizing warning signs

It is important to recognize postoperative headache due to intracranial hemorrhage or increased intracranial pressure. An at-risk procedure, appropriate co-morbidity, or the use of anticoagulants may alert suspicion. Risk factors for headaches from serious secondary causes among medical patient populations may be described and remembered by the acronym SNOOP: Systemic features (fever, myalgias, malignancy), Neurological signs, abrupt Onset, Onset beyond age 40 years, Progressive symptoms, or Pattern change of headache are worrisome signs.[2] The presence of SNOOP signs should prompt the clinician to investigate for serious secondary causes of headache. Unfortunately, the SNOOP acronym is poorly adaptable to the perioperative setting. However, perioperative headache associated with focal neurological findings or papilledema, fever, or an alteration in mental status should raise clinical suspicion for a more serious underlying process.

Primary headaches after surgery

Primary headaches may present after surgery and anesthesia. The influence of the perioperative period on chronic primary headache is inadequately studied. Tension headaches present as band-like circumferential headaches and are more common after surgery and anesthesia. Migraine headache is not reported to occur more frequently after anesthesia and surgery, but interruption of prophylactic medications and intravascular dehydration would be expected to exacerbate these.[4] Cluster headaches appear as periorbital headaches (ice pick). There is usually a history of current or former smoking, and male predominance. Although cluster headaches are not reported to be caused by surgery or anesthesia, a Valsalva-induced variant has been described which theoretically could be caused by airway manipulation and mechanical ventilation.[31]

References

1. Headache Classification Committee of the International Headache Society (IHS). The International Classification of Headache Disorders, 3rd edition (beta version). *Cephalalgia* 2013; 33:629–808.

2. D.W. Dodick. Clinical clues and clinical rules: primary versus secondary headaches. *Adv Stud Med* 2003; 3:S550–S555.

3. J.N. Blau, C.A. Kell, J.M. Sperling. Water-deprivation headache: a new headache with two variants. *Headache* 2004; 44:79–83.

4. J.N. Blau. Water deprivation: a new migraine precipitant. *Headache* 2005; 45:757–759.

5. D.C. Mitchell, C.A. Knight, J. Hockenberry, R. Teplansky, T.J. Hartmann. Beverage

caffeine intakes in the US. *Food Chem Toxicol* 2014; 63:136–142.

6. R.R. Griffiths, S.M. Evans, S.J. Heishman, et al. Low-dose caffeine physical dependence in humans. *J Pharmacol Exp Ther* 1990; 255:1123–1132.

7. L.M. Juliano, R.R. Griffiths. A critical review of caffeine withdrawal: empirical validation of symptoms and signs, incidence, severity, and associated features. *Psychopharmacology* 2004; 176:1–29.

8. M. Fennelly, D.C. Galletly, G.I. Purdie. Is caffeine withdrawal the mechanism of postoperative headache? *Anesth Analg* 1991; 72:449–453.

9. L. Nikolajsen, K.M. Larsen, O. Kierkegaard. Effect of previous frequency of headache, duration of fasting and caffeine abstinence on perioperative headache. *Br J Anaesth* 1994; 72:295–297.

10. K.L. Hampl, M.C. Schneider, U.R. Uttimann, W. Ummenhofer, J. Drewe. Perioperative administration of caffeine tablets for prevention of postoperative headaches. *Can J Anaesth* 1995; 42:789–792.

11. J.G. Weber, J.T. Klindworth, J.J. Arnold, D.R. Danielson, M.H. Ereth. Prophylactic intravenous administration of caffeine and recovery after ambulatory surgical procedures. *Mayo Clin Proc* 1997; 72:621–626.

12. Practice guidelines for preoperative fasting and the use of pharmacologic agents to reduce the risk of pulmonary aspiration: applicationto healthy patients undergoing elective procedures. *Anesthesiology* 2011; 114:495–511.

13. J. R. Couch. Rebound-withdrawal headache (medication overuse headache). *Curr Treat Options Neurol* 2006, 8:11–19.

14. R. Stalnikowicz. Nicotine gum withdrawal and migraine headaches. *Eur J Emerg Med* 2006; 13:247–248.

15. L. T. Sørensen. Wound healing and infection in surgery: the pathophysiological impact of smoking, smoking cessation, and

16. D.O. Warner, C.A. Pattern, S.C. Ames, K.P. Offord, D.R. Schroeder. Effect of nicotine replacement therapy on stress and smoking behavior in surgical patients. *Anesthesiology* 2005; 102:1138–1146.

17. C.A. Paciullo, M.R. Short, D.T. Steinke, H.R. Jennings. Impact of nicotine replacement therapy on postoperative mortality following coronary artery bypass graft surgery. *Ann Pharmacother* 2009; 43:1197–1202.

18. T.J. Gan, P. Diemunsch, A.S. Habib, et al. Consensus guidelines for the management of postoperative nausea and vomiting. *Anesth Analg* 2014; 118:85–113.

19. M. Venezian, M. Framarino Dei Malatesta, A.F. Bandiera, et al. Ondansetron-induced headache. Our experience in gynecological cancer. *Eur J Gynaecol Oncol* 1995; 16:203–207.

20. V. Singh, A. Sinha, N. Prakash. Ondansetron-induced migraine-type headache. *Can J Anaesth* 2010; 57:872–873.

21. J.H. Ye, R. Ponnudurai, R. Schaef. Ondansetron: A selective 5-HT3 receptor antagonist and its applications in CNS-related disorders. *CNS Drug Rev* 2001; 7:199–213.

22. M.R. Tramèr, C. Phillips, D.J.M. Reynolds, H.J. McQuay, R.A. Moore. Cost-effectiveness of ondansetron for postoperative nausea and vomiting. *Anaesthesia* 1999; 54:226–234.

23. J.L. Johnson, M.R. Hutchinson, D.B. Williams, P. Rolan. Medication-overuse headache and opioid-induced hyperalgesia: a review of mechanisms, a neuroimmune hypothesis and a novel approach to treatment. *Cephalalgia* 2013; 33:52–64.

24. E.R. Viscusi, M. Siccardi, C.V. Damaraju, D.J. Hewitt, P. Kershaw. The safety and efficacy of fentanyl iontophoretic transdermal system compared with morphine intravenous patient-controlled analgesia for postoperative pain

management: an analysis of pooled data from three randomized, active controlled clinical studies. *Anesth Analg* 2007; 105:1428–1436.

25. R. Gaiser. Postdural puncture headache. *Curr Opin Anaesthesiol* 2006; 19:249–253.

26. T.T. Horlocker, D.G. McGregor, D.K. Matsushige, D.R. Schroeder, J.A. Besse. A retrospective review of 4767 consecutive spinal anesthetics: central nervous system complications. *Anesth Analg* 1997; 84:578–584.

27. R.W. Evans, C. Armon, E.M. Frohman, D.S. Goodin. Assessment/prevention of post-lumbar puncture headaches. Report of the Therapeutics and Technology Assessment Subcommittee of the Academy of Neurology. *Neurology* 2000; 55:909–914.

28. C.L. Stella, C.D. Jodicke, H.Y. How, U.F. Harkness, B.M. Sibai. Postpartum headache: is your work-up complete? *Am J Obstet Gynecol* 2007; 196:318.e1–318.e7.

29. P.D. Berry, D.I. Sessler, M.D. Larson. Severe carbon monoxide poisoning during desflurane anesthesia. *Anesthesiology* 1999; 90:613–616.

30. J.C. Lane, D.B. Arciniegas. Post-traumatic headache. *Curr Treat Options Neurol* 2002; 4:89–104.

31. J.I. Ko, T.D. Rozen. Valsalva-induced cluster: a new subtype of cluster headache. *Headache* 2002; 42:301–302.

Delayed emergence

Jon Zhou and James W. Heitz

- Modern anesthetics allow for rapid emergence from anesthesia.
- Individual variability plays a major role in emergence from anesthesia.
- Residual neuromuscular blockade is common after surgery.
- Residual medication effects and metabolic disturbances account for most cases of delayed emergence.

Modern anesthetics have been developed to have a rapid onset and offset of action. Most patients recover from anesthesia quickly after the end of the procedure. Typically, they should be awake, responsive to simple commands, and be able to control their airway. Approximately 90% of patients regain consciousness within 15 minutes of admission to the Post-Anesthesia Care Unit (PACU).[1] Delayed emergence may be defined as when a patient fails to regain consciousness 30 to 60 minutes after the end of a surgical procedure. Time to emergence depends on the type and duration of anesthesia, as well as specific patient factors.

There are a myriad of potential causes of delayed emergence from anesthesia; however, the most frequent causes are medication effects, metabolic and respiratory disorders, or neurological abnormalities (see Figures 28.1, 28.2).

Medication effects

General anesthesia often includes the use of inhalational anesthetics, sedatives, opioids, and neuromuscular blocking agents. Delayed emergence may be due to overdose of medications, use of longer-acting anesthetics, drug–drug interactions causing potentiation of anesthetics, or prolonged neuromuscular blockade.

Significant individual variability to anesthetic medications makes optimal dosing of medications clinically challenging. Relative overdosing of anesthetics will prolong awakening time from anesthesia. Elderly and debilitated patients are more susceptible to medication overdose than are younger and healthier patients. Minimum alveolar concentration (MAC) of an inhaled anesthetic is the alveolar concentration at which 50% of patients will not show a motor response to surgical incision. MAC decreases approximately 6% per decade after age 40. Thus, the MAC of an 80-year-old would be roughly 25% lower than the MAC of a young adult. Patients with renal or hepatic insufficiency will have delayed drug metabolism or drug clearance and require dose reduction of some anesthetic

Post-Anesthesia Care: Symptoms, Diagnosis, and Management, ed. James W. Heitz. Published by Cambridge University Press. © Cambridge University Press 2016.

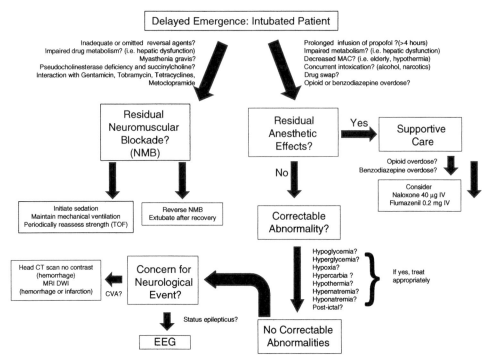

Figure 28.1 Differential diagnosis of delayed emergence for the intubated patient. TOF, train-of-four; CVA, cerebrovascular accident; EEG, electroencephalogram.

medications. Patients with certain co-morbidities (e.g. myasthenia gravis) are much more sensitive to neuromuscular blocking agents.

Although modern anesthetic agents have short durations of action when administered by intravenous (IV) bolus, some may display markedly different pharmacokinetics when administered by continuous IV infusion. Context-sensitive half-life is the time required for plasma concentration of a medication to decrease by 50% and varies by the context (bolus or infusion) of administration. Saturation of body compartments by certain medications may serve to sustain plasma levels and therefore exert prolonged drug effects. Lipid-soluble agents such as fentanyl will demonstrate an increased half-life after 2 hours of continuous infusion. Similarly, propofol will display an increased half-life after 3 to 4 hours of infusion.

Preoperative sedatives may prolong emergence. Benzodiazepines such as midazolam or lorazepam are frequently administered prior to surgery. Sedation may prolong emergence, particularly for short procedures or individuals very sensitive to their effects.[2] This effect may be particularly important in the elderly population. The scopolamine patch or diphenhydramine may be administered for nausea and vomiting prophylaxis, but may sometimes contribute to prolonged sedation. The sedating side effects of other medications, such as β-blockers and antihypertensives, may have synergistic effects with anesthetics.

The concurrent use of recreational narcotics or acute alcohol intoxication will also interact synergistically with anesthetics and may profoundly delay emergence. This may be observed frequently in trauma and emergency surgery, as traumatic injury and acute intoxication often co-exist. Patients undergoing elective procedures may also be successful

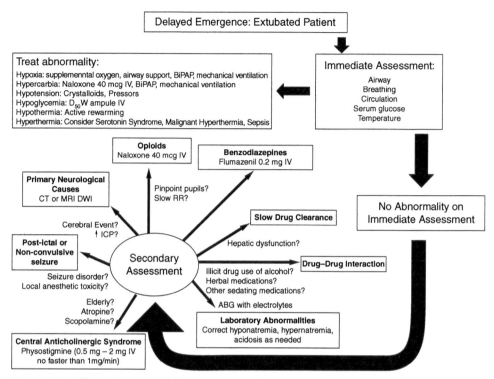

Figure 28.2 Differential diagnosis of delayed emergence for the extubated patient. BiPAP, bilevel positive airway pressure; ICP, intracranial pressure; RR, respiratory rate.

in concealing drug use. Occasionally, patients will self-medicate with controlled substances the morning of surgery, either to control for anxiety or to attempt to mitigate the anticipated discomfort.

Interaction between herbal supplements and anesthetic medications has the potential to delay emergence from anesthesia. The effect of perioperative herbal supplement usage is inadequately studied and complicated by the fact that commercially available herbal supplements lack standardization, so significant dosing differences exist between brands or even between batches of the same brand. Herbal medications can cause prolonged sedation after surgery.[3] A survey published in 2000 showed that 63% of surgical patients at one institution were taking some form of dietary supplement, and the majority of these patients did not disclose them.[4] Although the American Society of Anesthesiologists recommends discontinuation of herbals 2 to 3 weeks prior to surgery, this does not always occur. Perioperative herbal medications, such as valerian root and kava kava, may have sedative effects that may prolong the effect of anesthetics.[5] St. John's wort contains hypericin and hyperforin, which are believed to inhibit neuronal reuptake of serotonin, norepinephrine, and dopamine.[6] St. John's wort could contribute to delayed emergence from anesthesia by several mechanisms, and there are reports of delayed emergence where St John's wort usage was believed to be a factor.[7]

Residual effects of neuromuscular blockers (NMB) can delay the emergence of patients from anesthesia.[8] While delayed emergence more typically refers to the patient who has failed to awaken from anesthesia, residual neuromuscular blockade may give the appearance of delayed awakening in a fully conscious individual. Residual neuromuscular blockade should be considered for *every* case of delayed emergence. The causes of prolonged paralysis may be drug overdose, incomplete reversal, or pseudocholinesterase deficiency if succinylcholine was administered as part of the anesthetic.[9] Patients with disorders of the neuromuscular junction such as myasthenia gravis are acutely sensitive to non-depolarizing NMB. Aminoglycosides, such as gentamicin, have a synergistic effect with NMB and can potentiate their effects. Likewise, inhalational agents and local anesthetics have the potential to prolong the duration of action of NMB. If the anticonvulsant phenytoin is given acutely, then there may be augmentation of neuromuscular blocking potency.[10] Metoclopramide can also inhibit plasma cholinesterase and prolongs the action of succinylcholine.

Respiratory failure

Respiratory failure may cause impaired consciousness in the PACU. Risk factors for postoperative respiratory failure include: underlying respiratory disease (sleep apnea, chronic obstructive pulmonary disease), excessive opiates, residual NMB, and baseline airway obstruction.[11] Patients who do not ventilate effectively during the immediate postoperative period may become hypercarbic to a level that will produce sedation or unconsciousness. Hypercapnia may initially stimulate spontaneous respiration, but excess CO_2 buildup will depress the central respiratory centers. Routine plethysmography is insufficient in detecting hypercarbia. It is important to note that patients may have a normal SpO_2 despite having an elevated CO_2. Patients should be evaluated for respiratory rate and adequacy of ventilatory effort. If hypercarbia is a clinical concern, arterial blood gas analysis should be performed.

Hypoxia will also impair consciousness. Postoperative hypoxemia is most frequently caused by V/Q mismatch, intrapulmonary shunt, and impaired ventilatory effort, but may also be related to airway obstruction in patients making adequate ventilatory effort. Altered mental status combined with hypoxia is a medical emergency requiring immediate intervention.

Metabolic disturbances

A number of underlying metabolic imbalances may be responsible for delayed emergence.[12] Hypoglycemia will cause delayed emergence because the brain is dependent on glucose as the source of energy. Patients with chronic alcoholism or poorly controlled diabetics are more susceptible to the detrimental effects of low blood sugar, but hypoglycemia should be considered in all patients with delayed emergence. *De novo* hypoglycemia may present after certain procedures, particularly of the pancreas. Unintentional insulin administration (drug swap) is a rare, but potentially catastrophic medication error which must be considered. Drug–drug interactions are numerous for patients taking oral hypoglycemic agents (see Chapter 16, Table 16.1). Conversely, severe hyperglycemia may also contribute to delayed emergence and often occurs in decompensated diabetics (diabetic ketoacidosis and hyperosmotic hyperglycemic diabetic coma).

Severe electrolyte imbalances may occur as a consequence of a surgical procedure or secondary to an underlying disease process. Mild hyponatremia (<120 mmol/l) is usually asymptomatic, but severe hyponatremia (<110 mmol/l) will cause confusion, irritability, or even coma. Hyponatremia may occur in transurethral resection of the prostate owing to the use of large amounts of glycine or other hypotonic fluids for irrigation. High ammonia levels secondary to glycine metabolism can lead to confusion, agitation, or obtundation. Patients undergoing intracranial procedures can develop syndrome of inappropriate antidiuretic hormone (SIADH), which will cause fluid retention and possibly severe hyponatremia.

Hypothermia may lead to delayed emergence by several mechanisms. A core temperature below 33 °C has an anesthetic effect, but will also potentiate the effects of IV sedatives used in the case. Hypothermia also decreases the MAC of inhalational agents and slows drug metabolism.

Neurological complications

Neurological complications can cause delayed emergence. Some examples are cerebral hypoxia of any cause and intracerebral events including hemorrhage and embolic events. These complications are more common in neurosurgery, cardiac, vascular, and orthopedic procedures. Cerebral autoregulation functions within a mean arterial pressure (MAP) of 50 to 150 mmHg. Extended intraoperative periods of low MAP may increase the risk of cerebral ischemia. Mental status changes and delayed emergence can be attributed to cerebral anoxia from hypoperfusion, cerebral thromboembolism from air or fat, or cell injury from rapid correction of hyponatremia causing central pontine myelinolysis. Patients with atlanto-axial cervical spine instability (e.g. rheumatoid arthritis, Down's syndrome, trauma) are more susceptible to spinal cord trauma, especially during direct laryngoscopy, and may fail to follow commands at the conclusion of surgery.

Consideration must also be given to central anticholinergic syndrome (CAS) and serotonin syndrome when evaluating delayed emergence. The signs of CAS are identical to atropine poisoning and include central nervous system manifestations ranging from excitatory symptoms (agitation, delirium) to depressive effects (coma, unconsciousness).[13] Although rarely encountered, CAS is more common in individuals receiving perioperative scopolamine or atropine. Glycopyrrolate, an anticholinergic which does not cross the blood–brain barrier, is preferred clinically to atropine for adult patients partly because of its decreased propensity to cause CAS. However, many perioperative medications have some anticholinergic effect and in combination may cause CAS in susceptible individuals. It is a diagnosis of exclusion and when suspected can be treated with a central-acting cholinesterase inhibitor such as physostigmine.[14] Physostigmine 0.5 mg to 2 mg IV may be administered no faster than 1 mg/min, since too rapid administration may be associated with seizure, asystole, or death. Side effects include bronchospasm and bradycardia, and physostigmine is contraindicated for patients with seizure disorders, reactive airway disease, or existing bowel obstruction.

Serotonin syndrome should also be considered in the differential diagnosis of delayed emergence. Patients taking chronic tricyclic antidepressants, selective serotonin reuptake inhibitors, or serotonin-norepinephrine reuptake inhibitors are at increased risk. Some anesthetics have serotonin potentiation, including fentanyl, methadone, and oxycodone. Although these effects are weak, when combined with other more strongly serotonin-potentiating medications they may cause overt serotonin syndrome. The manifestations are protean and diagnosis may be difficult, but altered mental status and coma may be observed in severely affected individuals. These individuals will usually display hemodynamic instability, muscular rigidity, and hyperthermia. Treatment is cessation of the causative medications, but very severe cases may be treated with cyproheptadine 2 mg PO (titrate to effect) or chlorpromazine 50 mg IV.[15] A recent case of successful treatment with intralipid rescue therapy was recently reported.[16]

Management

The evaluation of delayed emergence in the PACU should begin with an immediate assessment to exclude life-threatening conditions requiring rapid intervention. The immediate assessment includes basic vital signs and blood glucose measurement. Hypoxia, hypotension, or diminished cardiac output if present should be immediately corrected. Blood glucose should be rapidly determined in all patients with delayed emergence or mental status change in the PACU, since failure to recognize hypoglycemia can have profound consequences. Significant hyperglycemia with diabetic ketoacidosis or hyperglycemic hyperosmolar non-ketotic coma should also be included in the differential diagnosis. Significant hypothermia requires active rewarming measures including forced air blankets. Hyperthermia should raise suspicion for possible serotonin syndrome, malignant hyperthermia, or sepsis.

The patient with stable vital signs, euglycemia, and delayed emergence requires a secondary assessment for other causes. Arterial blood gas and electrolytes are helpful for further work-up. Acidosis, hyponatremia, or hypernatremia should be appropriately treated if present. Opioid narcosis (i.e. pinpoint pupils, slow respiratory rate, hypercarbia) may be treated with incremental doses of naloxone 40 mcg IV. A titrated dose of naloxone is preferable in the postoperative setting to a larger bolus (i.e. 4 mg dose), because larger doses increase the risk of side effects including chest pain or seizures and unwanted reversal of analgesia. The duration of naloxone is only 20 minutes, so patients responding to opioid antagonism require extended observation since sedation may reoccur.

If benzodiazepine overdose is suspected, reverse with incremental doses of flumazenil 0.2 mg IV. Caution is advised on administering flumazenil in the PACU as it may cause hypertension, and it increases the risk of seizures, particularly among patients taking benzodiazepines chronically.

Residual neuromuscular blockade can be assessed using a peripheral nerve stimulator in the unresponsive patient. If the patient has residual neuromuscular blockade, more reversal agent may be needed. Alternatively, mechanical ventilation with sedation may be needed for some patients with profound residual weakness who cannot have their NMB adequately reversed. Administration of sedative drugs is rarely appropriate for delayed emergence, but is necessary in the setting of residual weakness.

Additionally, the possibility of slow drug metabolism or elimination from hepatic or renal insufficiency should be considered. Drug–drug interactions may also prolong emergence. A post-ictal state can present as delayed emergence, particularly in patients with pre-existing seizure disorder or receiving larger perioperative doses of local anesthetics, such as required for upper extremity nerve blocks. Central anticholinergic syndrome should be considered, particularly among elderly patients receiving scopolamine or atropine.

The timing of neurological imaging needs to be individualized. If no other etiology for delayed emergence can be found, or for patients with focal neurological signs or a history of increased intracranial pressure, brain scanning should not be delayed. A head CT scan without contrast is usually rapidly obtainable and will reveal an acute intracranial hemorrhage, but will fail to demonstrate ischemic stroke. If available, a diffusion-weighted MRI (MRI DWI) may reveal both acute hemorrhagic and ischemic intracranial processes.

References

1. R. Hines, P.G. Barash, G. Watrous, T. O'Connor. Complications occurring in the postanesthesia care unit: a survey. *Anesth Analg* 1992; 74:503–509.

2. J. Radhakrishnan, S. Jesudasan, R. Jacob. Delayed awakening or emergence from anesthesia. *Update Anesthesia* 2001; 13:4–6.

3. P. Posadzki, L. Watson, E. Ernst. Herb–drug interactions: an overview of systematic reviews. *Br J Clin Pharmacol* 2013; 75:603–618.

4. A.D. Kaye, R.C. Clarke, R. Sabar, *et al.* Herbal medicines: current trends in anesthesiology practice – a hospital survey. *J Clin Anesth* 2000; 12:468–471.

5. M.K. Ang-Lee, J. Moss, C. Yuan. Herbal medicines and perioperative care. *JAMA* 2001; 286:208–216.

6. S.J.S. Bajwa, A. Panda. Alternative medicine and anesthesia: implications and considerations in daily practice. *Ayu* 2012; 33:475–480.

7. S. Crowe, K.F. McKeating. Delayed emergence and St. John's wort. *Anesthesiology* 2002; 96:1025–1027.

8. G.S. Murphy, S.J. Brull. Residual neuromuscular block: lessons unlearned. Part I: definitions, incidence, and adverse physiologic effects of residual neuromuscular block. *Anesth Analg* 2010; 111:120–128.

9. L.I. Eriksson. The effects of residual neuromuscular blockade and volatile anesthetics on the control of ventilation. *Anesth Analg* 1999; 89:243–251.

10. A. Spacek, S. Nickl, F.X. Neiger, *et al.* Augmentation of the rocuronium-induced neuromuscular block by the acutely administered phenytoin. *Anesthesiology* 1999; 90:1551–1555.

11. D.K. Rose, M.M. Cohen, D.F. Wigglesworth, D.P. DeBoer. Critical respiratory events in the postanesthesia care unit. Patient, surgical, and anesthetic factors. *Anesthesiology* 1994; 81:410–418.

12. M.S. Arbous, A.E. Meursing, J.W. van Kleef, J.J. de Lange, H.H. Spoormans. Impact of anesthesia management characteristics on severe morbidity and mortality. *Anesthesiology* 2005; 102:257–268.

13. P. Meuret, S.B. Backman, V. Bonhomme, *et al.* Physostigmine reverses propofol-induced unconsciousness and attenuation of the auditory steady state response and bispectral index in human volunteers. *Anesthesiology* 2000; 93:708–717.

14. J. Link, G. Papadopoulos, D. Dopjans, *et al.* Distinct central anticholinergic syndrome following general anesthesia. *Eur J Anaesthesiol* 1997; 14:15–23.

15. R. Rastogi, R.A. Swarm, T.A. Patel. Case scenario: opioid association with serotonin syndrome: implications to the practitioners. *Anesthesiology* 2011; 115:1291–1298.

16. O. Dagtekin, H. Marcus, C. Müller, B.W. Böttiger, F. Spöhr. Lipid therapy for serotonin syndrome after intoxication with venlafaxine, lamotrigine and diazepam. *Minerva Anestesiol* 2011; 77:93–95.

Crying

Michelle Beam and James W. Heitz

- Crying is frequently observed after surgery and anesthesia.
- Non-emotional crying that occurs among adult patients after surgery is poorly understood and inadequately researched.
- The crying patient should be assessed for pain and postoperative delirium.
- Pain should be suspected as a cause of crying among patients with language or cognitive barriers to communication.
- The majority of tearful patients require only reassurance.

Crying may be defined as the expression of tears in the absence of ocular irritation. It is typically accompanied by changes in breathing and phonation. Crying is often observed after surgery. While crying is culturally considered an expression of sadness, postoperative crying may occur in the absence of emotional upset. The tearful postoperative patient often denies sadness and is unable to articulate a reason for crying. Although frequently observed in the clinical setting and casually discussed by healthcare providers and patients alike, the phenomenon of postoperative crying has been inadequately studied. Very little medical research has been conducted on this subject, and the causes of non-emotional postoperative crying are inadequately understood.

Anesthesia and crying

Although some patients report episodes of crying after anesthesia, the association between specific anesthetic agents and postoperative crying is poorly defined. Some agents typically administered for general anesthesia have been anecdotally associated with crying, but causality is unproven. The package insert for the inhalational anesthetic gas sevoflurane lists crying among its side effects,[1] but this effect is best documented among pediatric patient populations. Conscious sedation with midazolam has been reported to cause crying in adolescents[2] and adult patients.[3] The polypharmacy of the intraoperative period, with many medications exhibiting central nervous system effects, makes isolating the effect of a single medication problematic. Also, the effects of anesthetic agents in combination on mood or behavior are not known. The clinical impression that remifentanil infusion during general anesthesia is associated with more dysphoria and depression in the first postoperative day could not be validated in one small prospective randomized controlled study, although crying was not a measured outcome.[4]

Post-Anesthesia Care: Symptoms, Diagnosis, and Management, ed. James W. Heitz. Published by Cambridge University Press. © Cambridge University Press 2016.

Additionally, some anesthetics may affect lacrimation and cause passive tearing rather than crying. Ketamine is associated with both hyperlacrimation and hypersalivation. Although most commonly observed at the induction of general anesthesia, tearing from ketamine has also been reported on emergence from anesthesia. This appears as watery eyes possibly associated with pupillary dilation, but does not present as weeping or sobbing.

Anecdotal evidence implicating specific medications with actual crying is inadequate to guide therapy, and it is currently not possible to design an anesthetic plan to avoid crying in susceptible patients.

Evaluation: Prelanguage children or adults with communication barriers present a challenge in determining the cause of crying. The evaluation of prelanguage children is discussed in Chapter 44. Most adults can indicate severity of pain by use of a standardized pain scale even if unable to communicate directly. It is important that questioning about pain be directed at its presence or absence and its severity, and not the need for pain medication. Some patients may report not needing "more pain medication" despite the presence of severe pain, believing that requesting pain medication demonstrates weakness or that pain is inevitable, deserved, or untreatable.

Delirium is characterized by acute onset, inattention, altered level of consciousness, and disorganized thinking. Crying without explanation should elicit evaluation for postoperative delirium. The diagnosis and management of postoperative delirium is discussed in Chapter 26.

Once delirium and pain are excluded, most patients require only reassurance. Many crying patients deny dysphoria and cannot articulate a cause for their crying. Postoperative crying is usually self-limited, but distressed family members may also need explanation that their crying relative is not suffering.

Some postoperative patients may display emotional crying. There are many reasons for emotional crying after surgery, including fear, sadness, grief, guilt, or happiness. Fear of unfamiliar surroundings and people, or fear of diagnosis, pain, or disability may precipitate emotional crying. Others may experience feelings of guilt, shame, or embarrassment. Some patients may be happy that a feared event is behind them or that they have been cured. It is also important to note that some modern psychological theory also emphasizes *perceived helplessness* in causing crying.[5] The perioperative period is a time of profound helplessness for many patients who are able to exert little control over their disease or therapy. Efforts to empower patients as much as possible, such as by allowing self-positioning, actively engaging them in their care plan, and including appropriate patient controlled analgesia, might be beneficial in some patients.

Postoperative crying and emotional upsets are well documented in children and may be related to separation from their parents, fear of unfamiliar surroundings, pain, or emergence delirium. Bringing the parents to the Post-Anesthesia Care Unit (PACU) or into the operating room for induction reduces the prevalence of crying in pediatric patients,[6] but it is not known whether similar measures lessen crying among adult surgical patients. In a small randomized trial, postoperative feeding with milk as opposed to water reduced crying among infants having surgery.[7]

It is also important to determine that tear production is bilateral. Unilateral tear production should be differentiated from crying and requires evaluation for ocular or neurological etiology.

Unilateral tearing

In the postoperative period, epiphora or a watery eye will usually have an ocular cause. Corneal abrasion, which is typically associated with pain, foreign body sensation, photophobia, and conjunctival erythema, would be the most common type of ocular injury diagnosed after surgery. Chemical conjunctivitis from the accidental instillation of medication or skin preparation substance into the eye may also present as unilateral tearing, usually with other signs of ocular irritation. Less commonly, certain headache disorders including cluster headache and Short-lasting Unilateral Neuralgiform headache with Conjunctival injection and Tearing (SUNCT) may present with headache in association with conjunctival erythema and tearing. The conditions typically occur in mature adult men and would rarely be encountered *de novo* after surgery in a patient without a prior history of frequent episodic headaches. Each is associated with profound eye pain, which may cause clinical confusion with perioperative ocular injury. Patients experiencing cluster headache may describe the sensation of a sharp stick penetrating the globe or a sense that the globe is being pushed out of the eye socket from behind. Cluster headache pain typically lasts between 15 minutes and several hours. SUNCT produces stabbing pain in the eye, orbit, or temporal region, but generally lasts less than a minute.[8,9] The perioperative period has not been identified as a trigger for either of these syndromes, but recently a Valsalva-variant of cluster headache has been identified,[10] providing a possible mechanism for postoperative exacerbation in some individuals.

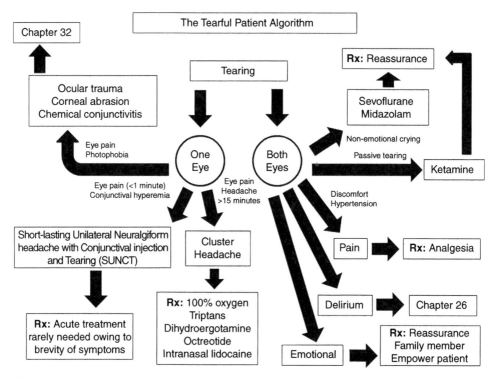

Figure 29.1 Diagnostic and treatment algorithm for postoperative crying or tearing.

Management: Postoperative crying has not been associated with adverse outcome or increased perioperative risk. Specifically, it is not known to be associated with either post-surgical depression or stress cardiomyopathy. There is a theoretical risk of increased postoperative bleeding after tonsillectomy in the crying patient, but there is little data to support this concern.

A high degree of clinical suspicion for pain should be held in the perioperative period, and many individuals should receive additional analgesia. In the absence of pain or another treatable underlying cause, management is supportive and entails calm and repeated reassurance, empowerment of the patient as much as possible in their own care, and the presence of a familiar person or family member, if available.

References

1. Package insert, Sevoflurane, Abbot Phamaceuticals, August 2012.

2. L. Lourenco-Matharu, G.J. Roberts. Effectiveness and acceptability of intravenous sedation in child and adolescent dental patients: report of a case series at King's College Hospital, London. *Br Dent J* 2011; 210(12):567–572.

3. C. Robin, N. Trieger. Paradoxical reactions to benzodiazepines in intravenous sedation: a report of 2 cases and review of the literature. *Anesth Prog* 2002; 49(4):128–132.

4. T.A. Crozier, D. Kietzmann, B. Döbereiner. Mood change after anaesthesia with remifentanil or alfentanil. *Eur J Anaesth* 2004; 21(1):20–24.

5. M. Miceli, C. Castelfranchi. Crying: discussing its basic reasons and uses. *New Ideas Psychol* 2003; 21(3):247–273.

6. D.R. Lardner, B.D. Dick, S. Crawford. The effects of parental presence in the postanesthetic care unit on children's postoperative behavior: a prospective, randomized, controlled study. *Anesth Analg* 2010; 110(4): 1102–1108.

7. R.H. Gunawardana, I.L.B. Ratnayaka. Postoperative crying in infants. *Anaesthesia* 2000; 55(2):197.

8. J.A. Pareja, A.B. Caminero, O. Siaastad. SUNCT syndrome: diagnosis and treatment. *CNS Drugs* 2002; 16(6):373–383.

9. J. Weaver-Agosoni. Cluster headache. *Am Fam Physician* 2013; 88(2):122–128.

10. J.I. Ko, T.D. Rozen. Valsalva-induced cluster: a new subtype of cluster headache. *Headache* 2002; 42(4):301–302.

Chapter

30

Rash

David Beausang and Michelle Beam

- Rash is frequently observed after surgery.
- Perioperative polypharmacy increases the risk of allergy and other drug reactions.
- Isolated rash in the absence of constitutional symptoms typically does not require treatment.

In the Post-Anesthesia Care Unit (PACU), a wide variety of skin conditions are often encountered (Figure 30.1). Some of these are minor and require no intervention, while others can be life-threatening problems. This review highlights the most common skin conditions encountered in the unit, their identifiable features, and their treatment. Rarely are providers of postoperative care to the surgical patient also experts in dermatology; in any skin condition that exceeds the normal bounds of postoperative care, a consult is always indicated. This review will help clarify situations where this consult may or may not be necessary.

Diffuse rashes

Red man syndrome: Red man syndrome results from vancomycin administration. The incidence increases at higher doses (>1 g) and faster rates of infusion (<1 hour).[1] The syndrome presents as an erythematous rash mainly of the face, neck, and upper chest. Pruritus often accompanies the rash, while hypotension and angioedema are less frequent. Onset usually appears 4 to 10 minutes following initiation of infusion, but can be delayed in patients on vancomycin for longer than 7 days.[1] When infusions are less than 1 hour, the incidence of the syndrome is 5% to 13%.[2] Healy and colleagues noted symptoms in 8 of 10 volunteers given 1 g over 1 hour, but in only 3 of 10 volunteers given the same dose over 2 hours.[3] Mast cell and basophil degranulation releases histamines, leading to the syndrome's signs and symptoms; thus, pretreatment with diphenhydramine will decrease the occurrence.[2] Upon diagnosis, the vancomycin infusion should be stopped immediately and oral or intravenous IV diphenhydramine (50 mg) administered. Upon resolution of the rash and pruritus, the infusion can be restarted at a slower rate. If the rash and pruritus are accompanied by significant hypotension, give fluids liberally and monitor for signs of anaphylaxis. In this instance, an alternative antibiotic should be selected instead of restarting the infusion.

Post-Anesthesia Care: Symptoms, Diagnosis, and Management, ed. James W. Heitz. Published by Cambridge University Press. © Cambridge University Press 2016.

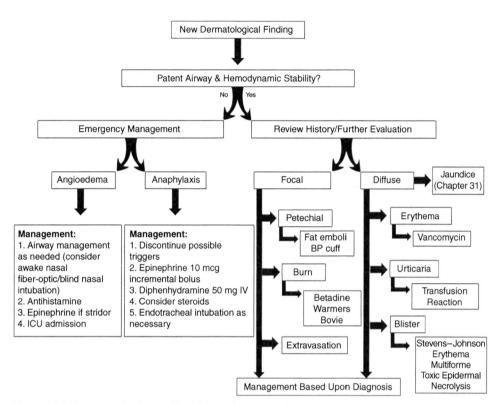

Figure 30.1 Common skin abnormalities of the early postoperative period.

Urticaria: The prevalence of drug rashes among hospitalized patients is 3.6 per 1,000. Fifty-five percent of these rashes are the result of antibiotics, most commonly amoxicillin, trimethoprim-sulfamethoxazole, and ampicillin. The two most common presentations of drug rashes are urticarial and maculopapular.[4]

The lesions of urticaria are smooth, erythematous, blanchable red papules that are often intensely pruritic. Regardless of the cause of urticaria, the lesions are established following the release of histamine and tryptase from basophils and mast cells.[5] Urticaria can be divided into two categories based upon presentation. Acute urticaria is IgE mediated and presents less than an hour following exposure to antigen. It can be accompanied by angioedema, bronchospasm, and anaphylaxis. Chronic urticaria is T-cell mediated, occurs at least an hour after exposure, and lasts up to a week.[5]

The prevalence of upper respiratory infection in acute urticaria is 28% to 62%. Other causes include aspirin, NSAIDs, vancomycin, quinolones, and radiocontrast, with antibiotics, radiocontrast, and NSAIDs also triggering chronic urticaria.[5]

Treatment for urticaria is second-generation H_1 blockers and observation for 4 to 6 hours to monitor the resolution of the rash.[5] If the rash is resolving appropriately, this observation can be continued, assuming that good communication and a designated physician for follow-up are available.

In 1993, Gadde *et al.* found that the result of penicillin skin testing performed on those with a stated history of penicillin allergy was positive in only 7.1%. Of note, 1.7% of patients with a negative history tested positive.[6] Owing to their shared β-lactam ring, it is recommended practice to avoid the administration of cephalosporins to patients with a known penicillin allergy. Cephalosporins will cause a reaction in 4.4% of people with a positive skin allergy test to penicillin.[4]

Blood transfusion also causes urticaria. Host mast cells degranulate in response to allergens in the donated plasma. Pretreatment with antihistamines is only indicated in those patients with a history of an allergic reaction to blood transfusion. Urticaria may be accompanied by pruritus and localized edema. In the event of a reaction, the blood transfusion should be stopped. If antihistamines lead to symptom resolution, the infusion can be restarted. Caution must be observed in patients with a known IgA deficiency as they are more prone to anaphylaxis from donor serum.

Blistering disorders: The spectrum of blistering skin disorders progresses in severity from erythema multiforme (EM) to Stevens–Johnson syndrome (SJS) to toxic epidermal necrolysis (TEN). The rash can result from drugs, graft-versus-host disease (GVHD), viral infection, usually herpes, or *Mycoplasma pneumoniae*.[7] Hundreds of drugs have been linked to this disease spectrum. The most commonly implicated medications are sulfona-mides, cephalosporins, imidazole, anticonvulsants, and NSAIDs. Differentiating between the types of blistering disorders is important because their treatment varies. In all of these cases, an early dermatology consult is recommended.

EM is a cell-mediated hypersensitivity that presents as acrally distributed, pleomorphic cutaneous eruptions, or target lesions. The major form of EM includes mucosal involvement, while the minor form does not. EM may also arise following radiation therapy in patients receiving phenytoin for seizure prophylaxis.[8] Early treat-ment of EM minor with systemic corticosteroids may prevent progression to the major form and SJS.

Differentiating SJS from the major form of EM is controversial, and overlap is inevit-able. Patients with SJS have a purpuric macular rash with more extensive blistering (up to 10%) of the trunk and oral mucosa. Ocular involvement is common. Systemic corticosteroid treatment is controversial. If initiated late (3 to 4 days after onset) it may assist in progression to TEN. TEN is a more significant form of SJS with over 30% blistering of the skin. Patients with TEN must be treated in a burn unit. Corticosteroids are contraindicated. Mortality is as high as 50%.[8]

Jaundice: Postoperative jaundice has an incidence of less than 1%. The majority of cases resolve spontaneously causing few, if any, ill effects. However, its presence requires evalu-ation as it may be a marker of massive hemolysis, hepatic hypoperfusion, or impending multi-organ failure. Severe hepatocellular dysfunction causes jaundice in 2% of patients following trauma-induced shock.[9]

Hereditary sources of jaundice can cause postoperative jaundice without the presence of severe hepatocellular dysfunction. Gilbert's syndrome affects 3% to 10% of the popula-tion.[10] Following surgical stress, it can cause an unconjugated hyperbilirubinemia with normal liver function tests and without overt hemolysis. Dubin–Johnson disorder is a rare autosomal recessive disorder of impaired hepatic storage and excretion of bromsulphalein, as well as impaired urinary excretion of coproporphyrin. It is most common in Israeli Jews of Iranian origin, 1:1,300.[9]

G6PD deficiency is an X-linked recessive disorder of red blood cell metabolism in which oxidative stress from drugs (aspirin, acetaminophen, diphenhydramine, sulfa, and vitamin K), metabolic derangement, or infection can lead to intraoperative and postoperative hemoly-sis. Infection is the most common trigger – an acute fall in hemoglobin occurred in 20% of

G6PD patients with pneumonia.[11] Acidosis and hyperglycemia may also precipitate hemolysis in those with G6PD.[12] In vitro, the inhaled anesthetics isoflurane and sevoflurane, inhibited G6PD enyzyme activity but its clinical significance is unknown.[13] Postoperative care of patients with G6PD is centered on avoiding oxidative stress. Pain and anxiety should be treated with benzodiazepines, codeine, and fentanyl, all of which are proven to be safe with G6PD. Acute hemolysis from G6PD deficiency is usually self-limited, but in rare instances will require blood transfusion.

With the discontinuation of halothane as an inhaled agent, anesthetic-induced postoperative jaundice has reduced markedly. Halothane was thought to have caused an immune-mediated hepatitis in patients. Two of today's commonly used agents, isoflurane and desflurane, are metabolized in the liver to a metabolite similar to that formed from halothane metabolism. The reduced incidence of hepatitis with these agents is due to their reduced hepatic metabolism (halothane 20% vs. isoflurane 0.2% and desflurane 0.01%). Patients with a history of a previous halothane anesthetic may be sensitized and prone to hepatitis from today's anesthetics.[14]

In patients with jaundice, liver function tests and blood counts should be ordered. If abnormal and/or no obvious cause for jaundice can be identified, a gastroenterology consult is recommended. If the cause is apparent and the patient is stable, continued supportive care is indicated.

Papulopustular rash: Since their approval by the FDA in 2003 for solid tumor chemotherapy, epidermal growth factor receptor inhibitors (EGFRIs) have gained in popularity. EGFRIs are less likely than their cytotoxic counterparts to cause myelosuppression, infection, nausea, vomiting, and diarrhea. They do, however, have an alarmingly high rate of papulopustular eruptions in a folliculocentric pattern. The incidence ranges from 44% in those treated with gefitinib, to 49% to 75% with erlotinib, and 90% with cetuximab and panitumumab. There is not an agreed treatment, but oral tetracyclines and mild to moderate topical steroids have been used. It is important to keep the skin clean and dry because the potential for staph superinfection is high.[15]

Focal rashes

Angioedema: Angioedema can affect any part of the body, but most commonly it consists of non-pitting, non-pruritic painless edema of the tongue, mouth, and periorbital area. Extension of the edema to supraglottic and laryngeal structures makes this condition potentially life-threatening. The incidence of angioedema is 0.1% to 0.7%. Renin–angiotensin–aldosterone system (RAAS) inhibiting drugs are the most common cause of angioedema, leading to bradykinin and angiotensin II accumulation. Malde et al. report that 25% of patients with ACE-inhibitor or ARB-induced angioedema had started the drugs within the month.[6] Patients with increased risk are females, African-Americans, those over age 65, and smokers.

Management of postoperative angioedema begins with an assessment of the airway, as it often requires intubation in the perioperative setting. Treatment with corticosteroids and antihistamines is indicated but often inadequate for cases of postoperative angioedema. Epinephrine (racemic, IV and/or SQ) should be given if stridor is present. In severe cases, fresh frozen plasma (FFP) is used to replenish enzymes. Icatibant, a B_2-receptor blocker used for hereditary angioedema, has efficacy for RAAS inhibitor-induced forms of angioedema. If time permits and intubation is indicated, an awake fiber-optic approach is preferred to prevent further airway trauma and maintain spontaneous breathing until the airway is secured. If intubation is not indicated, moderate to severe angioedema (edema of glottic, supraglottic, and laryngeal structures) still requires an admission to the Intersive Care Unit (ICU).

Petechiae: Fat embolism occurs with an impressively high frequency following pelvic or long bone fracture. Pulmonary artery blood samples contain fat in 70% of patients with these fractures.[16] Fat embolism syndrome refers to the presence of clinically significant intravasated fat. Patients will present with respiratory insufficiency, neurological changes, and petechial rash. The rash is present in 25% to 95% of cases of fat embolism syndrome.[16]

Oscillatory blood pressure cuffs can also create petechiae. Repeated or prolonged measurements in patients with increased capillary fragility may result in petechiae at the cuff site. Risk factors for capillary fragility include hypertension, diabetes, chronic kidney disease, thrombocytopenia, coagulopathy (warfarin therapy, von Willebrand disease, disseminated intravascular coagulation), and vitamin C deficiency. Capillary fragility may also cause petechiae surrounding an incision, created from the removal of an Ioband prep film. These petechiae are self-limited.

IV site: The incidence of IV infiltration and resultant extravasation of medication to the surrounding tissues is widely variable in the literature. Chemical properties, pH, osmolarity, and direct effects of the drug determine the likelihood of tissue damage. Phenytoin, anthracyclines, and promethazine are known to cause serious harm.

Fortunately, the extravasation of most drugs and fluids is relatively benign. The catheter responsible should be removed, followed by limb elevation. Warm and cold compresses may hasten recovery. Measurement of compartment pressures may be indicated in severe cases.

Promethazine, a vesicant with a pH of 4 to 5.5, is highly caustic to the intimal wall of the vein and surrounding tissues. Complications from its extravasation range from burning and phlebitis to tissue necrosis and gangrene. For this reason the drug should be dose limited (6.25 mg to 12.5 mg), diluted (10 to 20 ml normal saline, NSS), and slowly administered (10 to 15 minutes). The infusion must be stopped immediately following patient complaint.[17]

When given through an infiltrated catheter, vancomycin can result in a linear IgA bullous dermatosis.[18] IgA antibodies deposit on the basement membrane layer of the dermis, creating linear bullae at the catheter site that can later coalesce. Definitive differentiation from EM/SJS is with a skin biopsy.[8] Treatment requires only stoppage of the vancomycin and removal of the catheter.

Phenytoin, given intravenously, can cause purple glove syndrome (PGS) in the limb distal to the catheter, without extravasation. PGS is the development of progressive limb edema, discoloration, and pain following peripheral IV administration. In a study of 152 patients receiving IV phenytoin, 9 (5.9%) developed PGS. Of those 9, resolution occurred in 8 (88.8%) of them after one month with conventional treatment including, limb elevation, warm packs, and antibiotics. The ninth patient required a skin graft. The mechanism is thought to be due to the highly alkaline phenytoin solution. The prodrug fosphenytoin has yet to be cited as causing PGS.[19]

Burn injury: In an effort to avoid intraoperative and postoperative hypothermia, anesthesiologists commonly apply forced air warming blankets intraoperatively. Forced air warming blankets are the most common cause of intraoperative burns. In a case report, Siddik-Sayyid and colleagues reported first degree burns to a patient's upper extremity following the use of such a blanket during a 3-hour procedure.[20] They applied only a moisturizing cream, and the erythema resolved within 24 hours.

Though not the first to use electricity as a surgical tool, William Bovie is credited by many as the father of the electrosurgical devices used today. In 1926, Dr. Harvey Cushing was the first to use his device for the removal of a vascular myeloma from a patient's head. In the contemporary operating room, modern versions of Bovie's device are used almost ubiquitously. From the 1970s through the 1990s, electrosurgical injuries occurred in 2 to 5 in 1,000 patients. The grounding pad site, often placed on the patient's thigh intraoperatively, is a common location of iatrogenic electrosurgical burns. The burn is usually due to a failure in pad adhesion to the patient's skin. If only part of the pad is in contact with the patient, the current density to that area is increased and can cause a burn injury. A lack of grounding at this pad site may also create burns under the ECG pads.[21]

Povidone-iodine 10% (Betadine) solution gets its bactericidal properties from free iodine reacting with membrane proteins. Prolonged exposure to the skin, without drying, can lead to cell damage and iatrogenic burns. There are several case reports of patients who sustained severe full thickness burns beneath the tourniquet when Betadine prep was used as an antiseptic. In each instance, Betadine inadvertently soaked the "protective" gauze placed beneath the tourniquet and the damp gauze remained against the skin for a prolonged period. If severe, treatment will likely require wound excision and skin grafting.[22]

Betadine has also been implicated in burn injuries to the perineal and gluteal region. The burn occurs when Betadine pools between the legs and in gluteal folds. Because of their similarities the burn can be mistaken for a pressure ulcer. Both are erythematous, possibly blistering, and in the perineum. Pressure ulcers have blanchable erythema and are located only over bony prominences.[23]

Contact dermatitis: In present-day perioperative settings, adhesives are used to secure a wide variety of items to a patient's skin, including tape on IV lines, electrosurgical pads, ECG pads, warming devices, and surgical drapes. As such, many patients have discrete reactions to the adhesive. These reactions can be classified as contact dermatitis and are most often localized to the site of the adhesive. They can be identified by their distinct shapes (squares, lines, rectangles) in the locations of the attached devices. Commonly seen reaction sites are near the lips and cheeks, where the endotracheal tube was secured; over the eyes where the eyes were taped closed; on the arms; on the abdomen from the surgical draping; and, on the leg from the electrosurgical device pad. These irritations are usually self-limiting, but care should be taken to keep the area clean, as skin breakdown can occur, potentially leading to infection. Care should be made to rule out latex in the environment as another trigger associated with bandages and adhesives.

References

1. S. Sivagnanam, D. Deleu. Red man syndrome. *Crit Care* 2003; 7:119–120.

2. M. Wallace, J. Mascola, E. Oldfield. Red-man syndrome: incidence, etiology, and prophylaxis. *J Infect Dis* 1991; 164:1180–1185.

3. D.P. Healy, J.V. Sahai, S.H. Fuller, R.E. Polk. Vancomycin-induced histamine release and "red man syndrome": comparison of 1- and 2-hour infusions. *Antimicrob Agents Chemother* 1990; 34:550–554.

4. R. Gruchalla, M. Pirmohamed. Antibiotic allergy. *N Engl J Med* 2006; 354:601–609.

5. T. Limsuwan, P. Demoly. Acute symptoms of drug hypersensitivity (urticaria, angioedema, anaphylaxis, anaphylactic shock). *Med Clin North Am* 2010; 94:691–710.

6. M.J. Torres, M.B. Blanca. The complex picture of β-lactam hypersensitivity: penicillins, cephalosporins, monobactams, carbapenems and clavams. *Med Clin North Am* 2010; 94:805–820.

7. C. Leaute-Labreze, T. Lamireau, D. Chawki, J. Maleville, A. Taïeb. Diagnosis, classification, and management of erythema multiforme and Stevens–Johnson syndrome. *Arch Dis Child* 2000; 83:347–352.

8. R. Solensky, D.A. Khan. Drug allergy: an updated practice parameter. *Ann Allergy Asthma Immunol* 2010; 105:259–273.

9. D. Zamir, G. Groisman, C. Zamir, *et al.* Severe jaundice in a gunshot casualty due to the coexistence of Dubin–Johnson and glucose-6-phosphate dehydrogenase deficiency. *J Clin Gastroenterol* 1999; 28:383–385.

10. H. Nishi, T. Sakaguchi, S. Miyagawa, Y. Yoshikawa, Y. Sawa. Cardiac surgery in patients with Gilbert's syndrome. *J Card Surg* 2012; 27:60–61.

11. E.R. Burka, Z. Weaver, P.A. Marks. Clinical spectrum of hemolytic anemia associated with glucose-6-phosphate dehydrogenase deficiency. *Ann Intern Med* 1966; 64:817–825.

12. C.Q. Edwards. Anemia and the liver: hepato-biliary manifestations of anemia. *Clin Liver Dis* 2002; 6:891–907.

13. A.R. Elyassi, H.H. Rowshan. Perioperative management of the glucose-6-phosphate dehydrogenase deficient patient: a review of literature. *Anesth Prog* 2009; 56:86–91.

14. J.L. Martin, D.J. Plevak, K.D. Flannery, *et al.* Hepatotoxicity after desflurane anesthesia. *Anesthesiology* 1995; 83:1125–1129.

15. P.A. Wu, Y. Balagula, M.E. Lacouture, M.J. Anadkat. Prophylaxis and treatment of dematologic adverse events from epidermal growth factor receptor inhibitors. *Curr Opin Oncol* 2011; 23:343–351.

16. S. Akhtar. Fat embolism. *Anesthesiol Clin* 2009; 27:533–550.

17. M. Grissinger. Preventing serious tissue injury with intravenous promethazine. *Pharmacol Ther* 2009; 34:175–176.

18. N.M. Bohm, J.G. Wong. Bullous dermatosis associated with vancomycin extravasation. *Am J Med Sci* 2012; 343:177–179.

19. T.J. O'Brien, G.D. Cascino, E.L. So, D.R. Hannah. Incidence and clinical consequence of the purple glove syndrome in patients receiving intravenous phenytoin. *Neurology* 1998; 51:1034–1039.

20. S.M. Siddik-Sayyid, W.A. Saasouh, C.E. Mallat, M.T. Aowad. Thermal burn following combined use of forced air and fluid warming devices. *Anaesthesia* 2010; 65:646–656.

21. N.N. Massarweh, N. Cosgriff, D.P. Slakey. Electrosurgery: history, principles, and current and future uses. *J Am Coll Surg* 2006; 202:520–530.

22. D.J. Hubik, A. Connors, H. Cleland. Iatrogenic chemical burns associated with tourniquet use and prep solution *ANZ J Surg* 2009; 79:762–770.

23. E.G. Jones. Recognizing hospital-acquired burn injury in patients after coronary artery bypass surgery. *J Wound Ostomy Continence Nurs* 2011; 38:193–195.

Chapter

31

Jaundice

George Hsu and James W. Heitz

- Jaundice after surgery is rare.
- Hyperbilirubinemia may be divided into pre-hepatic, intra-hepatic, and post-hepatic causes.
- Management of postoperative jaundice is directed at treatment of the underlying cause.
- Many cases of postoperative jaundice are multifactorial.

The term jaundice is derived from *jaune*, the French word for yellow, and denotes yellowish discoloration (icterus) of skin or sclera. Bilirubin is the terminal product of heme catabolism and is the pigment responsible for the yellowing of old bruises; when it accumulates in large quantities in serum, systemic deposition produces jaundice. Normally, 80% of bilirubin is due to catabolism of hemoglobin, producing 250–400 mg of bilirubin daily in the average adult.[1] Unconjugated bilirubin is insoluble in water and undergoes conjugation with glucuronic acid in the liver to allow for excretion in aqueous bile. Hyperbilirubinemia may result from increased bilirubin production, decreased hepatic conjugation, decreased bilirubin excretion, or often a combination of these processes.[2] Serum bilirubin levels above 2 mg/dl may begin to produce jaundice, but it is rarely detected clinically until serum bilirubin levels exceed 3 mg/dl.[3]

Mild postoperative liver dysfunction in surgical patients is common, presumably owing to a combination of sympathetic stimulation, decreased hepatic blood flow, and direct surgical manipulation, but overt jaundice rarely develops. When jaundice is observed it may result from a new perioperative process in surgical patients without pre-existing liver disease or may be due to the exacerbation of pre-existing pathology. The overall incidence of clinical jaundice is less than 1% after general surgery. Abdominal and cardiac procedures have a substantially increased incidence of postoperative jaundice. The incidence of postoperative jaundice after major cardiac procedures ranges between 5% and 55% depending upon the procedure[4] and may average as high as 26.5%.[5]

Although often alarming to patient and family, jaundice is not itself harmful. Jaundice is a non-specific sign in the adult surgical patient that may alert the clinician to either benign or ominous pathology. Prognosis and management is critically dependent upon identification of the underlying pathology.

Post-Anesthesia Care: Symptoms, Diagnosis, and Management, ed. James W. Heitz. Published by Cambridge University Press. © Cambridge University Press 2016.

Table 31.1 Laboratory tests for the evaluation of jaundice

Test	Source	Significance
Bilirubin: total bilirubin, direct bilirubin	Blood	↑total bilirubin = jaundice ↑direct bilirubin = intra-hepatic or post-hepatic ↔direct bilirubin = pre-hepatic cause
Alanine transaminase (ALT) Aspartate transaminase (AST)	Blood	↑ALT & ↑AST = hepatocellular damage ↑ALT<↑↑AST = ethanol ↑↑↑ALT>↑↑AST = viral, shock liver
Alkaline phosphatase (ALP)	Blood	↑↑ALP = cholestasis Non-specific, also ↑ in bone disease
Lactate dehydrogenase (LDH)	Blood	↑LDH = hemolysis Non-specific, also ↑ with severe hepatocellular damage
Haptoglobin	Blood	↑haptoglobin = hemolysis
Coombs' test	Blood	+ in autoimmune hemolysis
Prothrombin time	Blood	Marker of hepatic synthetic function
Albumin	Blood	Marker of hepatic synthetic function
Urobilinogen	Urine	Requires conjugation of bilirubin

Diagnostic evaluation: Postoperative jaundice is evaluated by performing a directed physical exam and obtaining laboratory and additional studies, which need to be interpreted with attention to the individual medical history of the patient. Serum bilirubin levels with both direct (conjugated) and indirect (unconjugated) bilirubin levels confirm the diagnosis of hyperbilirubinemia and provide the first diagnostic clue between pre-hepatic and intra-hepatic or post-hepatic causes. Elevations of primarily unconjugated bilirubin suggest a pre-hepatic etiology. Elevations of the hepatic transaminases alanine transaminase (ALT) and aspartate transaminase (AST) may indicate the presence and degree of hepatic injury, while alkaline phosphatase is more specific to biliary dysfunction.

If pre-hepatic causes such as hemolytic anemias are suspected, additional laboratory testing including hemoglobin, hematocrit, direct and indirect Coombs' test, haptoglobin level, and reticulocyte count may help confirm the diagnosis. Viral serology testing could also establish the diagnosis of viral hepatitis. If biliary obstruction is suspected, right upper quadrant ultrasonography may confirm the initial suspicion from laboratory data.

Pre-hepatic hyperbilirubinemia: Pre-hepatic causes of jaundice occur as a result of an imbalance of bilirubin metabolism producing a relative overproduction of bilirubin. Hemolysis is the most common source of bilirubin overproduction. Bilirubin is produced primarily by the catabolism of hemoglobin from senescent red blood cells (with a small fraction derived from destruction of immature, defective red blood cells in the bone marrow). Only about 15% of bilirubin is derived from non-erythropoietic sources. Under normal circumstances around 1% of red blood cells are replaced daily. More rapid destruction of red blood cells as occurs with hemolytic anemia will therefore markedly increase bilirubin production in proportion to the quality of red blood cells that are hemolyzed.

Postoperative hemolysis may occur owing to a number of diverse etiologies. Hemolysis may be secondary to sickle cell disease or glucose-6-phosphate dehydrogenase (G6PD) deficiency among patients with pre-existing red blood cell pathology. Autoimmune medication-induced hemolysis may occur as a result of the introduction of new medications perioperatively. Although over 125 medications have been identified as causing autoimmune hemolysis, penicillins and cephalosporins are the most frequently encountered in the surgical patient.[6] If blood transfusion has occurred, acute hemolytic transfusion reaction or delayed hemolytic transfusion reaction may cause hemolysis, but delayed reactions are rarely implicated in causing jaundice. Rarely, massive blood transfusion could also overwhelm the conjugation mechanism by the liver and lead to jaundice without the overt transfusion reaction.[7] Mechanical destruction of red blood cells may occur because of stress upon the red blood cell during cardiopulmonary bypass, intra-aortic balloon pump counterpulsation, or passage through left ventricular assist devices, extracorporeal membrane oxygenators, and mechanical valves. Hemolysis is usually mild and peripheral blood smears typically show red blood cell fragments (schistocytes). Pre-existing hemoglobinopathies which are not typically associated with hemolytic crisis, such as thalassemias, may increase red blood cell fragility and hemolysis risk during major cardiac procedures.[8] Reabsorption of heme from large hematomas or gastrointestinal bleeding may also cause pre-hepatic jaundice. Lastly, unconjugated hyperbilirubinemia may produce kernicterus in infants characterized by icteric discoloration of the basal ganglia and bilirubin-mediated neurotoxicity. Kernicterus is very rarely observed in adults.[9]

Although clinically useful for categorizing and managing jaundice, the division between pre-hepatic, intra-hepatic, or post-hepatic is seldom mutually exclusive. Most cases of postoperative jaundice have components of each. Hemolysis often does not cause jaundice since the liver is able to compensate for increased bilirubin production. Hemolysis will cause jaundice if increased bilirubin production exposes diminished hepatic capacity. The clinical importance of the interrelationship between production, conjugation, and excretion and the difficulty it presents in neatly separating jaundice into pre-hepatic, intra-hepatic, or post-hepatic etiologies is best exemplified by Gilbert's syndrome.

Gilbert's syndrome: Familial non-hemolytic jaundice or unconjugated benign bilirubinemia is most commonly referred to by the eponym Gilbert's syndrome. An inherited defect of the *UGT1A1* gene leads to impaired production of the bilirubin uridine diphosphate glucuronosyltransferase (bilirubin-UGT) enzyme responsible for hepatic glucuronidation of unconjugated bilirubin. The syndrome is common and affects about 6% of the population.[10] Affected individuals typically have severely diminished glucuronosyltransferase activity (~30% normal) and develop jaundice with minor stress including fasting, fever, or emotional stress. Surgical patients with Gilbert's syndrome often have modest levels of unconjugated bilirubin prior to surgery but become symptomatic from perioperative stress. Jaundice without dark urine or elevated urobilinogen should raise suspicion for Gilbert's syndrome, and the diagnosis is confirmed by a moderately elevated level of unconjugated bilirubin in the absence of other laboratory abnormalities. Treatment is supportive and aimed at reversing the underlying precipitating factor such as fever and infection.[11,12] Although the actual pathophysiological lesion of Gilbert's syndrome is intra-hepatic, failure of the liver to increase the conjugation of bilirubin produces pre-hepatic pattern laboratory abnormalities with minimal increases in unconjugated bilirubin production, which would be otherwise trivial in unaffected individuals.

Intra-hepatic hyperbilirubinemia

Intra-hepatic causes of jaundice involve direct injury to the hepatocytes. Classic laboratory findings induced marked elevation of hepatic transaminases with modest elevation or normal values of alkaline phosphatase. Hypoperfusion due to prolonged hypotension, congestive heart failure, and sepsis may cause ischemic injury to the hepatocytes. Viral hepatitis is also associated with blood transfusion and IV drug users. Alcohol is a direct toxin to the liver, while a history of alcohol abuse may suggest chronic hepatic insult leading to cirrhosis. Acetaminophen is directly hepatotoxic and presents a unique risk to the surgical patient. Acetaminophen is frequently prescribed postoperatively and since it is also contained in other products in combination with codeine, hydrocodone, oxycodone, or tramadol, clinical caution must be exercised not to inadvertently prescribe acetaminophen from multiple products. Inhaled anesthetics have also been implicated in cases of postoperative jaundice.

Halothane hepatotoxicity and hepatitis: Very rarely, inhalational anesthetics can cause hepatitis leading to jaundice. Shortly after the introduction and widespread use of halothane, reports of hepatotoxicity related to its use appeared and led to the recognition of halothane hepatitis.[13–16] Two distinct types of hepatitis from inhalational agents have been described. The first form, also known as halothane hepatotoxicity, is more common, clinically mild, and thought to be related to the formation and accumulation of hepatotoxic intermediate metabolites (trifluoroacetyl acid). Elevations in AST and ALT are typically mild and the clinical progression self-limited. The other progressive and fulminant form of hepatic injury, commonly known as "halothane hepatitis," may be immune-mediated and is idiosyncratic. It is characterized by mass hepatic necrosis with marked elevation in AST, ALT, and bilirubin. The mortality rate is extremely high (50–75%) with an incidence of between 1:10,000 and 1:35,000. Risk factors include previous exposure to the inhalational agent, obesity, and female sex (two fold risk vs. male gender). The immunological nature of halothane hepatitis is supported by clinical symptoms of fever, rash, eosinophilia, and antibodies to hepatocytes.[17]

Hepatic injury from halothane has been reported more than 500 times, and halothane remains a source of potential hepatic injury in developing nations.[17] Fortunately, more modern volatile anesthetics have a lesser potential for hepatic injury. Nonetheless, there are sporadic reports of hepatitis from isoflurane,[18–25] desflurane,[26–31] and sevoflurane.[32–37]

It should be noted that "halothane hepatitis" is a diagnosis of exclusion. Other causes of hepatitis must be systematically excluded first. Definitive diagnosis is made by clinical suspicion and laboratory evidence of liver injury. A liver biopsy is usually not necessary for diagnosis, but the presence of centrilobular necrosis supports the diagnosis of halothane hepatitis.

Post-hepatic hyperbilirubinemia

Post-hepatic jaundice, or obstructive jaundice, includes instances of failure to excrete conjugated bilirubin. Cholestasis may be intra-hepatic and associated with elevations of alkaline phosphatase with minimal disturbance of hepatic transaminases. Intra-hepatic

Table 31.2 Differential diagnosis of postoperative jaundice

Pre-hepatic	Intra-hepatic	Post-hepatic (biliary)
Hemolytic anemia (hemolysis) Transfusion-related Hereditary spherocytosis Sickle cell Thalassemia G6PD deficiency Medication-induced Multiple/mass transfusion Blood reabsorption Hematoma Gastrointestinal bleeding Mechanical RBC destruction Cardiopulmonary bypass Intra-aortic balloon pump Left ventricular assist device ECMO Mechanical valve	Hypoperfusion/ischemia Perioperative hypotension Sepsis Surgical ligation of hepatic artery Congestive heart failure Budd–Chiari syndrome Infection Viral hepatitis (A, B, C) Hepatic abscess Drugs Acetaminophen overdose Medications Ethanol Alcoholic hepatitis Fatty liver Cirrhosis Fatty liver disease (non-alcoholic) Steatosis Fatty liver of pregnancy Genetic liver disease Gilbert' syndrome α-antitrypsin deficiency Hemochromatosis Wilson's disease Hepatitis from inhaled anesthetics Tumor Hepatocellular carcinoma Metastasis Systemic disease Sarcoidosis Amyloidosis	Biliary obstruction Postoperative cholecystitis Pancreatitis Retained common duct stone Bile duct injury Bile duct stricture Biliary stasis Cholestasis from TPN Cholestasis of pregnancy Immune/autoimmune hepatitis Sclerosing cholangitis Primary biliary cirrhosis

RBC, red blood cells; ECMO, extracorporporeal membrane oxygenation; TPN, total parenteral nutrition.

cholestasis is observed after major abdominal and cardiac procedures, several weeks of total parenteral nutrition, or with pregnancy-induced cholestasis. Cholestasis may also be extra-hepatic and associated with biliary obstruction. Biliary obstruction secondary to non-calculus cholelithiasis, choledocholithiasis, retained bile duct stone, and biliary stasis is common postoperatively from biliary and abdominal surgery. A mixed pattern of cholestasis and hepatocellular jaundice with elevation of both transaminases and alkaline phosphatase is often observed. Less frequently, common bile duct stricture secondary to recurrent pancreatitis or bile duct tumor may also cause jaundice.

Medications: Many medications, including those commonly used in the perioperative period, can trigger jaundice (Table 31.3). They cause jaundice via hemolysis, direct

Table 31.3 Perioperative medications associated with jaundice

Common perioperative medications causing hemolysis/hepatotoxicity/cholestasis
Acetaminophen
Alcohol
Allopurinol
Amiodarone
Aspirin
Calcium channel blockers
Captopril
Carbamazepine
Cephalosporins
Cyclosporine
Dantrolene
Enalapril
Erythromycin
Hydralazine
Insulin
Iron sulfate
Isoniazid
IV contrast dye
Niacin
Non-steroidal anti-inflammatory drugs
Penicillin and derivatives
Sodium thiopental
Steroid oral contraceptives
Sulfonamides
Tamoxifen
Tetracycline
Total parenteral nutrition
Valproic acid

hepatocellular toxicity, cholestasis, or a combination thereof. Penicillins, cephalosporins, and non-steroidal anti-inflammatory drugs (NSAIDs) such as ibuprofen have been associated with intravascular hemolysis. Others include insulin, hydralazine, sodium thiopental, and IV contrast. As mentioned, acetaminophen can unmask underlying hepatic insufficiency by causing direct hepatocellular toxicity, and it has also been associated with hemolysis.

Benign postoperative intra-hepatic cholestasis: Jaundice is frequently encountered on postoperative day 2 or 3. Marked elevations of bilirubin (direct > indirect) and alkaline phosphatase are common. Icterus may be pronounced, but other constitutional symptoms including fever are absent.[37] The etiology is probably multifactorial, but prognosis is usually good.

Postoperative jaundice is a non-specific sign caused by a variety of clinical entities. The division of pre-hepatic, intra-hepatic, and post-hepatic causes may help guide the clinician in obtaining appropriate laboratory and imaging studies in establishing the diagnosis, although pathology is often not mutually exclusive and sometimes multifactorial. Ultimately, identification of the underlying pathology will determine management and prognosis of the jaundice.

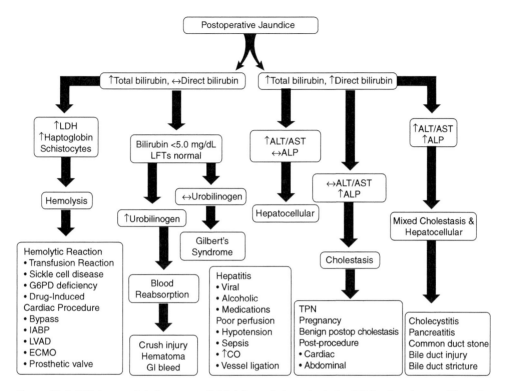

Figure 31.1 IABP, intra-aortic balloon pump; LVAD, left ventricular assist device; LFT, liver function test; CO, cardiac output.

References

1. P.D. Berk, R.B. Howe, J.R. Bloomer, N.I. Berlin. Studies of bilirubin kinetics in normal adults. *J Clin Invest* 1969; 48:2176–2190.

2. J.T. LaMoung, K.J. Isselbacher. Current concepts. Postoperative jaundice. *N Engl J Med* 1973; 288:305–307.

3. S.P. Roche, R. Kobos. Jaundice in the adult patient. *Am Fam Physician* 2004; 69:299–304.

4. E. Lockey, N. McIntyre, D.N. Ross, E.W.A. Brookes, M.F. Sturridge. Early jaundice after open-heart surgery. *Thorax* 1967; 22:165–169.

5. A. Mastoraki, E. Karatzis, S. Mastoraki, *et al.* Postoperative jaundice after cardiac surgery. *Hepatobiliary Pancreat Dis Int* 2007; 6:383–387.

6. G. Garratty. Immune hemolytic anemia associated with drug therapy. *Blood Rev* 2010; 24:143–150.

7. V. Bansal, V.D. Schuchert. Jaundice in the Intensive Care Unit. *Surg Clin N Am* 2006; 86:1495–1502.

8. V. Cokkinou, A. Katsiyanni, M. Orkopoulou, *et al.* Evidence of increased hemolysis after open heart surgery in patients heterozygous for beta-thalassemia. *Tex Heart Inst J* 1988; 15:35–38.

9. M. Waser, P. Kleihues, P. Frick. Kernicterus in an adult. *Ann Neurol* 1986; 19:595–598.

10. D. Owens, J. Evans. Population studies on Gilbert's syndrome. *J Med Genet* 1975; 12:152–156.

11. N.W. Quinn, J.L. Gollan. Jaundice following oral surgery: Gilberts

syndrome. *Br J Oral Surg* 1975;
12:285–288.

12. S. Taylor. Gilbert's syndrome as a cause of postoperative jaundice. *Anaesthesia* 1984; 39:1222–1224.

13. J. Lindenbaum, E. Leifer. Hepatic necrosis associated with halothane anesthesia. *N Engl J Med* 1963; 268:525–530.

14. G.L. Brody, R.B. Sweet. Halothane anesthesia as a possible cause of massive hepatic necrosis. *Anesthesiology* 1963; 24:29–37.

15. W.J. Heidenberg, I. Torio. Additional case of halothane hepatitis. *N Engl J Med* 1963; 268:1090–1091.

16. N.C. Kerbel, I.M. Hilliard. Halothane hepatotoxicity. *Can Med Assoc J* 1963; 89:944–946.

17. P. Habibollahi, N. Mahboobi, S. Esmaeli, S. Safari. Halothane-induced hepatitis: a forgotten issue in developing countries. *Hepat Mon* 2011; 11:3–6.

18. S.D. Malnick, K. Mahlab, J. Borchardt, N. Sokolowski, M. Attali. Acute cholestatic hepatitis after exposure to isoflurane. *Ann Pharmacother* 2002; 36:261–263.

19. D.J. Meldrum, R. Griffiths, J.G. Kenna. Gallstones and isoflurane hepatitis. *Anaesthesia* 1998; 53:905–909.

20. E. Ihtiyar, C. Algin, A. Haciolu, S. Isiksoy. Fatal isoflurane hepatotoxicity without re-exposure. *Indian J Gastroenterol* 2006; 25:41–42.

21. R.H. Thill, K.W. Millikan, A. Doolas. Isoflurane hepatitis. *Infect Med* 1996; 13:322–324.

22. G.B. Turner, D. O'Rourke, G.O. Scott, T.R. Beringer. Fatal hepatotoxicity after re-exposure to isoflurane: a case report and review of the literature. *Eur J Gastroenterol Hepatol* 2000; 12:955–959.

23. J.L. Martin, M.T. Keegan, G.M. Vasdev, *et al.* Fatal hepatitis associated with isoflurane exposure and CYP2A6 autoantibodies. *Anesthesiology* 2001; 95:551–553.

24. F. Hasan. Isoflurane hepatotoxicity in a patient with a previous history of halothane-induced hepatitis. *Hepatogastroenterology* 1998; 45:518–522.

25. L.J. Peiris, A. Agrawal, J.E. Morris, P.S. Basnyat. Isoflurane hepatitis-induced liver failure: a case report. *J Clin Anesth* 2012; 24:477–479.

26. J.S. Anderson, N.R. Rose, J.L. Martin, E.I. Eger, D.B. Njoku. Desflurane hepatitis associated with hapten and autoantigen-specific IgG4 antibodies. *Anesth Analg* 2007; 104:1452–1453.

27. J. Katz, J. Magee, B. Baker, E.I. Eger. Hepatic necrosis associated with herpesvirus after anesthesia with desflurane and nitrous oxide. *Anesth Analg* 1994; 78:1173–1176.

28. D. Tung, E.M. Yoshida, C.S. Wang, U.P. Steinbrecher. Severe desflurane hepatotoxicity after colon surgery in an elderly patient. *Can J Anaesth* 2005; 52:133–136.

29. J.L. Martin, D.J. Plevak, K.D. Flannery. Hepatotoxicity after desflurane anesthesia. *Anesthesiology* 1995; 83:1125–1129.

30. T.M. Berghaus, A. Baron, A. Geier. Hepatotoxicity following desflurane anesthesia. *Hepatology* 1999; 29:613–614.

31. T. Nelson. Desflurane-induced hepatitis. *Internet J Anesthesiol.* 2012; 30(3).

32. A. Reich, A.S. Everding, M. Bulla, *et al.* Hepatitis after sevoflurane exposure in an infant suffering from primary hyperoxaluria type 1. *Anesth Analg* 2004; 99:370–372.

33. Y. Jang, I. Kim. Severe hepatotoxicity after sevoflurane anesthesia in a child with mild renal dysfunction. *Paediatr Anaesth* 2005; 15:1140–1144.

34. E. Turillazzi, S. D'Errico, M. Neri, *et al.* A fatal case of fulminant hepatic necrosis following sevoflurane anesthesia. *Toxicol Pathol* 2007; 35:840–845.

35. A. Lehmann, M. Nehe, A.H. Kiessling, *et al.* Case report: fatal hepatic failure after aortic valve replacement and sevoflurane exposure. *Can J Anaesth* 2007; 54:917–921.

36. S. Shinghal, T. Gray, G. Guzman,
A. Verma, K. Anand. Sevoflurane
hepatotoxicity: a case report of sevoflurane
hepatic necrosis and review of the
literature. *Am J Ther* 2010; 1:219–222.

37. M. Schmid, M.L. Hefti, R. Gattiker,
H.J. Kistler, A. Senning. Benign
postoperative intrahepatic
cholestasis. *N Engl J Med* 1965;
272:545–550.

Chapter

32

Visual disturbance

James W. Heitz

- Ocular injury is uncommon after non-ophthalmological surgery.
- Corneal abrasions are the most common ocular injury.
- Severe eye pain associated with nausea or emesis requires urgent consultation.
- Postoperative visual loss may result in painless blindness.
- Cardiac surgery and spine surgery in the prone position are the most common procedures associated with postoperative visual loss.

Unless access is needed to the eyes or the immediately surrounding structures during surgery, eyes are typically taped shut during general anesthesia. This prevents desiccation and the resulting corneal disruption that accompanies drying, and limits the opportunity for direct mechanical trauma. However, the eyes are still vulnerable to direct mechanical trauma before and after the tape is removed or may still be injured even while taped by pressure upon the globe, changes in perfusion during disturbances in hemodynamics, changes in intraocular pressure caused by positioning, or the pharmacological effects of medications administered.

Ocular injuries during non-ophthalmological surgery are believed to be rare. A retrospective review of approximately 61,000 anesthetics identified only 31 ocular injuries for an incidence of only 0.056%.[1] However, because of the relative importance of vision, ocular issues are the fifth most common cause of litigation reflected in the American Society of Anesthesiologists (ASA)Closed Claimed Database, accounting for 4% of settlements against anesthesiologists, with the seventh highest median payout.[2] It is important that ocular problems be identified after surgery and properly managed to limit further injury, preserve vision, and avoid litigation when possible (Table 32.1).

Eye pain/foreign body sensation: Although an ocular foreign body sensation may be due to an actual foreign body, such as an errant eyelash, most postoperative foreign body sensation is caused by corneal abrasion or inflammation. The absence of a visible foreign body on inspection should raise the clinical suspicion for corneal abrasion. Signs and symptoms of corneal inclusion may include irritation, pain, burning sensation, blurred vision, grittiness, tearing, a foreign body sensation, or circumcorneal sclera hyperemia. The cornea may be mechanically abraded by contact of the unprotected globe with an

Post-Anesthesia Care: Symptoms, Diagnosis, and Management, ed. James W. Heitz. Published by Cambridge University Press. © Cambridge University Press 2016.

Table 32.1 Differential diagnosis of postoperative visual disturbance

	Eye pain	Redness	Foreign body sensation	Tearing	Photophobia	Change in acuity	Eye involvement	Key sign or symptom
Corneal abrasion	Yes	Yes	Yes	Yes	Yes	Variable	Typically unilateral	Foreign body sensation
Acute glaucoma	Yes	Yes	No	Yes	Yes	Yes	Unilateral, maybe bilateral	Anisocoria, emesis
Chemical keratitis	Yes	Yes	No	Yes	Often	Variable	Typically unilateral	Corneal discoloration, gray or white
Hemorrhagic retinopathy of Valsalva	No	No	No	No	No	Yes	Unilateral, maybe bilateral	Patient sees red
Cortical blindness	No	No	No	No	No	Blindness	Bilateral	Patient may be indifferent
Central retinal artery occlusion	No	Maybe	No	No	No	Blindness	Unilateral	Pale retina, may have external signs of trauma
Anterior ischemic optic neuropathy	No	No	No	No	No	Yes, variable. Blurriness, scotoma, or blindness	Unilateral	May have optic changes on fundoscopic examination
Posterior ischemic optic neuropathy	No	No	No	No	No	Yes, variable. Blurriness, scotoma, or blindness	Bilateral, maybe unilateral in 1/3	Fundoscopic examination may be normal initially
Glycine infusion syndrome	No	No	No	No	No	Blindness	Bilateral	After transurethral prostate resection or myomectomy where glycine-containing infusions have been used
Posterior reversible encephalopathy syndrome	No	No	No	No	No	Yes	Bilateral	Hypertension, headache, altered mental status, and seizures

Figure 32.1 Corneal abrasion.

Drying   Mechanical abrasion

instrument (such as an identification badge worn by personnel leaning over the face, or the anesthetic facemask) or by epithelial injury caused by drying. Blinking serves to lubricate and protect the eyes, and the loss of the blinking reflex during anesthesia renders the eye vulnerable.

In a study of 200 patients having general anesthesia and non-ophthalmological surgery in the supine position, 100 patients were randomized to eye taping (standard care), and 100 patients were randomized to no eye care.[3] Of the 100 patients with no eye care, 41 had natural eye closure after induction of anesthesia. Of the 59 patients with eyes partially open during surgery, only 3 developed symptomatic corneal abrasions, although 26 had evidence of epithelial injury on slit lamp examination. None of the patients in the eye taping group had corneal injury. Although this study has been often cited inappropriately to support an incidence of corneal abrasion of 44% (26 of 59) during general anesthesia, the incidence of subclinical corneal injury even without routine eye care was only 26% and frank corneal abrasion only 3%. Longer surgeries or surgeries performed in positions other than supine would probably carry higher risk.

The diagnosis of corneal abrasion can be confirmed by either slit lamp examination or fluorescein staining and Wood's lamp examination, if the prerequisite equipment is available. The presence of abrasion is diagnostic and its pattern suggestive of the etiology of the abrasion. Corneal abrasions caused by incomplete eye closure and drying tend to be complete or incomplete semicircular linear disruptions below or along the lower aspect of the pupil, mechanical abrasions are typically straight or irregularly shaped abrasions anywhere on the globe (see Figure 32.1). A confused and sleepy patient rubbing his/her eyes after surgery may inadvertently self-inflict a corneal abrasion, particularly if a pulse oximeter is worn on the first finger of the dominant hand. It should be emphasized that pupil size should be equal in the setting of corneal abrasion. Eye pain, unequal pupil size, and photophobia should raise suspicion for acute glaucoma.

Corneal abrasion management: Although prevention is preferable to treatment, most corneal abrasions heal spontaneously within 48 hours without sequela. Ophthalmological treatment may consist of antibiotic drops (to prevent bacterial infection), topical analgesics, lubricants, or patching of the affected eye. Deeper abrasions or abrasions that become frank corneal ulcerations may cause scarring and permanent visual impairment and require consultation.

Blurry vision: Blurry vision after surgery is common. This may be caused by the purposeful installation of lubricants onto the surface of the eye to retard drying or from the pharmacological effects of perioperative medications upon focus and ocular accommodation. A scopolamine patch applied prior to surgery for prophylaxis against postoperative nausea and vomiting may be causative, but many perioperative medications may affect vision. Blurred vision occurring in a patient with a history of diabetes mellitus or pancreatic surgery warrants exclusion of acute hyperglycemia.

Blurry vision lasting more than 3 days occurs at approximately 1 in 20,000 patients when measured retrospectively,[1] but many patients may not report visual changes so retrospective databases may underestimate the incidence. When followed prospectively, 28 of 671 patients (4.2%) had blurred vision lasting at least 3 days after various surgical procedures, with most of the affected patients having resolution at 1 to 2 months.[4] For the patients in this study with blurred vision at 3 days, 25% still had changes at 18 months and required either new or different corrective lenses. The etiology of persistent visual changes after non-ophthalmological surgery is poorly understood. Treatment is supportive care with particular focus on preventing a sedated patient from causing ocular injury by eye rubbing. Persistent blurry vision lasting more than a few days may require consultation.

Anisocoria: Unequal pupil size (if not present prior to surgery) and eye pain may be acute glaucoma, a true ophthalmological emergency. Medications with anticholinergic effects may precipitate closed angle glaucoma. The pupil in the affected eye is typically mid-range size and poorly or non-reactive to light. In addition to pain and blurry vision, the patient may experience severe headache, nausea and vomiting, or loss of peripheral vision, or may see a halo around light sources. Treatment requires urgent ophthalmological consultation.

Inflammation: Inflammation of the cornea (keratitis) or cornea and conjunctiva (keratoconjunctivitis) has a variety of etiologies, but when it occurs acutely after surgery it is typically secondary to installation of irritant substances into the eye. Many substances may be inadvertently splashed into the eye, with acidic or alkaline substances having the greatest potential to cause irritation. Skin preparations including alcohol-based compounds and chlorhexidine can cause chemical keratitis when applied around the face if pooling is allowed to occur around the eye. Povidone–iodine (Betadine) is relatively innocuous when in contact with the eye. Treatment requires consultation.

Seeing red: An unusual ocular injury is hemorrhagic retinopathy (Valsalva retinopathy) caused by forceful exhalation against closed glottis causing the affected individual to see "red." This may also occur from "bucking" during mechanical ventilation if the patient attempts to exhale while a mandatory positive pressure breath is being delivered. Fundoscopic examination will reveal hemorrhage and the lesion should be suspected for patients complaining of "seeing red" or reddish discoloration of vision after general anesthesia. Ophthalmological consultation is prudent, but treatment is usually supportive.

Diplopia: Diplopia (double vision) may occur after surgery. Residual neuromuscular blockade may interfere with extraocular muscle movement, causing diplopia. Aggressive hydration with crystalloid solutions has been implicated in transient postoperative diplopia in cardiac surgery patients.[5] Diplopia in a single eye is indicative of an ocular cause (retinal detachment, lens dislocation), and treatment requires ophthalmological consultation. Diplopia in both eyes suggests an extraocular muscle etiology. Raising the head of the bed to facilitate edema resolution and ensuring adequate neuromuscular blockade reversal is adequate for most patients.

Blindness: Transient blindness may occur from systemic absorption of glycine used in irrigation solutions during transurethral prostate resection or procedures on the uterus, since glycine acts as an inhibitory neurotransmitter of the retina. Treatment is supportive and includes correction of other electrolyte abnormalities that may accompany irrigation solution absorption. Permanent blindness may occur after surgery owing to damage to the eye, optic nerve, or visual cortex of the brain. Cortical blindness has occasionally been reported owing to embolic cerebrovascular accident,[6–10] and patients may present with bilateral blindness without visual abnormalities of the external eye or retina. Patients with cortical blindness may not report their blindness and may deny being blind when questioned.

Central retinal vein or artery occlusion may occur after surgery, particularly if pressure is exerted upon the globe during the procedure. Procedures performed in prone or lateral position carry increased risk. Often there may be signs of external ocular trauma.[11,12] Although the eyes are vulnerable to compression injury any time the procedure is performed in other than supine position, direct ocular compression is an atypical cause of postoperative blindness.

Most postoperative visual loss (POVL) is due to injury of the optic nerve. The etiology is still incompletely understood, but disturbances in nerve perfusion appear to be responsible. Anterior ischemic optic neuropathy (AION) occurs within the intraorbital portion of the optic nerve. Perioperative AION is most commonly seen after procedures requiring cardiopulmonary bypass and among patients with risk factors for vascular disease. It is typically monocular and only a portion of the visual field may be affected. Although pressure on the globe could theoretically be causal, AION is most often seen after surgery in the supine position. Perioperative posterior ischemic optic neuropathy (PION) occurs because of ischemia of the optic nerve after it has exited the orbit. Spine surgery in the prone position is particularly high risk. Pressure on the globe is not believed to be able to cause PION. The American Society of Anesthesiologists Task Force of Postoperative Visual Loss found no evidence to implicate pressure on the globe as causing perioperative AION or PION, although it is a substantiated risk factor for central retinal artery occlusion.[13] Compared with AION, patients experiencing PION tend to be younger, healthier, and undergoing procedures that are longer and associated with greater blood loss. However, hypotension and anemia do not seem to be causative,[14] and disturbances in microperfusion and venous drainage from intravascular volume expansion may be associated. Although spine surgery in the prone position and cardiac procedures requiring cardiopulmonary bypass are considered higher risk, POVL may occur after any surgical procedure, and there is some more recent evidence that total hip replacement and, to a lesser extent, total knee replacement procedures also carry increased risk for visual loss.[15]

Retinal changes may be seen fundoscopically earlier in the course of AION than PION. Treatment of POVL requires ophthalmological consultation, and cases of POVL occurring in the United States should be reported to the ASA POVL Registry (http://depts.washing ton.edu/asaccp/projects/postoperative-visual-loss-registry).

Posterior reversible encephalopathy syndrome (PRES) is a rare syndrome characterized by visual loss associated with headaches, confusion, and seizures. Magnetic resonance imaging reveals edema in the occipital lobes and sometimes parietal lobes and pons. PRES is classically associated with malignant hypertension and eclampsia, but has been associated with nephrotic syndrome, immunosuppressant medications used in organ transplantation (especially cyclosporine and tacrolimus), sepsis, and systemic lupus erythematosus.[16] The incidence and exact pathophysiology of PRES is not known, but there have been an increasing number of reports of PRES presenting in the PACU in both print literature and presentation at national anesthesiology meetings. Several of these early reports have occurred in patients with seemingly mild elevations of systemic blood pressure. Visual disturbance associated with altered mental status and seizures should raise suspicion for PRES. While a CT scan without contrast may be clinically appropriate to exclude subarachnoid hemorrhage, it is important to note that the CT scan is normally unremarkable in patients with PRES. Magnetic resonance imaging should be obtained. Blood pressure reduction of 20% to 25% is indicated when PRES is identified. Short-acting agents that can be administered by intravenous infusion (see Chapter 3) and continuous blood pressure monitoring by arterial line should be instituted.

References

1. S. Roth, R.A. Thisted, J.P. Erickson, S. Black, B.D. Schreider. Eye injuries after non-ocular surgery: a study of 60,945 anesthetics from 1988 to 1992. *Anesthesiology* 1996; 85:1020–1027.

2. R.A. Caplan, L.A. Lee, K.B. Domino. *ASA Closed Claims Project and Its Registries: Value to Patients and Pocketbook.* ASA Refresher Courses, 2008, p. 433.

3. Y.K. Batra, I.M. Bali. Corneal abrasions during general anesthesia. *Anesth Analg* 1977; 56:363–365.

4. M.E. Warner, P.J. Fronapfel, J.R. Hebl, *et al.* Perioperative visual changes. *Anesthesiology* 2002; 96:855–859.

5. M.A. Abbott, A.D. McLaren, T. Algie. Intra-ocular pressure during cardiopulmonary bypass: a comparison of crystalloid and colloid priming solutions. *Anaesthesia* 1994; 49:343–346.

6. J.J. Gelinas, R. Cherry, S.J. MacDonald. Fat embolism syndrome after cementless total hip arthroplasty. *J Arthroplasty* 2000; 15:809–813.

7. E.T. Crosby, R. Preston. Obstetrical anesthesia for a parturient with preeclampsia, HELLP syndrome and acute cortical blindness. *Can J Anaesth* 1998; 45:452–459.

8. S. Della Sala, H. Spinnler. Anton's (-Redlich-Babinski's) syndrome associated with Dide–Botcazo's syndrome: a case report of denial of cortical blindness and amnesia. *Schweiz Arch Neurol Psychiatr* 1998; 139:5–15.

9. A.P. Amar, M.L. Levy, S.L. Giannotta. Iatrogenic vertebrobasilar insufficiency after surgery of the subclavian or brachial artery: review of three cases. *Neurosurgery* 1998; 43:1450–1457.

10. T. Chaudhry, M.C. Chamberlain, H. Vila. Unusual case of postoperative blindness. *Anesthesiology* 2006; 106:869–870.

11. N. Kumar, S. Jivan, N. Topping, A.J. Morrell. Blindness and rectus muscle damage following spinal surgery. *Am J Ophthalmol* 2004; 138:889–891.

12. M.J. Halfon, P. Bonardo, S. Valiensi, *et al.* Central retinal artery occlusion and ophthalmoplegia following spinal surgery. *Br J Ophthalmol* 2004; 88: 1350–1352.

13. Practice Advisory for Perioperative Visual Loss Associated with Spine Surgery: an updated report by the American Society of Anesthesiologists Task Force on Perioperative Visual Loss. *Anesthesiology* 2012; 116:274–285.

14. M.A. Myers, S.R. Hamilton, A.J. Bogosian, C.H. Smith, T.A. Wagner. Visual loss as a complication of spine surgery: a review of 37 cases. *Spine* 1997; 22:1325–1329.

15. Y. Shen, M. Drum, S. Roth. The prevalence of perioperative visual loss in the United States: a 10-year study from 1996 to 2005 of spinal, orthopedic, cardiac, and general surgery. *Anesthesiology* 2009; 109:1534–1545.

16. J.E. Fugate, D.O. Claassen, H.J. Cloft *et al.* Posterior reversible encephalopathy syndrome: associated clinical and radiologic findings. *Mayo Clin Proc* 2010; 85:427–432.

Neuropathy

Brian Lai and John T. Wenzel

- Postoperative neuropathy has a variety of etiologies in the perioperative period, both surgical and non-surgical.
- Neuropathy may present as pain, weakness, or sensory deficits, often paresthesia with numbness or "pins and needles" sensation.
- History and physical exam may help to localize the level of the injury and suggest a specific etiology.
- Management and prognosis will depend on the etiology and extent of the nerve injury, and may necessitate the involvement of other consultants or intervention.

Peripheral nerve injury with neuropathy following a surgical procedure is a known complication, and may present as pain, weakness, or sensory deficits. Paresthesia is a common symptom, defined as an unpleasant alteration in sensation that produces a feeling of pain or tingling commonly described as "pins and needles."[1] If large-diameter neural axons are primarily involved, the perception is typically tingling; if small-diameter axons are involved, the perception is typically pain.[2]

Common etiologies of postoperative neuropathy include ischemic, compressive, stretch, contusion, transection, and inflammatory insults.[3] Depending on the location of the lesion, symptoms may follow dermatomal/myotomal patterns or the distribution of individual peripheral nerve(s). Inflammatory neuropathy may be a common yet poorly understood and difficult to recognize etiology; symptoms may be spatiotemporally separated from the surgical site and may be focal, multifocal, or diffuse.[3] In the surgical patient, nerve injury may be the result of surgical, non-surgical, positioning, or medication-related influences. Diagnosis and management of neuropathic symptoms include a focused history and physical exam to determine the likely etiology, which will influence prognosis, patient counseling, and possible consultant involvement (see Figure 33.1).

Postoperative neuropathy

When a patient complains of pain, weakness, or numbness/paresthesia, the first question is whether the symptom began before or after surgery. A thorough preoperative history is necessary for any known preoperative neuropathy to be able to discern new from prior symptoms. If present prior to surgery, the diagnosis and management is beyond the scope

Post-Anesthesia Care: Symptoms, Diagnosis, and Management, ed. James W. Heitz. Published by Cambridge University Press. © Cambridge University Press 2016.

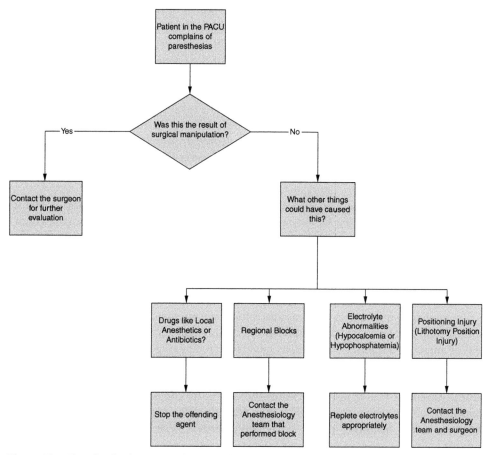

Figure 33.1 Algorithm for determining the cause of postoperative paresthesia.

of this chapter. A new-onset symptom, however, requires a thorough stepwise assessment that begins with a physical exam. The exam should elucidate the nature of the complaint (e.g. numbness, weakness, tingling) as well as the distribution. Symptoms in a specific dermatome or in the distribution of one or more peripheral nerves may aid in localization of the insult. The next step is to attempt to determine whether the paresthesia was caused by surgical manipulation or by some other event in the operating room.

Surgically related postoperative neuropathy

Certain surgical procedures have known implications for neuropathy, and it is helpful to have a high-yield summary of some known associations. For any patient work-up, a discussion with the surgical team regarding their exposure, retraction, and surgical manipulation would likely be of benefit.

In cardiac cases, sternal retraction during median sternotomy has been associated with brachial plexus injuries of variable severity based on location and extent of retraction.[4] Sensory deficits may occur in the leg after saphenous vein harvesting during coronary artery bypass graft (CABG).[5]

During a neck lift, the great auricular nerve can be injured, resulting in decreased sensation in the lower ear with or without paresthesias.[6] During mandibular osteotomies/genioplasty, the mental nerve can be injured, resulting in paresthesias affecting the skin in the anterior aspects of the chin and oral mucosa of the inferior lip.[6,7] For reconstructive surgery for sleep-disordered breathing including uvulopalatopharyngoplasty (UPPP), uvulopalatal flap (UPF), uvulopalatopharyngoglossoplasty (UPPGP), and laser midline glossectomy (LMG), paresthesias can be a complication of the surgical manipulation.[6]

For orbital blow-out fracture repairs, paresthesia due to infraorbital nerve dysfuction was a frequent complication noted.[8] For LeFort osteotomy, paresthesia of the forehead and upper cheek can be due to partial paralysis of cranial nerve II, and V1 and V2 as a result of displacement of bony fragments into the cavernous sinus. These symptoms resolved with a steroid taper.[9]

After dental work, oral paresthesia can be a presenting symptom and may be due to mechanical trauma resulting in damage to the inferior alveolar nerve, a pressure phenomenon due to obturation material or endodontic instruments within the inferior alveolar canal, neurotoxic effects related to solutions used to clear the root canal or solutions used as sealants, or thermal injury.[10] The paresthesia associated with these injuries usually resolves over time with conservative treatment, but in some cases microneurosurgical interventions may be appropriate.[11]

In lumbar spine surgery such as discectomy or microdiscectomy, paresthesias may occur owing to nerve-root irritation from the surgery that may be improved by analgesics and/or muscle relaxants.[6] In lumbar spine or hip surgeries, lateral femoral cutaneous nerve (LFCN) injury may result in an altered sensation known as meralgia paresthetica, described as persistent pain referred to the lateral thigh caused by direct nerve injury or neural ischemia.[12,13] If physical examination suggests compression of the LFCN, then neurolysis of this nerve may be all that is needed. If block of the LFCN eliminates all the pain, both a neurolysis of the LFCN and resection of its posterior branch would be indicated.[13]

This is by no means an exhaustive list, but highlights how surgical manipulation or retraction may risk peripheral nerve injury. Communication with the surgeon may be important in revealing a surgical etiology for a new postoperative neuropathy. In rare cases, the patient may need to return to the operating room to prevent permanent neurological damage.

Non-surgically related postoperative neuropathy

Non-surgically related postoperative neuropathy refers to all other causes that are not directly related to the surgical procedure. Occasionally, these can be related to anesthetic procedures. Transient hypoglossal nerve paralysis has been reportedly caused by endotracheal tube cuff compression.[14] Difficult placement of intravenous or intraarterial catheters may result in direct nerve trauma. As with surgical manipulation, any procedure performed on the patient has the potential for causing a nerve injury. Other non-surgical causes can be due to neuraxial/regional anesthesia blocks, patient positioning, medications, and electrolyte abnormalities.

Neuraxial/regional anesthesia and postoperative neuropathy: Neuropathic issues following neuraxial anesthesia (i.e. epidural, spinal, combined spinal–epidural) may include backache that can be persistent and is possibly related to needle trauma, local anesthetic irritation, or ligamentous strain. Patients may present with postdural puncture headache requiring possible medical management or epidural blood patch. Symptoms concerning for spinal hematoma require prompt diagnosis as emergent spinal decompression increases odds of a good prognosis.[15]

Regional anesthesia blocks may be performed for a variety of surgical procedures as the primary anesthetic or as an adjunct for postoperative analgesia. Assessment of paresthesia in this setting requires knowledge of the intended effects of the regional blockade and identification of any abnormal or unanticipated effects. For upper extremity procedures, where a brachial plexus block is performed, persistent paresthesia can be a complication of the block itself and may last 6 weeks or more.[6] An association has been noted between incidental elicitation of paresthesias and postoperative neurological complications; therefore, it is recommended that intentional elicitation of paresthesia as a neurolocalization technique should be avoided.[16] Nerve injuries in this setting are often multifactorial and involve nerve anatomy, needle insertion site, bevel type, needle tip location, injection pressures, and underlying patient nerve pathology.[17] Regional anesthesia techniques may have further undesired neurological complications due to accidental intravenous, intraarterial, intraneural, or neuraxial injections.

Positioning and postoperative neuropathy: Patient positioning is a collaborative effort between the surgical, anesthesia, and nursing teams in the operating room. Patients under anesthesia are unable to safely adjust their own position, rendering them susceptible to positional nerve injury.

In the supine position, the brachial plexus may be injured at various levels by stretching or compression at the axilla based on head and arm position, especially if the head is abnormally rotated or arms abducted >90 degrees. Padding is required to prevent ischemia from point pressure at bony prominences (e.g. occiput, elbows, heels, sacrum) that may lead to radial, ulnar, or median nerve dysfunction. Appropriate mattress pads are required to disperse point pressure and support the spine, where loss of lumbar curvature or hyperlordosis may result in backache and spinal nerve ischemia, respectively.[15]

In the lateral position, improper positioning may lead to compression of the common peroneal nerve by the legs, poor alignment of the head with the cervical and thoracic spines, or compression of the shoulder and neurovascular bundle in the axilla. Injury to the long thoracic nerve by positioning may lead to serratus anterior muscle dysfunction and winged scapula. Inadequate chest support in the lateral position may lead to suprascapular nerve injury causing shoulder pain.[15]

In the prone position, the eyes and ears are susceptible to injury. Neck pain or limitation of cervical motion can result from unnatural stretch of neck muscles and ligaments. Inappropiate head flexion/extension can compromise cerebral vascular flow. Brachial plexus injuries remain a concern, as is compression of the chest and abdomen.[15]

The lithotomy position, common in urological and gynecological procedures, is associated with paresthesias in the distribution of the obturator, lateral femoral cutaneous, sciatic, and peroneal nerves that were noted within 4 hours of surgery and resolved within 6 months.[18] A motor symptom of common peroneal nerve involvement may be foot drop. Prevention measures that can be taken include minimizing the time in the lithotomy position; using two assistants to coordinate the simultaneous movement of both legs to and from the lithotomy position; avoiding excessive flexion of the hips, extension of the knees, or torsion of the lumbar spine; and avoiding excessive pressure on peroneal nerve at the fibular head.[18]

In any patient position, hemodynamic influences can contribute to ischemic neuropathy. Poor perfusion to a peripheral nerve can be caused by systemic hypotension, compression of an extremity or point pressure at a bony prominence, or a raised limb where arterial pressure is unable to sufficiently perfuse the distal extremity.[15]

Drug-induced postoperative neuropathy: Local anesthetics have been implicated in instances of postoperative neuropathy. Articaine and prilocaine have been associated with persistent paresthesia of the lips, tongue, and oral tissues with slow, incomplete, or no recovery; studies are inconclusive as to the cause.[19] Theories include neurotoxicity from the local anesthetic and needle trauma resulting in nerve injury.[19,20] Systemic local anesthetic toxicity results from systemic absorption, possibly by accidental intravenous or intra-arterial injection, and has a dose-dependent range of symptoms that may begin with circumoral numbness, facial tingling, and tinnitus. Central nervous system (CNS) symptoms progress from irritability, restlessness, vertigo, and slurred speech to tonic-clonic seizures.[20] CNS effects may progress to cardiovascular effects with cardiac arrest that can be refractory to treatment. Vigilance during block placement, frequent aspirations during injection, and close patient monitoring are essential to diagnose local anesthetic toxicity and intervene early to minimize CNS or cardiovascular complications. The American Society of Regional Anesthesia and Pain Medicine Practice Advisory (ASRA) emphasizes primary prevention in reducing the frequency and severity of local anesthetic toxicity.[21]

Nitrofurantoin is another medication that has been associated with paresthesia as reported in case studies. Patients had normal nerve conduction studies, but skin biopsies showed normal intra-epidermal nerve fiber density but with clustered swellings of terminal nerve fibers. Medications such as gabapentin and duloxetine provided some relief.[22]

Immunosuppression is present in many patients undergoing surgical procedures, and may be associated with viral-induced neuropathies. Anesthetics, blood products, and other medications (e.g. antibiotics) have been shown to result in varying degrees of immunosuppression in some patients.[15]

Electrolyte abnormalities and postoperative neuropathy: After a total thyroidectomy or parathyroidectomy, hypocalcemia (total calcium <8.4 mg/dl) in the immediate postoperative period can present with paresthesias as one of the signs and symptoms in addition to muscle spasms, Trousseau's sign, Chvostek's sign, tetany, laryngospasm, bronchospasm, and apnea. Treatment of the hypocalcemia includes 10 to 20 ml calcium gluconate 10% over 10 minutes. Following blood levels and repeating therapy until the clinical signs of hypocalcemia are controlled are key to treating this condition. Continuous positive airway pressure is effective for associated airway obstruction.[6,23]

Severe hypophosphatemia (serum phosphorus <2 mg/dl) is another common postoperative electrolyte abnormality. The two most common causes are intravenous glucose administration and septicemia.[24,25] Symptoms, in addition to paresthesia, can include muscle weakness, lethargy, confusion, disorientation, generalized or Guillain–Barré-like ascending paralysis, seizures, coma, and even death. Treatment involves treating hypocalcemia first, if present, and considering the patient's renal function. The dose of intravenous phosphate should be decreased by 50% if serum creatinine is >2.5 mg/dl. For serum phosphate <2.5 mg/dl, administer 2 mmol/hr over 6 hours. For serum phosphate <0.5 mg/dl, administer 4 mmol/hr over 6 hours. For serum phosphate <1 mg/dl, administer 8 mmol/hr over 6 hours. While treating hypophosphatemia, one needs to monitor serum levels of both phosphate and calcium.[25]

Management of postoperative neuropathy

History and physical exam may point to an etiology for a postoperative paresthesia. Occasionally, the etiology will be unclear. Where possible, vigilance toward prevention is key. The patient may be counseled that most paresthesias are transient and self-limiting.[3] Some cases may require operative intervention and some may require formal neurology consultation for nerve conduction studies, imaging, blood work, or even nerve biopsy.[3] Any patient with a postoperative neuropathy should be followed after discharge for resolution of symptoms and/or continued appropriate management.

New-onset neuropathy, commonly paresthesia, in the postoperative period can be very distressing for the patient and can be very difficult for the healthcare provider to diagnose and manage. Work-up requires a thorough history and physical exam and an understanding of all possible influences in the perioperative period. A stepwise approach can help to elucidate the etiology of the symptom(s), allowing the provider to appropriately counsel the patient or involve other consultants as needed.

References

1. NT Aggarwal, DC Bergen, PA Calbresi, et al. Neurology for the Non-Neurologist. 6th edn. Weiner WJ, Goetz CG, Shin RK, Lewis SL, editors. Philadelphia, PA: Lippincott Williams & Wilkins; 2010.

2. RB Daroff, GM Fenichel, J Jankovic, JC Maziotta. Bradley's Neurology in Clinical Practice. 6th edn. Philadelphia, PA: Elsevier; 2012.

3. NP Staff, JE Engelstad, CJ Klein, et al. Post-surgical inflammatory neuropathy. Brain. 2010; 133: p. 2866–2880.

4. S Healey, B O'Neill, H Bilal, et al. Does retraction of the sternum during median sternotomy result in brachial plexus injuries? Interact Cardiovasc Thorac Surg. 2013 July; 17(1): p. 151–157.

5. UR Nair, G Griffiths, RA Lawson. Postoperative neuralgia in the leg after saphenous vein coronary artery bypass graft: a prospective study. Thorax. 1988 Jan; 43(1):p. 41–43.

6. VJ Adams, JR Adler, C Albanese, et al. Anesthesiologist's Manual of Surgical Procedures. 4th edn. Jaffe RA, Samuels SI, editors. Philadelphia, PA: Lippincott Williams & Wilkins; 2009.

7. KL Moore, AF Dalley. Clinically Oriented Anatomy. 5th edn. Sun B, Scogna KH, Glazer J, Odyniec C, editors. Baltimore, MD: Lippincott Williams & Wilkins; 2006.

8. M Brucoli, F Arcuri, R Cavenaghi, A Benech. Analysis of complications after surgical repair of orbital fractures. J Craniofac Surg. 2011 July; 22(4): p. 1387–1390.

9. JW Kim, BR Chin, HS Park, SH Lee, TG Kwon. Cranial nerve injury after Le Fort I osteotomy. Int J Oral Maxillofac Surg. 2011 March; 40(3): p. 327–329.

10. TMS Marques, JM Gomes. Decompression of inferior alveolar nerve: case report. J Can Dent Assoc. 2011 March; 77: p. b34.

11. MA Pogrel, R Jergensen, E Burgon, D Hulme. Long-term outcome of trigeminal nerve injuries related to dental treatment. J Oral Maxillofac Surg. 2011 September; 69(9): p. 2284–2288.

12. T Kiyama, M Naito, K Shiramizu, T Shinoda, A Maeyama. Ischemia of the lateral femoral cutaneous nerve during periacetabular osteotomy using Smith-Petersen approach. J Orthop Traumatol. 2009 September; 10(3): p. 123–126.

13. AL Dellon, M Mont, I Ducic. Involvement of the lateral femoral cutaneous nerve as source of persistent pain after total hip arthroplasty. J Arthroplasty. 2008 April; 23(3): p. 480–485.

14. S Al-Benna. Right hypoglossal nerve paralysis after tracheal intubation for

aesthetic breast surgery. *Saudi J Anaesth.* 2013 July; 9(3): p. 341–343.

15. P Barash, BF Cullen, RK Stoelting *et al.*, editors. *Clinical Anesthesia.* 7th edn. Philadelphia, PA: Lippincott Williams & Wilkins; 2013.

16. MJ Fredrickson, DH Kilfoyle. Neurological complication analysis of 1000 ultrasound-guided peripheral nerve blocks for elective orthopaedic surgery: a prospective study. *Anaesthesia.* 2009 August; 64(8): p. 836–844.

17. CL Jeng, MA Rosenblatt. Intraneural injections and regional anesthesia: the known and the unknown. *Minerva Anestesiol.* 2011 January; 77: p. 54–58.

18. DR Cummings, DDR Yamashita, JP McAndrews. Complications of local anesthesia used in oral and maxillofacial surgery. *Oral Maxillofac Surg Clin North Am.* 2011 August; 23(3): p. 369–377.

19. OE Ogle, G Mahjoubi. Advances in local anesthesia in dentistry. *Dent Clin N Am.* 2011 July; 55(3): p. 481–499.

20. RD Miller, MC Pardo. Local anesthetics. Ch. 11 in *Basics of Anesthesia.* 6th edn. Goolsby J, editor. Philadelphia, PA: Saunders; 2011.

21. JM Neal, CM Bernards, JF Butterworth, *et al.* ASRA Practice Advisory on Local Anesthetic Systemic Toxicity. *Reg Anesth Pain Med.* 2010 March/April; 35(2): p. 152–161.

22. IL Tam, MJ Polydefkis, G Ebenezer, P Hauer, JC McArthur. Peripheral nerve toxic effects of nitrofurantoin. *Arch Neurol.* 2012 February; 69(2): p. 265–268.

23. JE Jesus, A Landry. Images in clinical medicine: Chvostek's and Trousseau's signs. *N Engl J Med.* 2012 September; 367 (11): p. e24.

24. J Halevy, S Bulvik. Severe hypophosphatemia in hospitalized patients. *Arch Intern Med.* 1988 January; 148(1): p. 153–155.

25. DL Longo, AS Fauci, DL Kasper, *et al.*, editors. *Harrison's Principles of Internal Medicine.* 18th edn. New York: McGraw-Hill; 2012.

Shivering

James W. Heitz

- Shivering is very common in the early postoperative period.
- Shivering is frequently a source of discomfort, but rarely the cause of morbidity.
- Meperidine is very efficacious in small doses in the treatment of shivering.
- Many alternative pharmacological agents are available for the patient for whom meperidine is not appropriate.

Shivering after surgery is very common. The incidence has been reported to be an extraordinary 60% after general anesthesia with volatile agents[1] and 55% after neuraxial anesthesia.[2] Many elements of how general anesthesia is administered may influence the incidence of postoperative shivering, including medication selection, opioid dosing, and active warming. With spinal anesthetics, the incidence of shivering increases as the level of the block reaches higher dermatomes.[3]

Risk factors commonly attributed to causing postoperative shivering include longer surgery duration, male sex, anticholinergic premedication (e.g. atropine), spontaneous ventilation, higher American Society of Anesthesiologists (ASA) physical status, general versus orthopedic surgery, and the administration of blood.[4] Male sex is often cited as a risk factor for postoperative shivering. A more recent observational study was only able to validate three risk factors, specifically younger age, endoprosthetic surgery, and hypothermia.[5] Hypothermia was a very weak risk factor for postoperative shivering, but greatly increased the duration when shivering occurred.

Shivering has well-demonstrated adverse physiological effects. It may increase oxygen consumption as much as 200%[6] to 500%.[7] Shivering may contribute to increased cardiac output, tachycardia, hypertension,[6,8] and intraocular pressure.[9] Shivering in the surgical patient is concerning because of its potential to contribute to more serious adverse outcomes. However, the role of shivering in actually contributing to adverse outcome is poorly demonstrated.

Cardiac patients would seem to be particularly vulnerable to the adverse effects of shivering on blood pressure, cardiac output, and oxygen consumption. While hypothermia contributes to adverse cardiac outcomes, little evidence implicates shivering in causing cardiac ischemia.[10–12] Elderly patients may be at increased perioperative risk for cardiac ischemia, but shivering appears to be less common among elderly surgical patients than

Post-Anesthesia Care: Symptoms, Diagnosis, and Management, ed. James W. Heitz. Published by Cambridge University Press. © Cambridge University Press 2016.

among younger surgical patients.[13–15] Increased oxygen consumption raises clinical concern for exacerbating hypoxia in the delicate postoperative setting, but hypoxia appears to inhibit shivering in humans[16] and animal models.[17] Similarly, although the muscular activity involved in shivering would be expected to exacerbate perioperative hypoglycemia, hypoglycemia also has an inhibitory effect on shivering.[18]

Although one of the top 10 common postoperative complications by frequency, shivering ranks only 21 of 33 postoperative complications by severity in a survey of anesthesiologists.[19] This is attributable to its lack of demonstrated impact on perioperative morbidity and mortality. Shivering is a transient complication with no known potential to become chronic. While it seems to exert only a small effect upon outcome, postoperative shivering still requires treatment. It causes patient discomfort which may be particularly severe if shivering stretches surgical incisions. Additionally, shivering may interfere with postoperative monitoring including blood pressure[20] and pulse oximetry.[21] While patient comfort is adequate reason to treat shivering, it is equally important that clinical efforts to control shivering should not unnecessarily contribute to adverse outcomes.

Management

Prevention is preferable to treatment. The ASA Task Force on Postanesthetic Care previously recommended intraoperative active warming for the prevention of postoperative shivering,[22] but in the most recent version of these guidelines the recommendation was weakened to reflect the fact that the evidence of efficacy is equivocal.[23] Since a variety of neurotransmitters are involved in causing shivering, a variety of pharmaceutical agents with different mechanisms of action are effective for either prevention or treatment of shivering (Table 34.1).

Meperidine: Meperidine is first-line treatment of postoperative shivering owing to its combination of high efficacy and low side-effect profile. When administered as meperidine 25 mg IV, the number-needed-to-treat (NNT) to terminate shivering is very low. The NNT to terminate shivering at 1 minute after administration is 2.7; at 5 minutes the NNT falls to 1.3.[24] Meperidine effectively terminates postoperative shivering and returns oxygen consumption to near baseline levels.[7] Most opioids have some efficacy in the prevention and/or treatment of shivering, owing to μ-receptor agonist activity. Meperidine is an atypical opioid since it also has other distinctive pharmacodynamic properties. Meperidine displays α_2-agonist activity which appears to be important in shivering cessation[25] and is consistent with the fact that other α_2-agonists (dexmedetomidine, clonidine) also inhibit shivering. Additionally, neuronal norepinephrine reuptake inhibition, cholinergic antagonism, and N-methyl-D-aspartate (NMDA) receptor antagonism all may contribute to anti-shivering efficacy. Naloxone in low dose poorly antagonizes the anti-shivering efficacy of meperidine, indicating that more than μ-receptor agonism may be involved.[26]

Meperidine is relatively contraindicated with concurrent renal insufficiency owing to the accumulation of the toxic metabolite, normeperidine. Low-dose meperidine for shivering is safe for most patients even with renal failure. Meperidine is strongly contraindicated if monoamine oxidase (MAO) inhibitors have been administered within 14 days. Serotonin syndrome, with sometimes fatal consequences, has been observed between interactions of meperidine and MAO inhibitors, so this contraindication is best considered absolute. The risk cannot be clinically justified when the benefit of therapy does not reduce morbidity and alternate effective therapy is readily available. Meperdine is unique

Table 34.1 Pharmacological treatment of shivering

Medication	Dose	Mechanism	Comments
Alfentanil	250 mcg	μ-receptor agonist	Not as efficacious as meperidine
Clonidine	30 mcg IV q 5 minutes (max 90 mcg) 150 mcg IV	α₂-agonist	Off-label use
Dexmedetomidine	0.5 mcg/kg	α₂-agonist	
Doxapram	100 mg 1.5 mg/kg	Dopaminergic	
Fentanyl	5 mcg IV q 5 minutes (max 25 mcg) 1.7 mcg/kg IV	μ-receptor agonist	Not as efficacious as meperidine
Ketanserin	10 mg IV	Antiserotonergic	
Magnesium sulfate	30 mg/kg IV 50 mg/kg IV	Central and peripheral effects	**Efficacious after spinal anesthesia**
Meperidine	6.25 mg IV q 5 minutes (max 25 mg) 12.5 mg IV 25 mg IV 0.12, 0.33, 0.35, 0.4, or 0.8 mg/kg IV 50 mg IV (after neuraxial anesthesia)	κ-receptor agonist α₂-agonist	**First-line treatment** Caution in renal failure owing to renally eliminated metabolite (normeperidine), but small doses probably safe. **Contraindicated with monoamine oxidase inhibitors**
Morphine	0.5 mg IV q 5 minutes (max 2.5 mg)	μ-receptor agonist	Not as efficacious as meperidine
Nalbuphine	0.08 mg/kg IV		
Nefopam	50 ng IV 100 ng IV	Reuptake of serotonin and norepinephrine in the spinal cord	Not available in the USA
Ondansetron	4 mg IV 8 mg IV	Antiserotonergic	8 mg necessary (4 mg dose efficacious in one study where average patient weight only 52 kg) **Not effective for neuraxial anesthesia-induced shivering**

Table 34.1 (cont.)

Medication	Dose	Mechanism	Comments
Tramadol	0.5 mg/kg IV 1 mg/kg IV 2 mg/kg IV	Reuptake of serotonin and norepinephrine in the spinal cord	Slower onset time with 0.5 mg/kg
Urapidil	25 mg IV	α_1-agonist and 5-HT$_{1A}$ agonist	Not available in the USA

in that it is recommended specifically by the ASA Task Force on Postanesthetic Care in the treatment of shivering,[22,23] but it is by no means unique in its ability to treat postoperative shivering.

Opioids: Other opioids including fentanyl, alfentanil, and morphine have been used to treat postoperative shivering by their μ-receptor agonist properties.[24] Remifentanil is exceptional among the opioids in that it has been implicated in causing postoperative shivering in a dose-dependent fashion when administered by intravenous (IV) infusion as part of the maintenance of anesthesia.[27] Activation of NMDA receptors by remifentanil has been implicated in causing post-infusion hyperalgesia and hypothesized to exacerbate shivering, a hypothesis seemingly confirmed by the clinical finding that simultaneous infusion of ketamine attenuates both postoperative shivering and hyperalgesia.[28]

Ketamine: Ketamine has been validated to treat shivering after general anesthesia. In one study, ketamine 0.5 mg/kg and 0.75 mg/kg IV demonstrated superior efficacy to meperidine, but with a significantly higher incidence of side effects.[29] Patients experienced nystagmus and dysphoria. The clinical usefulness of ketamine is limited by its unacceptable side-effect profile.

α2-agonists: Clonidine has established efficacy in the treatment of postoperative shivering in multiple randomized clinical trials.[24] Most trials have examined a dose of clonidine 150 mcg IV, but in one trial 37.5 mg IV had no benefit in adult patients, while 75 mg IV stopped shivering at 5 minutes.[30] More recently, dexmedetomidine administered as a slow push bolus (0.5 mcg/kg IV over 3 to 5 minutes) was demonstrated to stop shivering in a pediatric surgical population.[31]

Antiserotonergics: Ondansetron has some efficacy in the treatment of shivering, although the mechanism is unclear. Antiserotonergic effect may have some effect upon heat loss and the development of perioperative hypothermia. There is some evidence that ondansetron reduces heat loss from vasodilatation during neuraxial anesthesia.[32] Serotonin is involved in thermoregulation, and 5-HT$_3$ antagonism can induce hyperthermia in rodents.[33,34] However, there is little evidence that ondansetron prevents shivering by affecting human body temperature.[35] In meta-analysis, ondansetron does reduce the incidence of shivering after general anesthesia, probably through a central mechanism.[36] Optimal dosing is undetermined, since these various studies have differing patient weights, but 8 mg is probably necessary for most adult populations. Ondansetron 4 mg was effective in a patient population where the average weight was only 52 kg for adults.[32] Ondansetron is ineffective in preventing shivering during neuraxial anesthesia or for parturients undergoing cesarean section with combined spinal–epidural anesthesia.[37,38]

Treatment of shivering after neuraxial anesthesia: Shivering after spinal or epidural anesthesia is more difficult to treat clinically. The best results have been obtained with higher-dose meperidine (50 mg IV), tramadol (0.25, 0.5, or 1 mg IV), and clonidine (30, 60, 90, or 150 mcg IV).[2]

References

1. P.K. Bhattacharya, L. Bhattacharya, R.K. Jain, R.C. Agarwal. Post anaesthesia shivering (PAS): a review. *Indian J Anaesth* 2003; 47:88–93.

2. L.J. Crowley, D.J. Buggy. Shivering and neuraxial anesthesia. *Reg Anesth Pain Med* 2008; 33:241–252.

3. K. Leslie, D.I. Sessler. Reducing in the shivering threshold is proportional to spinal block height. *Anesthesiology* 1996; 84:1327–1331.

4. A.W. Crossley. Six months of shivering in a district general hospital. *Anaesthesia* 1992; 47:845–848.

5. L.H. Eberhart, F. Doderlein, G. Eisenhardt, *et al.* Independent risk factors for postoperative shivering. *Anesth Analg* 2005; 101:1849–1857.

6. J. Bay, J.F. Nunn, C. Prys-Roberts. Factors influencing arterial PO_2 during recovery from anesthesia. *Br J Anaesth* 1968; 40:398–407.

7. P.E. Macintyre, E.G. Pavlin, J.F. Dwersteg. Effect of meperidine on oxygen consumption, carbon dioxide production, and respiratory gas exchange in postanesthesia shivering. *Anesth Analg* 1987; 66:751–755.

8. D.I. Sessler, E.H. Rubinstein, A. Moayeri. Physiologic responses to mild perianesthetic hypothermia in humans. *Anesthesiology* 1991; 75:594–610.

9. R.P. Mahajan, V.K. Grover, S.L. Sharma, H. Singh. Intraocular pressure changes during muscular hyperactivity after general anesthesia. *Anesthesiology* 1987; 66:419–421.

10. J.Y. Dupuis, H.J. Nathan, L. DeLima, *et al.* Pancuronium or vecuronium for treatment of shivering after cardiac surgery. *Anesth Analg* 1994; 79:472–481.

11. S.M. Frank, L.A. Fleisher, M.J. Breslow, *et al.* Perioperative maintenance of normothermia reduces the incidence of morbid cardiac events: a randomized clinical trial. *JAMA* 1997; 277:1127–1134.

12. S.M. Frank, C. Beattie, R. Christopherson, *et al.* Unintentional hypothermia is associated with postoperative myocardial ischemia. The Perioperative Ischemia Randomized Anesthesia Trial Study Group. *Anesthesiology* 1993; 78:468–476.

13. K.J. Collins, C. Dore, A.N. Exton-Smith, *et al.* Accidental hypothermia and impaired temperature homeostasis in the elderly. *Br Med J* 1977; 1:353–356.

14. F. Carli, M. Gabrielczyk, M.M. Clark, V.R. Aber. An investigation of factors affecting postoperative rewarming of adult patients. *Anaesthesia* 1986; 41:363–369.

15. S.M. Frank, L.A. Fleisher, K.F. Olson, *et al.* Multivariate determinants of early postoperative oxygen consumption in elderly patients. *Anesthesiology* 1995; 83:241–249.

16. H. Gautier, M. Bonora, S.A. Schultz, J.E. Remmers. Hypoxia-induced changes in shivering and body temperature. *J Appl Physiol* 1987; 62:2477–2484.

17. H. Iwashita, T. Matsukawa, M. Ozaki, *et al.* Hypoxemia decreases the shivering threshold in rabbits anesthetized with 0.2 MAC isoflurane. *Anesth Analg* 1998; 87:1408–1411.

18. T.C. Passias, G.S. Meneilly, I.B. Mekjavić. Effect of hypoglycemia on thermoregulatory responses. *J Appl Physiol* 1996; 80:1021–1032.

19. A. Macario, M. Weinger, P. Truong, M. Lee. Which clinical anesthesia outcomes are both common and important to avoid?

The perspective of a panel of expert anesthesiologists. *Anesth Analg* 1999; 88:1085–1091.

20. J.G. De Courcy. Artefactual "hypotension" from shivering. *Anaesthesia* 1989; 44:787–788.

21. S.J. Barker, N.K. Shah. Effects of motion on the performance of pulse oximeters in volunteers. *Anesthesiology* 1996; 85:774–781.

22. Practice Guidelines for Postanesthetic Care. A report by the American Society of Anesthesiologists Task Force on Postanesthetic Care. *Anesthesiology* 2002; 96:742–752.

23. Practice Guidelines for Postanesthetic Care. An updated report by the American Society of Anesthesiologists Task Force on Postanesthetic Care. *Anesthesiology* 2013; 118:291–307.

24. P. Kranke, L.H. Eberhart, N. Roewer, M.R. Tramer. Pharmacological treatment of postoperative shivering: a quantitative systematic review of randomized controlled trials. *Anesth Analg* 2002; 94:453–460.

25. K. Takada, D.J. Clark, M.F. Davies, *et al.* Meperidine exerts agonist activity at the alpha(2B)-adrenoceptor subtype. *Anesthesiology* 2002; 96:1420–1426.

26. M. Kurz, K. Belani, D.I. Sessler, *et al.* Naloxone, meperidine, and shivering. *Anesthesiology* 1993; 79:1193–1201.

27. M. Nakasuji, M. Nakamura, N. Imanaka, *et al.* Intraoperative high-dose remifentanil increases post-anaesthetic shivering. *Br J Anaesth* 2010; 105:162–167.

28. Y.K. Song, C. Lee, D.H. Seo, *et al.* Interaction between postoperative shivering and hyperalgesia caused by high-dose remifentanil. *Korean J Anesthesiol* 2014; 66(1):44–51.

29. E.A. Kose, D. Dal, S.B. Akinci, F. Saricaoglu, U. Aypar. The efficacy of ketamine for the treatment of postoperative shivering. *Anesth Analg* 2008; 106:120–122.

30. J. Joris, M. Banache, F. Bonnet, D.I. Sessler, M. Lamy. Clonidine and ketanserin both are effective treatment for postanesthetic shivering. *Anesthesiology* 1993; 79:532–539.

31. E.R. Blaine, K.M. Brady, J.D. Tobias. Dexmedetomidine for the treatment of postanesthesia shivering in children. *Paediatr Anaesth* 2007; 17:341–346.

32. E. Kelsaka, S. Baris, D. Karakaya, B. Sarihasan. Comparison of ondansetron and meperidine for prevention of shivering in patients undergoing spinal anesthesia. *Reg Anesth Pain Med* 2006; 31:40–45.

33. P. Mazzola-Pomietto, C.S. Aulakh, D.L. Murphy. Temperature, food intake, and locomotor activity effects of a 5-HT3 receptor agonist and two 5-HT3 receptor antagonists in rats. *Psychopharmacology (Berl)* 1995; 21:488–493.

34. S.B. Kandasamy. Effect of ondansetron and ICS 205–930 on radiation-induced hypothermia in rats. *Radiat Res* 1997; 147:741–746.

35. R.M. Powell, D.J. Buggy. Ondansetron given before induction of anesthesia reduces shivering after general anesthesia. *Anesth Analg* 2000; 90:1423–1427.

36. H-T. Tie, G-Z. Su, S-R. Lian, H-W. Yuan, J-Z. Mou. Efficacy and safety of ondansetron in preventing postanesthesia shivering: a meta-analysis of randomized controlled trials. *BMC Anesthesiol* 2014; 14:12. doi:10.1186/1471-2253-14-12.

37. R.M. Browning, W.H. Fellingham, E.J. O'Loughlin, N.A. Brown, M.J. Paech. Prophylactic ondansetron does not prevent shivering or decrease shivering severity during cesarean delivery under combined spinal epidural anesthesia: a randomized trial. *Reg Anesth Pain Med* 2013; 38:39–43.

38. S.S. Joshi, A. Arora, A. George, R.V. Shidhaye. Comparison of intravenous butorphanol, ondansetron and tramadol for shivering during regional anesthesia: a prospective randomized double-blind study. *Anaesth Intensive Care Med* 2013; 17:33–39.

Chapter

35

Oliguria and postoperative urinary obstruction

James W. Heitz

- Oliguria is common after surgery.
- Prerenal causes predominate for postoperative oliguria.
- Intravenous fluid challenges treat most oliguria after surgery.
- Do not overlook retention, urinary catheter obstruction, syndrome of inappropriate antidiuretic hormone (SIADH), abdominal compartment syndrome in the postoperative patient.

Broadly defined, oliguria refers to a sustained decrease in urine production. Although a myriad of differing definitions exist in the medical literature attempting to provide a quantified definition, none is entirely adequate for the postoperative patient. The Acute Dialysis Quality Initiative (ADQI) defines oliguria as urine output less than 0.3 ml/kg/hr over a 24-hour interval.[1] The ADQI definition is insufficient for perioperative usage, since it is important to recognize oliguria early and intervene before renal injury occurs. Postoperative renal failure is associated with high mortality, as much as 80% in some series.[2,3] Although no universal definition of perioperative oliguria has been accepted, 0.5 ml/kg/hr for 2 hours is a widely used definition useful in many clinical situations. For the majority of adult patients, a urinary output of 1 ml/kg/hr is considered adequate, although greater urinary output might be desired for patients with electrical burn injuries, rhabdomyolysis, or perioperative exposure to potentially nephrotoxic agents including intravenous(IV) contrast dye. It is important to emphasize that oliguria does not mean renal injury has occurred or is occurring, but it should raise suspicion that there may be renal injury.

Etiology

Oliguria may be caused by prerenal, intrarenal, or postrenal factors. (See Table 35.1.)[4] The incidence of prerenal factors in postoperative oliguria may be as high as 90%, warranting a high degree of clinical suspicion.[5]

Prerenal oliguria

Numerous factors contribute to relative intravascular volume depletion in the surgical patient, including: anesthetic effects (vasodilatation), inability to take oral liquids, blood loss, third spacing of fluids, insensible losses, nasogastric suction or emesis, or sepsis.

Post-Anesthesia Care: Symptoms, Diagnosis, and Management, ed. James W. Heitz. Published by Cambridge University Press. © Cambridge University Press 2016.

Table 35.1 Causes of oliguria

Prerenal oliguria
a. Decreased intravascular volume: hemorrhage, third spacing
b. Decreased cardiac output: shock, tamponade
c. Decreased renal perfusion: sepsis, pharmacological, ↑ intraabdominal pressure

Intrarenal oliguria
a. Ischemic acute tubular necrosis: hypotension, prolonged prerenal oliguria
b. Nephrotoxic acute tubular necrosis: drugs (vancomycin, gentamicin), IV contrast, rhabdomyolysis
c. Acute interstitial nephritis: drugs (nafcillin, furosemide)

Postrenal oliguria
a. Obstruction: bilateral hydronephrosis, prostatic hypertrophy, urinary catheter obstruction

Adapted from ref. [4].

Intrinsic cardiac shock or cardiac tamponade may occasionally present as oliguria in the postoperative patient.

If present, transduction of a central venous catheter allows for assessment of a central venous pressure (CVP), which is often used clinically as a marker of intravascular volume status, although the reliability of this sign is questionable.[6] A CVP <5 mmHg or downward trending CVP values may suggest intravascular volume depletion. An arterial catheter, if present, may be utilized to determine pulse pressure variation (PPV), a measure of the variation in pulse pressure (SBP – DBP) between inspiration and expiration during mechanical ventilation. PPV has been validated as a predictor of fluid responsiveness of hypotension, with a PPV ≥15 mmHg predicting a greater likelihood of blood pressure response to fluid challenge. The significance of increased PPV in the absence of hypotension is unclear, but may be associated with decreased intravascular volume. Oliguria, hypotension, and increased PPV should be treated with IV fluids; PPV might be one of the clinical signs used to guide fluid challenge in the normotensive and oliguric patient. While the majority of postoperative patients will not have either central venous or arterial access, all patients in the PACU should have pulse oximetry monitoring. Respiratory variation during plethysmography, while less sensitive or specific than PPV, may be a marker of hypovolemia.[7]

Ultrasound may be used to determine intravascular volume status by determining absolute inferior vena cava (IVC) diameter as well as respirophasic variation in diameter. An IVC of normal diameter with <50% respirophasic variation suggests euvolemia. Progressively diminishing vessel diameter and great respirophasic variation are correlated with lesser CVP values. Although the accuracy of this technique has been well validated by several decades of experience, the measurements obtained are influenced by the precision of the ultrasound view. Its reliability in the hands of inexperienced operators or under emergency conditions has been disappointing. More recently, respirophasic variation in carotid artery peak velocity as determined by ultrasound has been correlated with fluid responsiveness of hypotension.[8] As of yet, it is undetermined whether this technique will prove advantageous under clinical conditions.

Abdominal compartment syndrome after surgery is rare, but deserves special mention. Acute compartment syndrome occurs when intraabdominal pressure exceeds 20 mmHg and should be considered after intraabdominal procedures and large volumes of IV crystalloid. Ventilatory difficulties due to interference with diaphragmatic function are typical, but this syndrome may present as oliguria from decreased renal perfusion. Fluid administration aimed at treating the oliguria may exacerbate the underlying pathology. In one interesting case report, intraabdominal compartment syndrome developed owing to postoperative ileus. Pain caused the patient to over-utilize the patient-controlled analgesia (PCA), exacerbating the underlying ileus and the compartment syndrome.[9]

Intrarenal oliguria

Intrarenal oliguria may be caused by a variety of renal insults occurring in the perioperative period. Intraoperative hypotension may cause renal hypoperfusion, and the embolic phenomenon including cholesterol emboli may cause renal injury. Rhabdomyolysis in trauma patients, electrical burn patients, or patients experiencing malignant hyperthermia, or rhabdomyolysis from other causes (e.g. succinylcholine and Duchenne's muscular dystrophy) causes a heme-pigment-induced tubular toxicity. The polypharmacy of perioperative period also carries the risk of renal injury since numerous medications have the potential for renal toxicity. Many antibiotics (including penicillins, cephalosporins, ciprofloxacin, and sulfonamides) used for surgical prophylaxis may cause an allergic interstitial nephritis, as may non-steroidal anti-inflammatory drugs (NSAIDs) utilized as part of a multimodal analgesic regimen. IV contrast dye, NSAIDs, and angiotensin-converting enzyme inhibitors may decrease renal perfusion, causing injury, an effect which may be exacerbated by perioperative hypotension.[10]

Prerenal and intrarenal causes of oliguria can usually be differentiated clinically. However, laboratory analysis may be helpful in some cases. A fraction excretion of sodium (FENa) may be calculated from the serum sodium, serum creatinine, urinary sodium, and urinary creatinine using the formula:

$$FENa = 100 \times (Urinary\ sodium \times Plasma\ creatinine)/(Plasma\ sodium \times Urinary\ creatinine)$$

A FENa $<1\%$ is associated with prerenal causes and a FENa $>2\%$ is associated with intrarenal causes. A FENa between these values is indeterminate. Similarly, a fractional excretion of urea may be calculated by the formula:

$$Fractional\ excretion\ of\ urea\ (FEUrea) = (Urinary\ urea\ Cr \times Plasma\ creatinine)/$$
$$(Plasma\ urea \times Urinary\ creatinine)$$

A FEUrea $<35\%$ is associated with prerenal causes while a FEUrea $>35\%$ is associated with intrarenal causes. A summary of the interpretation of urinary electrolytes is provided in Table 35.2.[4] The presence of hyaline casts on microscopic urinalysis may be indicative of

Table 35.2 Urinalysis

	Prerenal	Intrarenal
Urine osmolality (mOsm/kg)	>500	<400
Urine Na (mEq/l)	<20	>40
Fractional excretion Na (%)	<1	>2
Fraction excretion urea (%)	<35	>35

Adapted from ref. [4].

acute tubular injury and an intrarenal process. Urine eosinophilia, although rarely seen, strongly suggests intrarenal etiology (drug reaction or atheromatous emboli).

Oliguria associated with mild hyponatremia should raise suspicion for the syndrome of inappropriate antidiuretic hormone secretion (SIADH). SIADH is associated with pain, mechanical ventilation, and some medications commonly utilized perioperatively including morphine. Mild hyponatremia is common after surgery, particularly after intracranial and spine procedures. Most SIADH after surgery is mild and self-limited to about 24 hours, but recognition is important since attempts to increase urine output with fluid challenges may exacerbate the hyponatremia without improving urinary output. Direct therapy is rarely needed, but volume restriction, loop diuretics, and rarely hypertonic 3% saline are needed when hyponatremia becomes severe.

Postrenal oliguria

Although uncommonly implicated in postoperative oliguria, postrenal causes are often easily treated and should not be overlooked. If a urinary catheter is present, is it functioning? Is it properly positioned: has it ever produced urine? If not, it may be malpositioned and not in the bladder. A defective urinary catheter may not be able to drain urine from the bladder even if properly positioned.[11] A properly positioned catheter that no longer drains urine may have become occluded or kinked. Anuria which occurs abruptly should raise the clinical suspicion for a problem with the urinary catheter. Urinary catheters may be occluded by sediment, stone, or clot when associated with hematuria. Irrigation of the catheter or replacement will usually resolve this.

Manual palpation of the bladder may reveal urinary retention which is particularly common in older men. Spinal anesthesia, pain, and opioid administration may exacerbate this. Some patients will complain of bladder discomfort or low abdominal pain, but others may present with hypertension, confusion, agitation, or delirium.

Bilateral ureteral obstruction (unilateral in the case of solitary kidney) may still exist, but unless suggested by surgical procedure (major gynecological or intraabdominal procedures) or history is unlikely and probably requires a renal ultrasound or CT scan to diagnose.

Management: Treatment of oliguria is directed at the underlying cause. In adults, a 500 ml fluid bolus of crystalloid is appropriate for prerenal oliguria in the absence of signs of congestive failure (rales, presacral edema). Volume is also appropriate for intrarenal oliguria due to IV contrast dye or rhabdomyolysis. Postrenal causes are treated by relieving the obstruction. Most intrarenal oliguria is treated supportively by optimizing hemodynamics and volume status. Renal dose dopamine or routine diuretic use does not improve outcome, although diuretics are appropriate as part of the therapy of oliguria associated with congestive heart failure.

Postoperative urinary retention

As opposed to oliguria which is a problem of urination (passage of urine from kidney to bladder), postoperative urinary retention (POUR) is a problem of micturition (bladder voiding). Each may be initially recognized as a poor urine output. However, each requires different therapy, so proper diagnosis is essential (see Figure 35.3).

In the adult, the urge to void is first felt with a bladder volume of approximately 150 ml, and voiding normally occurs by a bladder volume of 300 ml[12] with a maximal bladder volume of 400 to 500 ml.[13] No definition has been universally agreed upon, but a bladder volume greater than 600 ml for 30 minutes or a post-void residual volume of 200 ml suggests a diagnosis of POUR. Bladder volume can be accurately determined by bladder scanning for bladder volumes between 100 ml and 1000 ml. At the extremes, bladder scanning is less accurate quantitatively, but still gives a good qualitative estimate of bladder volume. Alternatively, low abdominal percussion may approximate bladder volume with a bladder extending to the umbilicus holding as much as 500 ml, a bladder extending above the umbilicus as much as 1000 ml. Deep palpation should be avoided for severely distended bladders, both because of patient discomfort and the possibility of severe vagal reactions and profound bradycardia.

POUR is common, affecting 3.8% to 16% of patients having general surgery, with a male sex predominance.[14,15] The incidence after some procedures is much higher, with an incidence of 34% after hemorrhoidectomy[16] and incidence ranging from 10.7% to 84% after total joint replacement.[17–20] While POUR may occur after any anesthetic, spinal and epidural anesthetics carry increased risk.[12] Detrusor contraction is abolished in 2 to 5 minutes after intrathecal injection of local anesthesia and does not return until the sensory block regresses to S2–S3. Normalization of detrusor strength occurs 1 to 3.5 hours *after* the ability to ambulate returns.[21] Patient risk factors include age >50 years, intraoperative fluids >750 ml, and bladder volume >270 ml on arrival to PACU.[15]

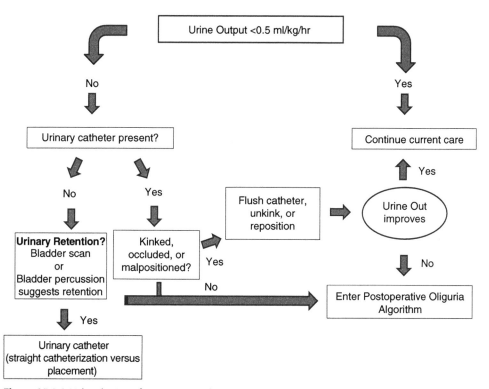

Figure 35.1 Initial evaluation of postoperative oliguria.

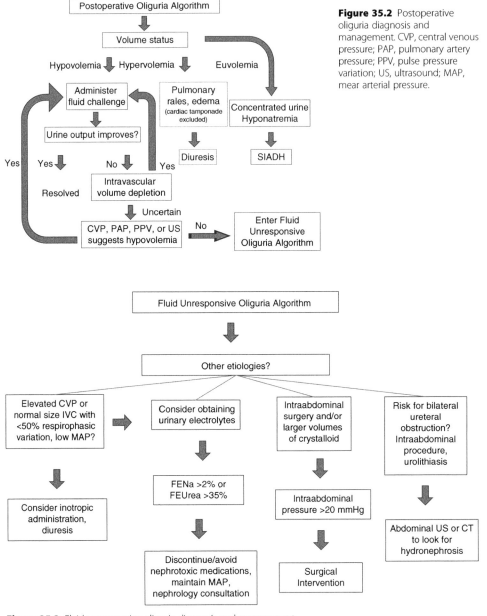

Figure 35.2 Postoperative oliguria diagnosis and management. CVP, central venous pressure; PAP, pulmonary artery pressure; PPV, pulse pressure variation; US, ultrasound; MAP, mear arterial pressure.

Figure 35.3 Fluid unresponsive oliguria diagnosis and management.

Treatment: POUR may be effectively treated by urinary catheterization with the associated benefits and risks being determined for an individual patient. Bladder over-distension has been associated with pain, emesis, hypertension, bradycardia, and postoperative delirium and carries a risk to detrusor function if it persists for more than 2 hours. Indwelling urinary catheters are a significant risk factor for bacteriuria, bacteremia, or urosepsis; but even a single straight catheterization carries some risk. The incidence of bacteremia may be as high as 8% after a single catheterization,[22] and more than 1 in 5 women requiring catheterization after laparoscopic surgery will have persistent bacteriuria at postoperative day 6.[23] Therefore, the decision to place a urinary catheter should be individualized to the patient. Protocols requiring catheterization due to procedure or anesthetic are discouraged.

References

1. R. Bellomo, C. Ronco, J.A. Kellum, R.L. Mehta, P. Palevsky. Acute renal failure—definition, outcome measures, animal models, fluid therapy and information technology needs: the second International Consensus Conference of the Acute Dialysis Quality Initiative (ADQI) Group. *Crit Care* 2004; 8:R204–R212.

2. B.K. Novis, M.F. Roizen, S. Aronson, R.A. Thisted. Association of preoperative risk factors with postoperative acute renal failure. *Anesth Analg* 1994; 78:143–149.

3. G. Zanardo, P. Michielon, A. Paccagnella, *et al.* Acute renal failure in the patient undergoing cardiac operations: prevalence, mortality rate, and main risk factors. *J Thorac Cardiovasc Surg* 1994; 107:1489–1495.

4. R. Verhataraman, J.A. Kellum. Treatment of acute oliguria. *Perioperative Medicine: Managing for Outcome* (ed. Newman MF, Fleisher LA, Fink, MP), Philadelphia, Saunders Elsevier, 2008.

5. E. Cordes-Behringer. Oliguria: perioperative management. *Rev Mex Anest* 2006; 29:S21–S26.

6. P.E. Marik, M. Baram, B. Vahid. Does central venous pressure predict fluid responsiveness? A systematic review of the literature and the tale of seven mares. *Chest* 2008; 134:172–178.

7. A. Murray, G.B. Drummond, S. Dodds, L. Marshall. Low frequency changes in finger volume in patients after surgery, related to respiration and venous pressure. *Eur J Anaesthesiol* 2009; 26:9–16.

8. Y. Song, Y.L. Kwak, J.W. Song, Y.J. Kim, J.K. Shim. Respirophasic carotid artery peak velocity variation as a predictor of fluid responsiveness in mechanically ventilated patients with coronary artery disease. *Br J Anaesth* 2014; 113:61–66.

9. B.A. Van Noord, P. Roffey, D. Thangathurai. Abdominal compartment syndrome following opioid-induced postoperative ileus. *J Clin Anesth* 2013; 25:146–149.

10. R. Thadhani, M. Pascual, J.V. Bonventre. Acute renal failure. *N Engl J Med* 1996; 334:1448–1460.

11. B.D. Bergman, J. Sprung. Unusual cause of intraoperative urinary retention. *Anesthesiology* 2003; 4:1030–1031.

12. G. Baldini, H. Bagry, A. Aprikian, F. Carli. Postoperative urinary retention: anesthetic and perioperative considerations. *Anesthesiology* 2009; 110:1139–1157.

13. G.M. Coombes, R.J. Millard. The accuracy of portable ultrasound scanning in the measurement of residual urine volume. *J Urol* 1994; 152:2083–2085.

14. T. Tammela, M. Kontturi, O. Lukkarinen. Postoperative urinary retention: I. Incidence and predisposing factors. *Scand J Urol Nephrol* 1986; 20:197–201.

15. H. Keitz, E. Diouf, F. Tubach, *et al.* Predictive factors of early postoperative urinary retention in the postanesthesia care unit. *Anesth Analg* 2005; 101:592–596.

16. S. Zaheer, W.T. Reilly, J.H. Pemberton, D. Ilstrup. Urinary retention after operations for benign anorectal diseases. *Dis Colon Rectum* 1998; 41:696–704.

17. N. Waterhouse, A.R. Beaumont, K. Murray, P. Staniforth, M.H. Stone. Urinary retention after total hip replacement. A prospective study. *J Bone Joint Surg Br* 1987; 69:64–66.

18. C.S. Oishi, V.J. Williams, P.R. Hanson, *et al.* Perioperative bladder management after primary total hip arthroplasty. *J Arthroplasty* 1995; 10:732–736.

19. K. Lingaraj, M. Ruben, Y.H. Chan, S.D. Das. Identification of risk factors for urinary retention following total knee arthroplasty. A Singapore hospital experience. *Singapore Med J* 2007; 48:213–216.

20. J.A. O'Riordan, P.M. Hopkins, A. Ravenscroft, J.D. Stevens. Patient-controlled analgesia and urinary retention following lower limb joint replacement: prospective audit and logistic regression analysis. *Eur J Anaesthesiol* 2000; 7:431–435.

21. E.T. Kamphuis, T.I. Lonescu, P.W. Kuipers, *et al.* Recovery of storage and emptying functions of the urinary bladder after spinal anesthesia with lidocaine and with bupivacaine in men. *Anesthesiology* 1998; 88:310–316.

22. M.M. Sullivan, V.I. Sutter, M.M. Mims, V.H. Marsh, S.M. Finegold. Clinical aspects of bacteremia after manipulation of the genitourinary tract. *J Infect Dis* 1973; 127:49–55.

23. M.S. Akhtar, D.M. Beere, J.T. Wright, K.D. MacRae. Is bladder catheterization really necessary before laparoscopy? *Br J Obstet Gynaecol* 1985; 92:1176–1178.

Polyuria

James W. Heitz

- Iatrogenic overhydration is a common cause of polyuria after surgery.
- Diabetes insipidus and cerebral salt wasting syndrome may cause polyuria after craniotomy or head injury.
- Hyperglycemia may cause postoperative polyuria and may occur in the absence of a prior history of diabetes mellitus.

Polyuria is a condition of excessive production of urine. Polyuria may be defined as an output exceeding 3 l/day in adults and 2 l/m^2/day in children. This definition is not entirely adequate for the perioperative period, since it is often necessary to recognize and treat polyuria before 24 hours of urine has been collected. Although no single definition of perioperative polyuria has been universally accepted, urine output exceeding 4 to 5 ml/kg/hr is excessive. The differential diagnosis of polyuria is unique after surgery and relatively narrow (see Table 36.1).

Iatrogenic overhydration

Polyuria is often merely the appropriate response of the kidney to volume overload. Polyuria may be noted in the early postoperative setting owing to intravenous crystalloid infusion during surgery. Perioperative care includes the attempt to replace fluid deficits due to preoperative fasting, bowel preparation, preoperative emesis, diarrhea, or nasogastric tube suctioning. Inaccurate estimation of preoperative fluid deficit may lead to clinically excessive volume resuscitation. Additionally, intraoperative fluid losses including insensible losses due to evaporation are highly variable between patients and dependent upon ambient environmental conditions. Overestimation of operative fluid loss may also cause excessive volume replacement and resulting polyuria.

The timing of polyuria in the postoperative setting may be affected by the extensiveness of surgical resection. The surgical stress response may increase a number of hormones that favor perioperative fluid retention including aldosterone, antidiuretic hormone (ADH), and renin–angiotensin II.[1,2] Mobilization of infused crystalloids after extensive surgical procedures is delayed and most typically observed on postoperative Day 3.

The detrimental effect of iatrogenic overhydration on outcome is controversial, but may include impairment of wound healing, pulmonary edema, and cardiac complications.[3]

Post-Anesthesia Care: Symptoms, Diagnosis, and Management, ed. James W. Heitz. Published by Cambridge University Press. © Cambridge University Press 2016.

Table 36.1 Differential diagnosis of polyuria

	Central diabetes insipidus	Cerebral salt wasting syndrome
Urine output	High	Variable, may be high
Serum sodium	High >145 mEq/l	Low <135 mEq/l
Urinary sodium	Normal <20 mmol	High >25 mmol
Serum osmolality	High >295 mOsm/kg	Low <275 mOsm/kg
Urine osmolality	<100 mOsm/kg	>200 mOsm/kg
Urine color	Clear	Dark

In contrast, the polyuria secondary to overhydration is typically benign, self-limiting, and not associated with significant electrolyte abnormality.

Hyperglycemia

Glucose is not normally present in urine. Elevated plasma glucose causes glomerular filtration of glucose which may exceed the ability of the renal tubule to reabsorb glucose. Glucosuria results when plasma glucose exceeds this critical reabsorption capacity (renal threshold), which is approximately 180 mg/dl. The renal threshold is variable, and glucosuria may present only at markedly higher plasma glucose levels in some individuals.[4]

Hyperglycemia may develop in the postoperative period in surgical patients with known or undiagnosed diabetes mellitus, as well as in non-diabetic individuals secondary to the surgical stress response or glucocorticoid administration. Postoperative polyuria should raise suspicion for possible hyperglycemia. Hyperglycemia does not cause polyuria in the absence of glucosuria, so polyuria caused by hyperglycemia may be detected by either testing serum glucose level or urine for the presence of glucose. Left uncorrected, the osmotic diuresis of hyperglycemia will cause volume depletion and hypokalemia. If diabetic ketoacidosis or hyperglycemic hyperosmolar non-ketotic coma (HHNK) develops, surgical mortality is increased.

Diuretics

Mannitol is a monosaccharide which causes an osmotic diuresis. It is most typically administered for reduction of intracranial pressure by cerebral dehydration or to increase urine production for renal protection from toxins such as myoglobin. The duration of action of a typical bolus dose of mannitol is about 1.5 to 3 hours, so recent administration of mannitol may be associated with polyuria in the very early postoperative setting. Acute administration of mannitol causes increased serum osmolality, serum hyponatremia and hypokalemia, although serum hyperkalemia has been reported with high dose mannitol administration.[5] Glycerin, urea, or isosorbide are osmotic diuretics, particularly useful for acute reduction of intraocular pressure, but are not typically encountered in the perioperative setting. Other diuretics are less commonly administered perioperatively, but may have comparatively longer duration of actions. Intravenous furosemide and bumetanide may each exhibit a duration of action of up to 6 hours.

Diabetes insipidus

Polyuria and serum hyperosmolality (>285 mOsm/kg) should raise suspicion for diabetes insipidus (DI). DI can either be caused by a deficiency of ADH release by the pituitary (neurogenic DI) or unresponsiveness of the kidney to ADH (nephrogenic DI).

Neurogenic DI: DI may be caused by pituitary insufficiency of any etiology. Neurogenic DI is recognized most frequently after procedures around the pituitary fossa, traumatic brain injury, craniotomies, and patients with pituitary infarction after postpartum hemorrhage (Sheehan's syndrome). The development of DI may be temporally distant from the inciting trigger. A triphasic pattern of polyuria, recovery, and return of polyuria is sometimes observed. Patients with traumatic brain injury often have a brief period of neurogenic DI in the first 4 or 5 days after injury while ADH release is inhibited followed by a week or more of improvement while stored ADH is released from the partially recovering pituitary.[5–8] A third phase of DI may return if greater than 80% of the vasopressin-secreting neurons have been damaged and may present weeks, months, or occasionally years after the initial injury. Transsphenoidal pituitary adenoma resection may also rarely present with a triphasic DI presentation, although only a very small minority of these patients display polyuria after resection.[9] Transient DI may be a positive prognostic variable and may correlate with successful resection of adenoma and decreased neuroendocrine levels after surgery.[10]

Management: The polyuria of DI may be severe and the resultant urine colorless. Serum hyperosmolality, hypernatremia, and low urine osmolality are commonly observed. Decreased urine output after administration of desmopressin (DDAVP) is diagnostic and therapeutic. Carbamazepine and chlorpropamide both increase the renal sensitivity to ADH and may be useful clinically in the treatment of central DI.[11]

Nephrogenic diabetes insipidus: DI may occur despite normal ADH secretion by the pituitary. Aquaporins are cell membrane proteins, which allow for cellular water passage. Aquaporin-2 allows for reabsorption of water in the collecting tube of the nephron when bound to ADH. If circulating ADH cannot bind normally to aquaporin-2, nephrogenic DI ensues. Nephrogenic DI may be inherited or acquired. Acquired etiologies are more common, particularly in the postoperative setting. A variety of medications have been implicated in causing nephrogenic DI, but lithium is implicated more than any other medication.[12] Lithium needs to be considered in the differential diagnosis of polyuria, particularly for patients taking lithium or for trauma patients when medications are not known. Other medications associated with nephrogenic DI are infrequently encountered in the perioperative environment or rarely associated with nephrogenic DI.

Nephrogenic DI has been reported from infiltrative or granulomatous processes (amyloid, sarcoid, Wegener's, tuberculosis), which would be unlikely to be initially recognized in the perioperative setting. However, four interesting presentations of perioperative nephrogenic DI warrant special mention. Craniopharyngioma resection results in transient postoperative DI in as many as 90% of patients after resection.[13] Although most patients experience central DI due to surgical disruption of ADH release, a small subset of patients produce a defective form of ADH which competitively binds to aquaporin-2 without stimulating water resorption.[14] These patients display an ADH-unresponsive nephrogenic DI after surgery. Gestational DI may be observed in the third trimester by a number of mechanisms both central and nephrogenic. Placental production of the enzyme vasopressinase metabolizes ADH and produces an ADH-

Table 36.2 Postoperative polyuria

Etiology	Frequency	Examples	Laboratory abnormalities	Management
Iatrogenic overhydration	Common	Crystalloid infusion Absorption of irrigation fluids	Urine osmolality <250 mOsm/kg Serum hyponatremia *Variably present*	Observation
Hyperglycemia	Common	Diabetes mellitus Stress hyperglycemia Steroid administration	Glucosuria Pseudohyponatremia Hypokalemia Acidosis (DKA) ↑osmolality (HHNK)	Insulin, potassium supplementation
Mannitol	Occasional	Reduction of intracranial pressure (ICP), renal protection during rhabdomyolysis	Serum hyponatremia, increased osmolality, hypokalemia; rarely hyperkalemia	Self-limited
Post-obstruction diuresis	Common	Bilateral ureteral obstruction causing hydronephrosis		Supportive
Other diuretics	Unusual	Loop ● bumetanide ● ethacrynate ● furosemide ● torsemide Potassium-sparing ● amiloride hydrochloride ● spironolactone ● triamterene Carbonic anhydrase inhibitors ● acetazolamide ● methazolamide Osmotic ● glycerin ● isosorbide ● urea	Variable	Self-limited

Condition	Frequency	Cause / Association	Findings	Treatment
Neurogenic diabetes insipidus	Unusual	Procedures of the pituitary, traumatic brain injury, craniotomy, Sheehan's syndrome	Hypernatremia, high serum osmolality, low urine osmolality	DDAVP, carbamazepine, chlorpropamide
Hypercalcemia	Unusual	Hyperparathyroidism, paraneoplastic syndrome (lung, breast carcinoma)	Calcium >14 mg/dl	IV normal saline, loop diuretic, calcitonin
Nephrogenic diabetes insipidus	Rare	Pregnancy, craniopharyngioma, medications: • lithium • demeclocycline • ofloxacin • aminoglycosides • cimetidine • amphotericin	Hypernatremia, hyperosmolality	Furosemide, NSAIDs
Cerebral salt wasting syndrome	Rare	SAH, traumatic brain injury, craniotomy	Hyponatremia, Low serum osmolality	IV normal saline
Acute thyrotoxicosis	Rare	Graves' disease, thyroid storm	Elevated T3 or T4	Supportive, treatment of hyperthyroidism
High protein enteral feeding	Rare	Jevity, Ensure	Increased urea	Decrease protein content of enteral feeding
Radiographic contrast dye	Unusual			Self-limited, hydration
Recovery from ATN	Rare		Decreasing blood urea nitrogen and creatinine	Supportive
Sevoflurane	Rare		None	Transient

DDAVP = desmopressin, NSAIDs = non-steroidal anti-inflammatory drugs, DKA = diabetic ketoacidosis, HHNK = hyperglycemic hyperosmolar non-ketotic coma, ATN = acute tubular necrosis, SAH = subarachnoid hemorrhage unresponsive nephrogenic DI.[15] Correction of bilateral ureteral obstruction will produce post-obstructive polyuria of mixed etiology in which nephrogenic DI may play a role. Hypercalcemia, either due to hyperparathyroidism or as a paraneoplastic process, may also cause polyuria via nephrogenic DI.

Management: Non-specific therapy for nephrogenic DI includes administration of thiazide diuretics. Administration of a diuretic in treatment of polyuria may seem paradoxical, but the increased urinary sodium losses limit free water loss. NSAIDs may limit renal free water loss by affecting renal prostaglandins. Lithium-induced DI may be specifically antagonized by amiloride. Parathyroidectomy may be curative of nephrogenic DI caused by hyperparathyroidism. Treatment of hypercalcemia will improve DI due to increased serum calcium.

Cerebral salt wasting syndrome (CSW)

CSW may develop after traumatic brain injury, craniotomy, or subarachnoid hemorrhage. Increased sympathetic outflow and inappropriate release of natriuretic proteins may lead to polyuria. The clinical presentation has significant overlap with neurogenic DI, but the volume loss includes salt wasting rather than free water. Neurogenic DI and CSW may be distinguished by laboratory findings. Management of CSW is supportive replacement of sodium and fluid losses.[16]

Miscellaneous

Thyrotoxicosis and/or thyroid storm will cause polyuria through down-regulation of aquaporin-2 and may be observed in the perioperative setting,[17] but polyuria is unlikely to be the predominate sign. Polyuria may be observed at intravenous contrast administration and rarely observed with protein-rich enteral feeds if excessive urea is produced. Urea is an osmotic diuresis if glomerular filtration rate is intact, although urea accumulates in chronic renal insufficiency without causing diuresis.

Sevoflurane

Sevoflurane is metabolized to fluoride ions in much the same way methoxyflurane was metabolized. Since methoxyflurane was associated with significant renal toxicity, much attention has been paid to the renal effects of sevoflurane. Sevoflurane now has two decades of established clinical safety and no reports of significant renal toxicity in humans. Sevoflurane does have a transient inhibitory effect upon aquaporin-2.[18] Reports of sevoflurane-induced polyuria are unusual.[19–21] These reports are generally not associated with the development of laboratory abnormalities and are self-limited to the time of administration of the volatile agent. While sevoflurane might in rare cases be the cause of intraoperative polyuria, its contribution to postoperative polyuria has not been observed.

References

1. D.W. Wilmore, R.J. Smith, S.T. O'Dwyer, et al. The gut – a central organ following surgical stress. *Surgery* 1988; 104:917–923.

2. J.P. Desborough. The stress response to trauma and surgery. *Br J Anaesth* 2000; 85:109–117.

3. K. Holte, N.E. Sharrock, H. Kehlet. Pathophysiology and clinical implications

of perioperative fluid excess. *Br J Anaesth* 2002; 89:622–632.

4. G.R. McAnulty, H. Robertshaw, G.M. Hall. Anaesthetic management of patients with diabetes mellitus. *Br J Anaesth* 2000; 85:80–90.

5. P.H. Manninen, A.M. Lam, A.W. Gelb, S.C. Brown. The effect of high-dose mannitol on serum and urine electrolytes and osmolality in neurosurgical patients. *Can J Anaesth* 1987; 34:442–446.

6. J. Rimal, S.V. Pisklakov, H. Boules, A. Patel. Acute hyperkalemia and hyponatremia following intraoperative mannitol administration. *J Anesth Clin Res* 2013; 4:294. doi:10.4172/2155-6148.1000294.

7. M. Nakasuji, M. Nomura, M. Yoshioka, *et al.* Hypertonic mannitol-induced hyperkalemia during craniotomy. *J Anesth Clin Res* 2013; 4:299. doi:10.4172/2155-6148.1000299.

8. J.P. Sharma, R. Salhotra. Mannitol-induced intraoperative hyperkalemia, a little-known clinical entity. *J Anaesthesiol Clin Pharmacol* 2012; 28:546–547.

9. J. Hensen, A. Henig, R. Fahlbusch, *et al.* Prevalence, predictors and patterns of postoperative polyuria and hyponatraemia in the immediate course after transsphenoidal surgery for pituitary adenomas. *Clin Endocrinol (Oxf)* 1999; 50:431–439.

10. G. Zada, W. Sivakumar, D. Fishback, P.A. Singer, M.H. Weiss. Significance of postoperative fluid diuresis in patients undergoing transsphenoidal surgery for growth hormone-secreting adenomas. *J Neurosurg* 2010; 112:744–749.

11. C. Saifan, R. Nasr, S. Mehta, *et al.* Diabetes insipidus: a challenging diagnosis with new drug therapies. *ISRN Nephrol* 2013: 797620. doi:10.5402/2013/797620.

12. H. Bendz, M. Aurell. Drug-induced diabetes insipidus. Incidence, prevention, and management. *Drug Saf* 1999; 21:449–456.

13. S. Ghirardello, N. Hopper, A. Albanese, M. Maghnie. Diabetes insipidus in craniopharyngioma: postoperative management of water and electrolyte disorders. *J Pediatr Endocrinol Metab* 2006; 19:413–421.

14. J.R. Seckl, D.B. Dunger, J.S. Bevan, *et al.* Vasopressin antagonist in early postoperative diabetes insipidus. *Lancet* 1990; 335:1353–1356.

15. S. Ananthakrishnan. Diabetes insipidus in pregnancy: etiology, evaluation, and management. *Endocr Pract* 2009; 15:377–382.

16. A.H. Yee, J.D. Burns, E.F.M. Wijdicks. Cerebral salt wasting: pathophysiology, diagnosis, and treatment. *Neurosurg Clin N Am* 2010; 21:339–352.

17. W. Wang, C. Li, S.N. Summer, S. Falk, R.W. Schrier. Polyuria of thyrotoxicosis: down regulation of aquaporin water channels and increased solute excretion. *Kidney Int* 2007; 72:1088–1094.

18. K. Morita, T. Otsuka, T. Ogura, *et al.* Sevoflurane anaesthesia causes a transient decrease in aquaporin-2 and impairment of urine concentration. *Br J Anaesth* 1999; 83:734–739.

19. S.Y. Lee, H.Y. Kim, H.W. Shin, *et al.* Transient polyuria during sevoflurane anesthesia: a report of two cases. *Anesth Pain Med* 2006; 1:139–143.

20. S.H. Kim, C.H. Kim, Y.J. Kim, *et al.* Polyuria during sevoflurane anesthesia for parotidectomy patient. *Ewha Med J* 2013; 36:72–76.

21. L. Schirle. Polyuria with sevoflurane administration: a case report. *AANA J* 2011; 79:47–50.

Abnormal urine color

James W. Heitz

- Abnormal urine color *may* indicate serious pathology.
- Green or blue urine is typically benign.
- Propofol infusion may result in green, white, pink, or red discoloration of the urine.
- Red or green urine may be associated with propofol **AND** when associated with metabolic acidosis, bradycardia, hypotension, or ketonuria should raise suspicion for propofol infusion syndrome.
- Rhabdomyolysis, transfusion reaction, hemolysis, and hypovolemia are the most serious disorders likely to be visually detectable in the urine after surgery.

Hippocrates emphasized the importance of examining urine for color, odor, and consistency. While abnormal urine color (Table 37.1) is infrequently the sole cause of concern in the postoperative patient, it still provides diagnostic insight and is often readily visible in the collection bag when the patient has an indwelling bladder catheter. Abnormal urine color may be benign even when extreme, or may indicate serious pathology even when mild. Despite more than two millennia of observation by physicians, there is still no standardized nomenclature for describing urine color.

Yellow urine

The presence of urochrome in urine imparts its characteristic normal yellow hue. Deviation from this color is produced by either increasing or decreasing the concentration of urochrome or by the presence of additional pigments.

Dark or bold yellow urine: The term "dark" may be applied to urine that is a bolder than normal shade of yellow, brown, orange, or red. For purposes of discussion here, dark urine refers to bold yellow; other hues will be considered separately. In the postoperative patient, dark urine most commonly indicates abnormally concentrated urine with relatively increased urochrome. Concentrated urine may be confirmed on urinalysis by increased specific gravity and osmolality, but laboratory confirmation is seldom necessary. Dark urine and low urine output are typically associated with intravascular volume depletion. Intravascular hypovolemia is common after surgery and may be due to inadequate volume replacement, inappropriate vasodilatation, ongoing hemorrhage, or fluid loss into the third

Post-Anesthesia Care: Symptoms, Diagnosis, and Management, ed. James W. Heitz. Published by Cambridge University Press. © Cambridge University Press 2016.

Table 37.1 Causes of urinary discoloration

Color	Causes
Red	Chloroquine deferoxamine, hydroxobalamin, ibuprofen, phenazopyridine (pyridium), rifampin, warfarin, intravascular hemolysis, hematuria, propofol infusion syndrome, porphyria, beets, blackberries, carrots
Orange	Rifampin, isoniazid, riboflavin, sulfasalazine, conjugated bilirubin, blackberries, beets, rhubarb, senna herbs, dehydration, phenolphthalein, prochlorperazine, phenazopyridinc (pyridium)
Blue or green	Methylene blue, indigo carmine, biliverdin, propofol (bolus or infusion), amitriptyline indomethacin, cimetidine, flupirtine, food coloring, metoclopramide, methocarbamol, promethazine, thymol, pseudomonas infection, sildenafil, triamterene, asparagus, black licorice
Purple	Purple Urine Bag Syndrome, porphyria
Brown	Acetaminophen toxicity, propofol infusion syndrome, metronidazole, nitrofurantoin, hemolytic anemia, rhabdomyolysis, porphyria, fava beans, rhubarb, iodine contamination from perineal skin prep
Black	Alpha-methyldopa, cresol, iron, L-dopa, methocarbamol, metronidazole, nitrofurantoin, sorbitol, porphyria, malignant melanoma
White	Lipiduria, propofol infusion, proteinuria, chyluria, hypercalciuria, hyperoxaluria, phosphaturia

space. Improvement of urine output with an intravascular fluid challenge with 500 to 1000 ml of crystalloid for the typical adult patient is both diagnostic and therapeutic. Fluid challenge is an appropriate treatment for the majority of postoperative patients after intravascular volume overload has been excluded by physical examination.

Dark urine may occur in the euvolemic or hypervolemic patient owing to the syndrome of inappropriate antidiuretic hormone secretion (SIADH). SIADH is more typically recognized in the clinical setting by mild hyponatremia, but may be first suspected by dark urine from the postoperative patient without laboratory testing. Unlike dark urine caused by hypovolemia, SIADH will *not* respond appropriately to a fluid challenge with increased urine output or urinary dilution, and inappropriate fluid challenge also may exacerbate the severity of hyponatremia.[1]

Red urine

The differential diagnosis of red to reddish-brown urine is broad. Red discoloration of the urine may indicate hematuria. Hematuria may be due to tissue trauma which might be expected after urological surgery or may occur unexpectedly after other procedures of the abdomen or pelvis. Traumatic and infectious complications of bladder catheterization or urolithiasis may also present with hematuria. It is difficult to gauge the severity of bleeding by visual examination of urine color, with insignificant amounts of blood sometimes causing profound color alteration. As little as 1 milliliter of blood per liter of urine may cause visible reddening of the urine. Serial blood tests are necessary to monitor blood loss from hematuria. Contamination of urine from menstrual or hemorrhoidal bleeding may be mistaken for true hematuria.

Reddish or red to brown urine may also be due to hemoglobinuria caused by intravascular hemolysis. Hemolysis may occur postoperatively because of transfusion reaction in patients receiving blood products during or after surgery, in patients with glucose-6-phosphate deficiency (G6PD), or patients with sickle cell anemia, thalassemia, idiopathic thrombocytopenic purpura, or thrombotic thrombocytopenic purpura. Patients of African or Mediterranean descent are at increased risk for G6PD and may experience hemolysis when exposed to many of the medications used perioperatively.[2] Hereditary spherocytosis also results in hemolysis, with crisis being precipitated typically by systemic infection, but these patients may commonly present for splenectomy or cholecystectomy and hemolysis may be seen postoperatively. Discolored urine due to hemoglobinuria will test positive for the presence of heme.

The presence of myoglobin in the urine may cause similar reddish or red to brown discoloration. Myoglobinuria requires immediate treatment owing to the risk of nephrotoxicity. Rhabdomyolsis causing myoglobinuria may occur in the surgical patient for a variety of reasons; trauma with significant crush or electrical injury, as a complication of intraoperative positioning in long procedures, malignant hyperthermia, propofol infusion syndrome, or rarely as a complication of depolarizing neuromuscular blockers. Discolored urine due to myoglobinuria will also test positive for heme. Serum creatine kinase is usually elevated.

Additionally, red urine may also indicate the presence of porphyrin. Acute porphyria may occur in the postoperative patient through exposure to triggering medications. Porphyria is actually a group of diseases which may be caused by a number of enzymatic defects of heme synthesis and occurs in the general population at an incidence of approximately 1 in 25,000.[3] Abnormality of urine color is unlikely to be the sole presentation of illness, as most patients experience abdominal pain, symptoms of sympathetic excess including tachycardia and sweating, cutaneous manifestations, and/or psychosis. In the acute postoperative setting, some of these symptoms may be masked or the diagnosis otherwise complicated by the confounding effects of opioids, sedatives, and perioperative stress.

A variety of medications and foods have been associated with reddish urine, but none would be commonly encountered in the postoperative patient. Red or reddish brown urine has been described in propofol infusion syndrome, a rare but potentially fatal syndrome characterized by bradycardia, hypotension, lactic acidosis, rhabdomyolysis, serum hyperkalemia, elevated serum creatine kinase, and/or hepatomegaly.[4] Propofol may interfere with mitochondrial function, causing cellular death. Although initially described after prolonged infusion at high doses, it is now recognized that propofol infusion syndrome may be triggered after as little as 5 hours, so it may be seen during or after surgeries where propofol is used during maintenance of anesthesia. Of note, propofol infusion has also been reported to cause pinkish urine[5] and later examination of this urine by microscopy revealed apparent uric acid crystals as well as elevated uric acid levels in the urine,[6] but this abnormality is unrelated to propofol infusion syndrome.

Orange urine

Rifampin has been described as causing orange to red urine and may be seen in the surgical patient being concurrently retreated for tuberculosis. Conjugated bilirubin due to hepatic obstruction causes yellow-orange urine with yellow foam when agitated.[7] Concentrated urine from hypovolemia may sometimes be orange tinged. Prochlorperazine may cause orange urine as may the urinary analgesic pyridium (phenazopyridine).

Brown urine

Deep reddish urine may appear brown and the differential diagnosis of brown urine is the same as red. The presence of conjugated bilirubin in the urine manifesting from cholestasis may cause urine to appear brown. Mild icterus and clay-colored stools may accompany the urinary discoloration. Additionally, brown urine may be seen in the clinical setting with acetaminophen overdose owing to urinary p-aminophenol. Povidone-iodine contamination from perineal areas prep has been reported to falsely give the appearance of brown urine abnormality after surgery.[8]

Black urine

Urinary porphyrins may impart a black color to the urine as well as the red to reddish brown discoloration described above. Intramuscular supplementation of iron may cause black urine and may be observed in gynecological or colorectal surgery patients being concurrently treated for severe anemia. The antibiotics metronidazole and nitrofurantoin are other possible postoperative causes of black urine.

Blue/green urine

Blue or green urine is often encountered in the postoperative patient and is usually due to the intraoperative administration of methylene blue or indigo carmine, which may be administered intravenously during surgery for the explicit purpose of staining the urine to make it more easily recognized if a ureter becomes inadvertently disrupted. These blue pigments are renally excreted, but may appear green when combined with the yellow of urochrome. The ratio of blue pigment to urochrome determines whether urine appears blue, green, or blue-green. Methylene blue may be contained in other medications or prescribed primarily for therapeutic purposes (such as treatment of methemoglobinemia), but this would be unusual in postoperative setting.

Hepatic conjugation of the phenol ring of propofol during prolonged infusion has been associated with green discoloration of urine[9] as well as feces[10] and human breast milk.[11] Urine discoloration after a single bolus of propofol for induction of anesthesia is unusual, but has been reported and may last up to 2.5 hours after administration.[12,13] Alternatively, green urine may develop only after several days of continuous propofol infusion.[14] Normalization of urine color 6 hours after stopping the propofol infusion has been observed,[15] as has a lightening of the green urine color 6 hours after propofol infusion dose reduction.[16] However, it may take as long as 2 days for urine color to normalize after discontinuation of the propofol infusion.[17] Urinary discoloration from propofol is benign in the absence of symptoms suggestive of propofol infusion syndrome.

Green urine has been reported from other phenol-containing medications sometimes administered perioperatively including promethazine, thymol, and cimetidine. Additionally, some non-phenol-containing medications including metoclopramide and amitriptyline have also been associated with greenish urine discoloration. Urinary biliverdin accumulation from severe hepatic disease can cause green urine discoloration. Infection with *Pseudomonas* can cause green urine from the presence of the pigment pyocyanin.[18]

Purple urine

Indigo (blue) and indirubin (red) are sometimes secreted into urine. In urinary tract infection with a variety of gram-negative bacteria producing the enzyme indoxyl phosphatase, both pigments may be produced, imparting a purple discoloration to the urine. Often, this infection may be polymicrobial with one form of bacteria (often *Klebsiella* or *Providencia*) producing the blue pigment and another producing the red. This is most typically seen in patients with chronic indwelling bladder catheterization and sometimes referred to as Purple Urine Bag Syndrome.[19] Porphyrias may also cause purple urine, although red to reddish purple are more commonly observed.

White urine

Whitish discoloration of urine may be caused by pyuria and warrants urinalysis looking for white blood cells indicating infection. In the absence of white cells, hypercalciuria, hyperphosphaturia, or hyperoxaluria or chyluria may all present as whitish discoloration. Lipiduria, which may occur after the administration of total parenteral nutrition, also appears as whitish discoloration with the urine sometimes described as having a "milky" appearance. Although there are numerous case reports of prolonged propofol infusion causing milky white urine it is unclear whether this is caused by the lipid component or uric acid excretion.[7]

Colorless urine

Pale yellow to colorless urine is typically due to diuresis. It is commonly seen in patients receiving intravenous crystalloids. Although urine color by itself is a poorly reliable sign of volume status,[20] the appearance of pale or colorless urine often requires no further investigation or therapy. Sources of diuresis besides volume overload, which may also produce pale to colorless urine, include osmotic diuresis of any cause, including the administration of mannitol or the administration of loop, thiazide, and potassium-sparing diuretics. Osmotic diuresis from glycosuria may occur even in the absence of prior history of diabetes mellitus. Many diabetic patients may be undiagnosed at the time of surgery, or hyperglycemia may result from the surgical stress response (e.g. catecholamine-induced gluconeogenesis) or surgical resection involving the pancreas. Hypercalcemia or acute alcohol ingestion may also cause diuresis. Diabetes insipidus may produce colorless urine and should be suspected in any patient after an intracranial procedure or closed head trauma.

Standing urine

Standing urine may change color owing to pigment production by bacteria or exposure to light. The color changes of porphyria may first be noticed after urine is allowed to stand. Urine from patients with alcaptonia, a rare inherited metabolic disorder causing alkaptonuria in which urine turns dark-brown to black when exposed to air, also darkens when standing. Methocarbamol causes bluish discoloration in standing urine.

References

1. G.R. Bell, A.R. Gurd, J.P. Orlowski, *et al.* The syndrome of inappropriate antidiuretic-hormone secretion following spinal fusion. *J Bone Joint Surg Am* 1986; 68:720–724.

2. R.D. Aycock, D.A. Kass. Abnormal urine color. *South Med J* 2012; 105:43–47.

3. H. Puy, L. Gouya, J.C. Deybach. Porphyrias. *Lancet* 2010; 375:924–937.

4. A. Fudickar, B. Bein. Propofol infusion syndrome: update of clinical manifestation and pathophysiology. *Minerva Anestesiol* 2009; 75:339–344.

5. A. Masuda, K. Hirota, T. Satone, Y. Ito. Pink urine during propofol anesthesia. *Anesth Analg* 1996; 81:666–667.

6. A. Masuda, T. Asahi, M. Sakamaki, *et al.* Uric acid excretion increases during propofol anesthesia. *Anesth Analg* 1997; 85:144–148.

7. C.L. Foot, J.F. Fraser. Uroscopic rainbow: modern matula medicine. *Postgrad Med J* 2006; 82:126–129.

8. W.W. Noll, D.D. Glass. Cause of dark urine. *JAMA* 1980; 243:2398.

9. A. Bodenham, L.S. Culank, G.R. Park. Propofol infusion and green urine. *Lancet* 1987; 2:740.

10. A.W. O'Regan, M. Joyce-Brady. "Pond poop" from propofol. *Intensive Care Med* 2003; 29:2106.

11. T. Birkholz, G. Eckardt, S. Renner, A. Irouschek, J. Schmidt. Green breast milk after propofol administration. *Anesthesiology* 2009; 111:1168–1169.

12. C. Ananthanarayan, J.A. Fisher. Why was the urine green? *Can J Anaesth* 1995; 42:87–88.

13. D.W. Barbara, F.X. Whalen. Propofol induction resulting in green urine discoloration. *Anesthesiology* 2012; 116:924.

14. A.B. Pedersen, T.K. Kobborg, J.R. Larsen. Grass-green urine from propofol infusion. *Acta Anaesthiol Scand* 2015; 59:265–267.

15. B.D. Ku, K.C. Park, S.S. Yoon. Dark green discolouration of the urine after prolonged propofol infusion: a case report. *J Clin Pharm Ther* 2011; 36:734–736.

16. S.A. Blakey, J.A. Hixson-Wallace. Clinical significance of rare and benign side effects: propofol and green urine. *Pharmacotherapy* 2000; 20:1120–1122.

17. J. Lepenies, E. Toubekis, U. Frei. Green urine after motorcycle accident. *Nephrol Dial Transplant* 2000; 15;725–726.

18. P. Leclercq, C. Loly, P. Delanaye, C. Garweg, B. Lambermont. Green urine. *Lancet* 2009; 373:1462.

19. C.H. Lin, H.T. Huang, C.C. Chien, D.S. Tzeng, F.W. Lung. Purple urine bag syndrome in nursing homes: ten elderly case reports and a literature review. *Clin Interv Aging* 2008; 3:729–734.

20. S.J. Fletcher, A.E. Slaymaker, A.R. Bodenham, M. Vucevic. Urine colour as an index of hydration in critically ill patients. *Anaesthesia* 1999; 54:189–192.

Chapter

38

Pain

Benjamin Vaghari, Jaime Baratta, and Kishor Gandhi

- Pain is the fifth vital sign.
- Pain after surgery is often inadequately treated.
- Multimodal analgesia emphasizing non-opioid adjuvants improves analgesia while reducing side effects.

Pain occurring in the Post-Anesthesia Care Unit (PACU) setting is all too common and often an expected occurrence. Even the most thorough anesthetic plan may not properly provide the patient with adequate analgesia in recovery. This means that the clinician in the PACU must determine the type and severity of pain and formulate a treatment plan taking into account both patient and surgical factors.

Traditionally, opioids were the cornerstone of analgesic therapy despite their many unwanted and undesirable side effects. Recently, as more non-opioid medications have become available and regional techniques have gained prominence, opioids have become less cornerstones of therapy and more adjuncts to a successful analgesic strategy. This multimodal analgesic therapy is continuing to gain prominence by improving analgesia, reducing patient side effects, and improving both patient satisfaction and recovery times.

Clinicians need to be familiar with intravenous (IV) opioids as well as IV non-opioids such as acetaminophen. Additionally, many ambulatory patients will be prescribed oral analgesics, both opioid and non-opioid, which can be initiated in the PACU as well. Also, regional anesthesia with its benefits and risks can aid in improving analgesia and reducing opioid side effects. A clinician must be familiar with both rescue nerve blocks and existing neuraxial and peripheral catheters.

Pain assessment in the PACU

Accurately assessing a patient's pain in the postoperative period is often a very daunting task. Recent surveys suggest a patient's most common concern preoperatively is postoperative pain. Despite ever-improving technology and pharmacotherapy, the majority of patients still experience moderate to severe pain.[1] And although it is well known that uncontrolled pain may hinder rehabilitation, increase morbidity and mortality, decrease patient satisfaction, and be a risk factor for chronic pain, no single tool has been developed to assess pain 100% accurately.

Post-Anesthesia Care: Symptoms, Diagnosis, and Management, ed. James W. Heitz. Published by Cambridge University Press. © Cambridge University Press 2016.

Recently pain has been labeled as "the fifth vital sign" to ensure that it is appropriately addressed with every patient. However, pain is complex and subjective, and a clinician will benefit from having familiarity with the different types of pain. There are five accepted types of pain: nociceptive, neuropathic, psychogenic, mixed, and idiopathic.[2] Nociceptive pain may be described as aching, sharp, throbbing pressure, or stiffness. Neuropathic pain is often burning, tingling, crushing, or stabbing. Psychogenic pain entails complaints of pain that may not match the presenting symptoms. A mixed pattern of pain contains characteristics of neuropathic and nociceptive pathways, and idiopathic pain is that of unknown origin.

In order to assess pain accurately, one must delineate both quantitative and qualitative aspects of the pain in order to appropriately direct treatment, as no single therapeutic agent is effective in treating all types of pain. Numerous quantitative tools exist and have been proven effective, such as the Numeric Rating Scale (NRS), Verbal Rating Scale (VRS), Visual Analog Scale (VAS), and Faces Pain Scale (FPS), although no single tool has been deemed superior.[2] Assessment may be done via self-report or observer-based, but observer-based assessment should be reserved for those who are unable to communicate. The NRS is the most commonly used method as it is reliable and easy to use, while the VRS, although simple to use because of the limited number of descriptors, may lack sensitivity to treatment-induced changes. The VAS scale has proven to be effective in clinical and research settings, but is often time-consuming and may be difficult for the cognitively impaired. The FPS is commonly utilized in the pediatric population and likely may be useful for the cognitively impaired or those with language barriers.[2] Regardless of which method is utilized to quantitatively address pain, a proper pain assessment may only be done when identifying qualitative aspects as well. It is imperative to identify the character of a patient's pain (dull, stabbing, sharp, burning, spasm-like, etc.) in conjunction with the severity in order to appropriately guide therapeutic measures.[2]

Opioids

Opioids have long been used to treat pain and are a mainstay of providing analgesia to patients in a PACU setting. While highly effective in providing analgesia, opioid use is often limited by unwanted side effects. As such, guidelines from the American Society of Anesthesiologists (ASA) task force of 2012 have recommended using opioids more as adjuncts to supplement analgesia provided by other modalities such as non-opioids or regional techniques. By far the most frequently used opioids in the PACU are morphine, hydromorphone, and fentanyl.

Morphine is the most widely used opioid in the world. Morphine is relatively hydrophilic, which slows its time of onset, reaching its peak at around 30 minutes. With a half-life of approximately 2 hours, morphine lasts about 4 hours. Morphine is primarily metabolized in the liver into morphine-3-glucuronide and morphine-6-glucuronide. However, morphine-6-glucuronide is an active metabolite and is excreted primarily by the kidneys. Thus, morphine should be used with caution in patients with renal impairment, as they are more prone to potentially dangerous sedation and respiratory depression.[3] Morphine also causes dose-dependent histamine release, which can result in blood pressure decreases, although bronchospasm is unlikely.

Hydromorphone is a semisynthetic opioid. When compared with morphine, hydromorphone is about 5 times as potent, with a slightly decreased duration of action of 3 to

4 hours, and has a more rapid onset of 10 minutes. Hydromorphone undergoes primarily hepatic metabolization with no active metabolites and therefore is a better choice than morphine for patients with renal impairment. Given these characteristics, hydromorphone is useful in the PACU where rapid analgesia is desirable, especially in opioid-tolerant patients.

Fentanyl is a synthetic opioid that is up to 100 times as potent as morphine. Much of fentanyl's usefulness in a PACU setting is a result of its rapid onset: it acts in seconds, reaching peak activity within 6 minutes owing to its high lipid solubility. While fentanyl undergoes hepatic metabolism and has an upwards of 8 hour half-life, fentanyl's apparent clinical half-life appears much shorter because of redistribution to inactive sites. Typically a 100 mcg dose will have an analgesic effect for 1 to 1.5 hours. This relatively shorter duration means that it may require readministration. Like hydromorphone, fentanyl has no active metabolites and will not accumulate in patients with compromised renal function.

Each of the three above opioids has certain advantages and disadvantages. An appropriate treatment plan will take into account characteristics of each opioid but also the characteristics of the individual patient (e.g. renal failure, sleep apnea, opioid tolerant) as well as the setting (e.g. ambulatory). Disadvantages that all the opioids have in common are pruritus, nausea and vomiting, urinary retention, sedation, and respiratory depression. Each patient can react differently to each opioid medication with differences in analgesic efficacy and side-effect profile. If a patient cannot tolerate morphine owing to nausea, a change to hydromorphone may be beneficial.

In addition, learning to manage unwanted side effects of opioids is important in caring for surgical patients. Pruritus is common and though it is frequently treated with antihistamines such as diphenhydramine, the mechanism of opioid-induced pruritus does not appear to involve histamine release. Administration of naloxone will relieve pruritus with the downside of reduced analgesia. Opioid-induced nausea and vomiting occurs from stimulation of opioid receptors in the brainstem. About 25% of all patients receiving opioids will experience nausea and vomiting. Hence, postoperative nausea and vomiting (PONV) is a leading cause of delayed PACU discharge.[4] The most prophylactic medications are serotonin-3 (5-HT$_3$) inhibitors (e.g. ondansetron) and dexamethasone.[5,6] (PONV rescue therapy is discussed in Chapter 19 and the management of pruritus in Chapter 20.)

While PONV and pruritus can make suffering patients miserable, the most important opioid side effect to the clinician is respiratory depression. The incidence of opioid-induced respiratory depression is estimated to be between 0.09% and 0.5%.[7] While any patient is susceptible to opioid-induced respiratory depression, patient populations such as those with obstructive sleep apnea, the elderly, opioid tolerant, and infants up to 60 weeks postconceptual age are particularly at risk. The only effective therapy for opioid-induced respiratory depression is an antagonist such as naloxone. Always be aware that many of the commonly used opiates have half-lives that are longer than the antagonists, leading to the risk of the patient relapsing after the antagonist effect remits.

A treatment modality that will assist in reducing a patient's risk of significant respiratory depression is IV patient-controlled analgesia (PCA). While PCA is not useful for outpatient surgeries, it has been shown to improve patient satisfaction and lead to improved analgesia relative to nurse-administered dosing. PCA can often be started in the PACU, and a clinician should be familiar with PCA settings. Optimal usage of a PCA involves a loading dose of an opioid. Once the patient achieves a desired level of comfort, or further treatment is withheld because of respiratory depression, the PCA then functions as patient-directed maintenance. For this reason, basal infusions should be used with caution as they remove an important safety device inherent to PCA, i.e. the patient must be awake to self-administer an additional dose.

Non-opioids

Non-opioid analgesic medications are an important component of any analgesic plan in a PACU. Non-opioids are useful not only in reducing pain scores, but also in limiting the side effects of opioids. Often these unwanted opiate side effects such as pruritus, sedation, and respiratory depression are the major limiting factor in opiate use. Commonly used non-opioid analgesics such as acetaminophen and non-steroidal anti-inflammatory drugs (NSAIDs) such as ketorolac and ibuprofen have no such side effects and can be an effective supplement to or at times even a complete replacement for opioid-based analgesics. While many of these medications were traditionally available only in oral forms, thus limiting their use as rescue analgesics, recently IV formulations have become available and are important to be familiar with.

NSAIDs produce analgesia via inhibition of cyclooxygenase and have powerful peripheral anti-inflammatory properties. Commonly used IV ketorolac and the more recently approved IV ibuprofen are two valuable medications to use in a PACU setting. Ketorolac as a rescue medication is typically given in single doses of 30 to 60 mg, either IV or IM, and is very effective in reducing both pain and oral analgesic requirements. Typical maximal onset of analgesia occurs at 30 minutes, roughly similar to morphine. Additionally, 30 mg of ketorolac achieves pain relief similar to that of 4 mg of morphine. When compared with fentanyl, a commonly used PACU medication, ketorolac has a slower onset of analgesia. However, unlike smaller doses of fentanyl, ketorolac is effective in reducing pain 4 to 6 hours after administration.[8]

In terms of optimum dose and timing of ketorolac administration, the data are mixed. Some studies have suggested that ketorolac is much more effective when given preoperatively, implying that ketorolac is more effective when given as part of an analgesic plan as opposed to a rescue medication in the PACU.[9] Other data suggest that ketorolac is just as effective in reducing pain scores when given postoperatively in a PACU setting.[10] As for dosing, a meta-analysis examining perioperative single-injection ketorolac found that 60 mg had a clear postoperative benefit, while 30 mg of ketorolac displayed varied results.[11] At this time, based on the available data, ketorolac is an effective single-dose rescue medication in the PACU with doses of at least 30 mg, though 60 mg may be preferable.

IV ibuprofen is a second non-opioid analgesic that can be of use in a PACU setting. Dosing ranges and schedules are similar to oral dosing with a typical adult dose being 400 to 800 mg every 6 hours. The medication must be given as an infusion over 30 minutes. As IV ibuprofen was approved for use by the US Food and Drug Administration (FDA) in 2009, at the current time information on single-dose administration in the PACU is limited. However, good clinical evidence exists that demonstrates significant reductions in opiate use and pain scores when IV ibuprofen is administered around the clock for the first 24 postoperative hours.[12,13] For PACU use, based on the available information, 800 mg of IV ibuprofen appears to be a more effective analgesic than 400 mg.[13] As a note, both ibuprofen and ketorolac can cause gastrointestinal upset in patients and should be used with caution in those patients with significant renal impairment.

Both oral and rectal acetaminophen have a long history of use as rescue medications in the PACU. More recently, IV acetaminophen has become available and has certain advantages over the more traditional slower release forms. Acetaminophen, like NSAIDs, appears to function via inhibition of cyclooxygenase, but its activity appears to be primarily central acting with no peripheral anti-inflammatory properties. Common dosages range from 650 to 1000 mg for oral, 1000 mg vials for IV, and 1 to 2 g for rectal administration. In terms of safety profile and unwanted effects, acetaminophen has minimal side effects with the main concern being hepatotoxicity. Overall acetaminophen, especially oral and IV, has been shown to be very effective in reducing pain and sparing opioid use.[14,15]

In a PACU setting the rapidity of onset of an analgesic is critical to its effectiveness both as a pain reliever but also in improving patient flow through the recovery period. While oral acetaminophen can begin to alleviate pain within 15 minutes, the IV formulation onset time is even faster. At this time patients appear to report equal improvement in pain scores when either IV or oral acetaminophen is administered in a PACU, though the evidence is not yet robust.[16] When compared with either IV or oral routes, however, rectal acetaminophen can take hours to demonstrate significant plasma levels. This delay makes rectal acetaminophen simply impractical for use in a PACU setting. Both IV and oral acetaminophen are excellent choices for analgesia in a PACU setting, with IV having an edge in terms of speed of onset and ability to use in patients unable to take oral medications.

Oral analgesics

Pain in the PACU is often successfully treated with parenteral medications and/or regional anesthesia (Table 38.1). However, an ever-increasing number of patients will be discharged to home after an adequate recovery. Many of these patients will have some level of pain and will be prescribed any of a variety of oral analgesics. Often these medications can be administered in a PACU setting in lieu of parenteral medications.

Oral analgesics are most effective for mild to moderate pain. The World Health Organization Pain Ladder recommends non-opioid analgesics for mild pain and a weak opioid or weak opioid/non-opioid combination for moderate pain.[17] If patients are to be discharged with a prescription for a particular oral analgesic, that medication can be started in recovery. Otherwise an oral analgesic can be selected taking into account pain severity and patient-related factors such as allergies and co-morbidities. Oral analgesics have a range of effectiveness and significant patient-to-patient analgesic variability. Of note, codeine 60 mg, a frequently prescribed weak opioid, while an excellent antitussive agent is a poor analgesic when not used in combination with acetaminophen. Given the availability of other more effective agents, codeine should not be used for analgesia in the PACU.

Overall, there are numerous different oral medications, both as single or combination agents. One recommendation is to administer analgesics as single agents rather than in combination for increased flexibility in dosing. For example, oral non-opioids can be given as scheduled dosing while oral opioids are used for breakthrough pain. On the other hand, a benefit of combination agents is that they take advantage of the synergistic analgesic effect of combining opioids and non-opioids such as acetaminophen and oxycodone. An important note on combination agents: a downside of combination pills, while convenient, is that many non-opioids such as acetaminophen and ibuprofen have important toxicity limits that should be avoided. Many patients can unwittingly overdose on these non-opioids at home as they add these combination pills to their prior non-opioid regimen.

Table 38.1 Commonly used oral opioid analgesics

Drug	Dose in milligrams	Frequency in hours	Expected duration in hours
Hydrocodone	10–30	4–6	4–8
Oxycodone	10–20	4–6	3–4
Hydrocodone/ Acetaminophen	5/325 7.5/325 10/325	4–6	4–8
Oxycodone/ Acetaminophen	5/325 7.5/325	4–6	3–4
Acetaminophen/ Codeine	300/30	4–6	3–4
Hydromorphone	4–8	3–4	3–4

Regional analgesia in the PACU

As the 2012 ASA Task Force on Acute Pain Management guidelines clearly emphasize a multimodal approach to analgesia in the perioperative setting, regional analgesia has a clear role in reducing postoperative pain in the PACU and should be employed whenever possible.[18] It is well documented, especially in the orthopedic population, that regional analgesia is superior to opioids in managing pain postoperatively. For instance, brachial plexus continuous peripheral nerve blockade (CPNB), when used in the inpatient and outpatient setting, has demonstrated prolonged pain control of up to 72 hours, less opioid use, faster resumption of physical therapy, fewer sleep disturbances, and overall increased patient satisfaction.[19] Similar results have been demonstrated for the various types of regional analgesia when compared with opioids.

While the majority of regional anesthetics are performed preoperatively to assist in intraoperative pain management, it is imperative to assess the quality of the regional blockade in the PACU in an expedient manner and have a low threshold for rescue blockade following a block failure. Each patient who has received a regional anesthetic, including brachial plexus, lumbar plexus, femoral, saphenous, sciatic, and transversus abdominis plane block, should be assessed for adequacy of sensory as well as motor blockade and an overall pain assessment upon arrival in the PACU. If a continuous catheter is in place and the block is determined inadequate, a 10 ml bolus of ropivacaine 0.5% (or alternatively bupivacaine 0.25%) should be administered via the catheter, as an increase in volume and local anesthetic spread may sufficiently improve the block. If the bolus proves unsuccessful or the patient received a single-shot peripheral nerve blockade, a repeat block should strongly be considered. However, in the event of extensive surgery or combination peripheral nerve blockade, it is imperative to properly delineate the distribution of pain to appropriately determine which block may be necessary.

Familiarity with the different types of peripheral nerve blocks is essential as well. For instance, the interscalene approach of a brachial plexus block provides good analgesia following shoulder surgery, but a common complaint encountered in the PACU is persistent axillary pain. In order to properly address such pain, the provider must be familiar with the distribution of the brachial plexus, which encompasses C5–T1 nerve roots, while the dermatome of the axilla is innervated by the intercostobrachial nerve (T2) and is therefore missed. Treatment of persistent axillary pain may be achieved by a supplemental intercostobrachial nerve block or supplemental opioids. As the benefits of regional analgesia have clearly been documented in published research and its utilization continues to increase, familiarity with the various types of peripheral nerve blockade is essential in the postoperative setting.

With improving technology and the increasing utilization of ultrasound, the use of continuous peripheral nerve blockade is on the rise specifically with regards to ambulatory catheters. Interscalene, infraclavicular, and popliteal catheters have all been shown to lower pain scores at rest and with movement as well as lower oral opioid analgesic use.[20] However, when utilizing ambulatory catheters it is important to use a dilute solution of local anesthetic, such as ropivacaine 0.2% at a rate of 4–10 ml/hr depending on location, to maximize sensory blockade while minimizing motor blockade as well as the risk of local anesthetic toxicity. Patient selection and education is imperative and detailed discharge instructions with contact information and emergency instructions must be provided.

Managing epidural catheters in the PACU

Common reasons for epidural failure include incorrect placement, inadequate infusion, and migration of catheters.[21] Failure rates as high as 32% for thoracic epidurals and 27% for lumbar epidurals have been previously reported.[22] The management of patients with thoracic and lumbar epidurals requires close supervision by a dedicated acute pain management team.

Prior to usage, all epidural catheters should be given a test dose to rule out intrathecal or intravenous placement. In instances when the patient is given a combined spinal–epidural (CSE) for surgical anesthesia, the test dose should be given after resolution of the spinal anesthetic since an intrathecal placement of the catheter can be missed. A common test entails aspirating the catheter for continuous blood or cerebrospinal fluid flow; however, this test has a high false-negative rate. Once negative flow is confirmed, a test dose of 2% lidocaine with dilute epinephrine (10 mcg/ml) can further rule out a misplaced epidural catheter. Epinephrine, as an additive to a test dose, functions as a marker of intravascular catheter placement. Epinephrine will cause an increase in heart rate and blood pressure with intravascular locations of the catheter. However, this test is insensitive and false negatives can occur. Other symptoms of intravascular injection of test dose include perioral numbness, tinnitus, vertigo, and rare seizures.

An infusion of local anesthetic can be started at a rate of 10–14 ml/hr after ruling out intrathecal and intravascular placement of an epidural catheter. The ideal concentration and local anesthetic agent depend on the desired differential block. Most institutions utilize dilute ropivacaine (0.1%, 0.2%) or bupivacaine (0.15%) to minimize motor block and maximize sensory blockade. The main quality of analgesia is determined by the total dose of local anesthetic, which is dependent on both rate per hour and concentration. The addition of opioids (e.g. fentanyl, sufentanil, dilaudid) to the local anesthetic can allow for reduction in local anesthetic dose and increasing patient comfort. Epinephrine can be added to epidural infusion to decrease systemic absorption of local anesthetic.

Epinephrine also binds to α_2 adreno receptors, resulting in anti-nociceptive effects on the spinal cord.[21]

Postoperative control of pain in the PACU entails a multimodal approach. Clinicians will need to be familiar with IV opioids and non-opioids. Additionally, many ambulatory patients can be prescribed oral analgesics, which can be initiated in the PACU. Regional anesthesia with its benefits and risks can aid in improving analgesia, reducing opioid side effects, and decreasing overall PACU stay. A multimodal approach that combines the previously mentioned techniques will assist in improving patient care in the PACU.

References

1. J.L. Apfelbaum, C.M. Chen, S.S. Mehta, T.J. Gan. Postoperative pain experience: results from a national survey suggest postoperative pain continues to be undermanaged. *Anesth Analg* 2003; 97:534–540.

2. R. Sinatra, O.A. de Leon-Cassasola, B. Ginsberg, E.R. Viscusi. *Acute Pain Management.* New York, NY: Cambridge University Press; 2009; 147–616.

3. J.X. Mazoit, K. Butscher, K. Samii. Morphine in postoperative patients: pharmacokinetics and pharmacodynamics of metabolites. *Anesth Analg* 2007; 105:70–78.

4. R.P. Hill, D.A. Lubarsky, B. Phillips-Bute, *et al.* Cost-effectiveness of prophylactic antiemetic therapy with ondansetron, droperidol, or placebo. *Anesthesiology* 2000; 92:958–967.

5. P.S. Loewen, C.A. Marra, P.J. Zed. 5-HT$_3$ receptor antagonists vs. traditional agents for the prophylaxis of postoperative nausea and vomiting. *Can J Anaesth* 2000; 47:1008–1018.

6. P.J. Karanicolas, S.E. Smith, B. Kanbur, *et al.* The impact of prophylactic dexamethasone on nausea and vomiting after laparoscopic cholecystectomy: a systematic review and meta-analysis. *Ann Surg* 2008; 248:751–762.

7. A. Dahan, L. Aarts, T.W. Smith. Incidence, reversal, and prevention of opioid induced respiratory depression. *Anesthesiology* 2010; 112:226–238.

8. R. Twersky, A. Lebovits, C. Williams, *et al.* Ketorolac versus fentanyl for postoperative pain management in outpatients. *Clin J Pain* 1995; 11:127–133.

9. D. Fletcher, P. Zetlaoui, S. Monin, *et al.* Influence of timing on the analgesic effect of intravenous ketorolac after orthopedic surgery. *Pain* 1995;61:291–297.

10. C. Vanlersberghe, M.H. Lauwers, F. Camu. Preoperative ketorolac administration has no preemptive analgesic effect for minor orthopaedic surgery. *Acta Anaesthesiol Scand* 1996; 40(8 Pt 1):948–952.

11. G.S. De Oliveira Jr., D. Agarwal, H.T. Benzon. Perioperative single dose ketorolac to prevent postoperative pain: a meta-analysis of randomized trials. *Anesth Analg* 2012; 114:424–433.

12. P. Kroll, L. Meadows, A. Rock, *et al.* A multicenter, randomized, double-blind, placebo-controlled trial of intravenous ibuprofen (i.v. ibuprofen) in the management of postoperative pain following abdominal hysterectomy. *Pain Pract* 2011; 11:23–32.

13. S. Southworth, J. Peters, A. Rock, *et al.* A multicenter, randomized, double-blind, placebo-controlled trial of intravenous ibuprofen 400 mg and 800 mg every 6 hours in the management of postoperative pain. *Clin Ther* 2009; 31:1922–1935.

14. L. Toms, H. McQuay, S. Derry, *et al.* Single dose oral paracetamol (acetaminophen) for postoperative pain

in adults. *Cochrane Database Syst Rev* 2008; (4):CD004602.

15. R. Sinatra, J. Jahr, L. Reynolds, *et al.* Efficacy and safety of single and repeated administration of 1 gram intravenous acetaminophen injection (paracetamol) for pain management after major orthopedic surgery. *Anesthesiology* 2005; 102: 822–931.

16. C.N. Brett, S.G. Barnett, J. Pearson. Postoperative plasma paracetamol levels following oral or intravenous paracetamol administration: a double-blind randomized controlled trial. *Anaesth Intensive Care* 2012; 40:166–171.

17. World Health Organization (WHO) Stepwise Approach to Pain Management. 2012. http://www.who.int/cancer/palliative/painladder/en/. (Accessed November 05, 2012.)

18. American Society of Anesthesiologists Task Force on Acute Pain Management. Practice guidelines for acute pain management in the perioperative setting: an updated report by the American Society of Anesthesiologists Task Force on Acute Pain Management. *Anesthesiology* 2012; 116:248–273.

19. B.M. Ilfeld. Continuous peripheral nerve blocks: a review of the published evidence. *Anesth Analg* 2011; 113: 904–925.

20. B.M. Ilfeld, F.K. Enneking. Continuous peripheral nerve block at home: a review. *Anesth Analg* 2005;100:1822–1833.

21. J. Hermanides, M.W. Hollmann, M.F. Stevens, *et al.* Failed epidural: causes and management. *Br J Anaesth* 2012; 109:144–154.

22. L.B. Read. Acute pain: lessons learned from 25,000 patients. *Reg Anesth Pain Med* 1999; 24:499–505.

Chapter

39

Shoulder pain

Jordan E. Goldhammer

- Shoulder pain is common after non-shoulder surgery and requires special attention to identify the cause.
- Increased pain on movement suggests an intrinsic shoulder injury.
- No exacerbation on movement suggests referred pain from another region of the body.
- Pain is more commonly referred to the left shoulder after laparoscopy or with cardiac ischemia.

The shoulder is a complex joint composed of multiple bones and ligaments. The clavicle, scapula, and humerus converge to form four articular surfaces: sternoclavicular, acromioclavicular, glenohumeral, and scapulothoracic. The articular surfaces are stabilized by two major groups of connective tissue: the glenohumeral ligaments, and the rotator cuff, which is formed from the supraspinatus, infraspinatus, subscapularis, and teres minor ligament. This complex anatomy allows the shoulder the greatest range of motion of any joint in the human body.

Shoulder pain in the early postoperative period after non-shoulder procedures can be classified into two categories, intrinsic shoulder pain or extrinsic shoulder pain (Figure 39.1). Intrinsic pain is directly due to damage of the shoulder girdle structures. Extrinsic pain is referred from elsewhere in the body. Evaluation of the postoperative patient with shoulder pain should begin with a pertinent history and physical exam. Intrinsic shoulder pain is localized to the shoulder and exacerbated with movement. Extrinsic sources of pain will be poorly localized, and normal shoulder movement will not alter the character of the pain.

Intrinsic shoulder pain

Patients with intrinsic shoulder injury will present with pain, stiffness, weakness, and instability of the shoulder joint. Pain is most commonly at the anterolateral shoulder and is reproducible with specific shoulder movements. Postoperative intrinsic shoulder pain is most commonly due to patient positioning. Surgical positioning in the supine or lateral decubitus position may lead to neurological, vascular, or ligamentous compromise. The supine patient should have arms abducted no more than 90 degrees to limit brachial plexus

Post-Anesthesia Care: Symptoms, Diagnosis, and Management, ed. James W. Heitz. Published by Cambridge University Press. © Cambridge University Press 2016.

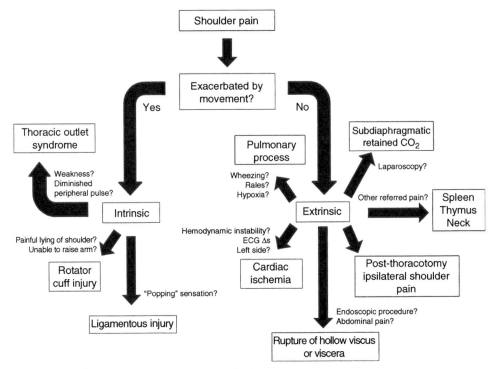

Figure 39.1 Differential diagnosis of postoperative shoulder pain.

stress or musculoskeletal injury. Ligamentous injury, labral or rotator cuff tear, or complete shoulder subluxation may occur because of trauma during positioning. Any patient moved from the supine to prone position is at risk for traumatic shoulder injury. Additionally, the particular placement of arm boards or arm board malfunction may contribute to intrinsic shoulder injury if not properly secured to the operating room table. Ligament injury presents as shoulder weakness, anterolateral shoulder pain, and a popping sensation when the shoulder is moved.[1] Complete shoulder subluxation will result in multidirectional instability of the shoulder, excessive range of motion, and crepitus over the shoulder joint. Symptoms are often vague and non-specific. If intrinsic musculoskeletal injury is suspected, specialty consultation should be sought.

Positioning in lateral decubitus position may cause compression of the shoulder structures and entrapment of the axillary neurovascular bundle. At the thoracic outlet, the subclavian vasculature and the brachial plexus exit the chest and enter the arm. The thoracic outlet is an anatomically small space confined by the clavicle, first rib, and scalene tendon. Subtle variations in the anatomy of the passage may cause compression and irritation of the nerves and vessels. Entrapment of the axillary neurovascular bundle at the thoracic outlet commonly presents as numbness, paresthesia, and pain radiating from the hand to the shoulder. A weak radial pulse may be palpated that diminishes with change in arm position.[2] Acute thoracic outlet syndrome may be due to venous obstruction (blue, swollen, painful arm) or arterial obstruction (pain, pallor, diminished pulse).[3] If acute thoracic outlet syndrome is suspected, urgent surgical consultation is recommended.

Extrinsic shoulder pain

Extrinsic shoulder pain is poorly localized to the shoulder joint and not exacerbated with shoulder movement. Range of motion is typically normal. The differential diagnosis of referred pain to the shoulder is robust, but a few causes are frequently observed after surgery.

Subdiaphragmatic gas: Laparoscopic surgery may cause extrinsic shoulder pain and has been reported to occur in up to 63% of laparoscopic cases.[4] The pain is often reported in the Post-Anesthesia Care Unit (PACU) and may peak at 24 hours after the surgery.[5] The pain is typically self-limited and resolves by 72 hours.[6] Carbon dioxide retention in the subdiaphragmatic region causes irritation of the phrenic nerve.[7] Additionally, the rapid overstretching of the diaphragm and peritoneum during insufflation may cause trauma to muscle fibers, blood vessels, and nerves, resulting in referred shoulder pain through the phrenic nerve.[4] Left shoulder pain is more common than right shoulder pain, since the liver protects against gas accumulation under the right hemi-diaphragm.[8] Specific neurons within the ventroposterolateral nucleus of the thalamus have been shown to have a dual response to both phrenic sensory stimulation and tactile stimulation of the shoulder, providing a mechanism for referred diaphragmatic pain.[9]

Subdiaphragmatic gas pain management: Although self-limited, this complication may be associated with significant patient discomfort and attempts have been made to decrease the incidence with attention to surgical technique. Decreased shoulder pain has been associated with low flow, low pressure pneumoperitoneum, as well as gasless exposure by mechanical lifting to allow surgical visualization.[10] The ability to decrease the incidence of postoperative shoulder pain is procedure specific. For laparoscopic cholecystectomy (performed in reverse Trendelenburg position), only low flow, low pressure pneumoperitoneum has been demonstrated to decrease the incidence and severity of shoulder pain.[11] Conversely, for gynecological laparoscopy (performed in Trendelenburg position), active gas drainage and pulmonary recruitment maneuvers are beneficial.[12] Attempts to relieve shoulder pain by local anesthetic infiltration of the diaphragm and aspiration of the pneumoperitoneum at the conclusion of surgery have been moderately successful. Postoperative phrenic nerve block has proven efficacious, but confers only transient pain relief.[13] Pain relief of post laparoscopic shoulder pain is most commonly achieved with non-steroidal anti-inflammatory drugs (NSAIDs), acetaminophen, or opioids. Typically, pain may be controlled with oral analgesics and home discharge, if desired, need not be delayed.

Visceral injury: Shoulder pain may also occur because of irritation, ischemia, compression, or rupture of visceral organs. Referred shoulder pain has been reported following esophageal, gastric, or intestinal rupture; surgery to the liver, biliary tree, or spleen; adrenal or pancreatic hematoma; and cholecystitis.[2] Pneumoperitoneum or hemoperitoneum secondary to viscus or vasculature injury may occur following trauma, endoscopy, laparotomy, lower extremity vascular access, or any surgical procedure involving the abdomen. In addition to shoulder pain, patients with pneumoperitoneum or hemoperitoneum may display hypotension and peritonitis. Shoulder pain after esophagoscopy should raise concern for esophageal rupture and may be accompanied by chest pain, throat pain, and fever. This is a surgical emergency and consultation should be sought.

Thoracotomy: Ipsilateral shoulder tip pain has been described following thoracotomy, and may occur in up to 50% of cases.[14] Pain is typically independent of movement, poorly localized, aching in quality, and described as moderate to severe.[15,16] Ipsilateral post-thoracotomy shoulder pain is not relieved with epidural analgesia.[15] Referred shoulder pain can be differentiated from incisional pain by dosing an epidural catheter. With a properly functioning catheter, incisional pain will be relieved; however, referred ipsilateral shoulder pain will persist. Classic ipsilateral post-thoracotomy shoulder pain will gradually decline over the first 4 to 6 postoperative hours, rarely extending until postoperative day 1.[15,17] Many hypotheses exist about the etiology of ipsilateral shoulder pain including excessive surgical retraction, brachial plexus positioning injury, transaction of a major bronchus, or pleural irritation secondary to thoracostomy tube. The phrenic nerve clearly plays a role in referred pain transmission as preoperative phrenic nerve infiltration with local anesthetic has been shown to reduce ipsilateral shoulder pain by nearly 50%.[18] Additionally, postoperative phrenic nerve blockade by an interscalene brachial plexus block has been shown to provide immediate pain relief lasting 6 to 10 hours.[16] The cornerstone of postoperative ipsilateral shoulder pain treatment is conservative management with NSAIDs or acetaminophen.[15] A postoperative interscalene brachial plexus block may be considered for pain relief; however, care must be taken in selecting patients, as blockage of the phrenic nerve and ipsilateral diaphragm may cause respiratory compromise. Ipsilateral shoulder pain does not respond well to intravenous opioids and care must be taken to avoid overmedication and respiratory depression in patients with compromised pulmonary function.[18]

Other referred pain: Other sources of extrinsic pain include neurological, vascular, pulmonary, and cardiac disease. Referred pain to the shoulder may arise from the neck, thymus, and spleen. Particularly important in the postoperative patient are pulmonary and cardiac insult.

The administration of anesthesia depresses airway reflexes and places the patient at risk for pulmonary aspiration of gastric contents. Aspiration occurs in approximately 1 in 8,000 general anesthetics in healthy patients and may occur in the presence of endotracheal intubation.[19] Aspiration pneumonia may present in the postoperative period with hypoxia, cough, bronchospasm, and pleuritic shoulder pain. Diagnosis can be confirmed by chest X-ray. Management includes supplemental oxygen and advanced airway management.

Classically, acute myocardial infarction may present as nausea, diaphoresis, shortness of breath, substernal chest pain, and referred left-sided shoulder, jaw, or neck pain. In the postoperative setting, associated chest and referred pain may be masked by systemic opioids and anesthetic recovery. Myocardial ischemia in the PACU typically presents as tachycardia and hypotension. Myocardial ischemia should be considered in postoperative patients with risk factors for cardiac disease displaying tachycardia, hypotension, and shoulder pain.

References

1. C.S. Neer. Impingement lesions. *Clin Orthop Relat Res* 1983;173:70–77.

2. S. Campbell. Referred shoulder pain: an elusive diagnosis. *Postgrad Med* 1983; 73:193–203.

3. B. Brooke, J. Freischlag. Contemporary management of thoracic outlet syndrome. *Curr Opin Cardiol* 2010; 25:535–540.

4. M.G. Cunniffe, O.J. McAnena, M.A. Dar, J. Calleary, N. Flynn. A prospective random trial of intraoperative bupivacaine irrigation for management of shoulder tip pain following laparoscopy. *Am J Surg* 1998; 176:258–261.

5. H. Tsai, Y. Chen, C. Ho, *et al.* Maneuvers to decrease laparoscopy-induced shoulder and upper abdominal pain: a randomized controlled study. *Arch Surg* 2011; 146:1360–1366.

6. M. Rosenblum, R.S. Weller, P.L. Conrad, E.A. Falvey, J.B. Gross. Ibuprofen provides longer lasting analgesia than fentanyl after laparoscopic surgery. *Anesth Analg* 1991; 73:255–259.

7. A. Nyerges. Pain mechanisms in laproscopic surgery. *Semin Laparosc Surg* 1994; 1:215–218.

8. P. Schoeffle, P. Diemunsch, L. Fourgeau. Coelioscopie ambulatoire. *Cah Anesthesiol* 1993; 41:385–391.

9. W. Zhang, P. Davenport. Activation of thalamic ventroposteriolateral neurons by phrenic nerve afferents in cats and rats. *J Appl Physiol* 2002; 94:220–226.

10. M. Berberoglu, O.N. Dilek, F. Ercan, *et al.* The effect of CO_2 insufflation rate on postlaparoscopic shoulder pain. *J Laparoendosc Adv Surg Tech A* 1998; 8:768–770.

11. A.M. Donatsky, F. Bjerrum, I. Gögenur. Surgical techniques to minimize shoulder pain after laparoscopic cholecystectomy. A systematic review. *Surg Endosc* 2013;27:2275–2282.

12. B. Taş, A.M. Donatsky, I. Gögenur. Surgical techniques to minimize shoulder pain after laparoscopic surgery for benign gynaecological disease. A systematic review. *Gynecol Surg* 2013;10:169–173.

13. K. Mats, M. Yoshida, Y. Maemura, *et al.* Significance of phrenic nerve block in the anesthetic management of laparoscopic cholecystectomy. *Masui* 1994; 43:1718–1721.

14. P. MacDougall. Postthoracotomy shoulder pain: diagnosis and management. *Curr Opin Anaesthesiol* 2008; 21:12–15.

15. M. Barak, A. Ziser, Y. Katz. Thoracic epidural local anesthetics are ineffective in alleviating postthoracotomy ipsilateral shoulder pain. *J Cardiothorac Anesth* 2004; 18:458–460.

16. N. Tan, N.M. Agnew, N.D. Scawn, *et al.* Suprascapular nerve block for ipsilateral shoulder pain after thoracotomy with thoracic epidural anesthesia: a double blind comparison of 0.5% bupivacaine and 0.9% saline. *Anesth Analg* 2002; 94:199–202.

17. S.H. Pennefather, M.E. Akrofi, J.B. Kendall, *et al.* Double-blind comparison of intrapleural saline and 0.25% bupivacaine for ipsilateral shoulder pain after thoracotomy in patients receiving thoracic epidural analgesia. *Br J Anaesth* 2005; 94:234–238.

18. N.D. Scawn, S.H. Pennefather, A. Soorae, *et al.* Ipsilateral shoulder pain after thoracotomy with epidural analgesia: the influence of phrenic nerve infiltration with lidocaine. *Anesth Analg* 2001; 93:260–264.

19. M.A. Warner, M.E. Warner, J.G. Weber. Clinical significance of pulmonary aspiration during the perioperative period. *Anesthesiology* 1993; 78:56–62.

Chapter

Anemia

40

Elizabeth Wolo and James W. Heitz

> - No single hemoglobin or hematocrit value should trigger transfusion for all patients.
> - The etiology of postoperative anemia is multifactorial and may occur in the absence of surgical blood loss.
> - Anemia disproportionate to the surgical blood loss necessitates a search for another cause of red blood cell loss or destruction.

Anemia is defined as a deficiency of circulating erythrocytes. Anemia may be expressed as low hemoglobin or hematocrit. Hemoglobin is the protein contained in erythrocytes that is primarily responsible for the delivery of oxygen to bodily tissues. Hematocrit measures the volume of erythrocytes compared with the total blood volume. Normal values vary by age and sex. Although some differences will exist between individual laboratories, hemoglobin ranges of 13.5 to 17.5 g/dl for men and 12.0 to 15.5 g/dl for women are considered normal. Hematocrit ranges from 40% to 50% for men and 36% to 44% for women.

Oxygen delivery to the body may be expressed by the equation:

$$DO_2 = CO \times (Hgb \times SaO_2 \times 1.34 + PaO_2 \times 0.003)$$

where DO_2 = oxygen delivery; CO = cardiac output; Hgb = hemgloloin;
SaO_2 = hemoglobin oxygen saturation; PaO_2 = partial pressure of oxygen in blood.

Oxygen delivery to the body is principally a function of cardiac output, hemoglobin content, and hemoglobin oxygenation saturation. A small amount of oxygen is freely dissolved in blood, but increasing the PaO_2 of arterial blood increases oxygen delivery only nominally.

Although blood oxygen content falls proportionately to hemoglobin concentration, the physiological significance of any degree of anemia varies between patients, thwarting the ability to establish a universal transfusion trigger. Differences in the ability to increase cardiac out put, basal oxygen consumption, and the efficiency of extraction of oxygen by the tissues will determine how well or how poorly the body can adapt to any given degree of anemia.

The adequacy of compensatory mechanisms also impacts the clinical significance of anemia. Increased production of 2, 3-diphosphoglycerate (2,3-DPG) by red cells decreases hemoglobin binding affinity for oxygen, effectively increasing the efficiency of oxygen

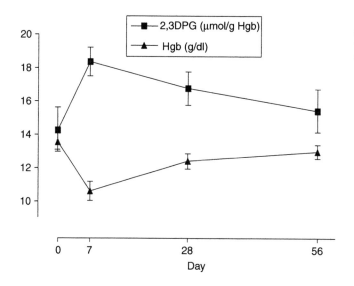

Figure 40.1 Levels of 2,3-DPG versus hemoglobin (Hgb) over time.

release to tissue from hemoglobin and occurs in response to postoperative anemia. Increased levels of 2,3-DPG begin almost immediately after the onset of anemia, and peak levels coincide with the nadir of the hemoglobin (Figure 5.1).[1]

Etiology of postoperative anemia

The incidence of preoperative anemia ranges from 11% to 76% depending upon the patient population studied,[2] and anemia will be even more prevalent after surgical blood wastage. Postoperative anemia is an anticipated outcome of surgery. Clinical concern ought to be elicited when the severity of anemia is out of proportion to the reported surgical blood loss. The differential diagnosis of postoperative anemia out of proportion to expectations is narrow, but determining the etiology is crucial to minimizing potential complications.

Inaccurate estimated blood loss (EBL): Surgical blood loss is typically estimated by visual inspection of visible blood loss, gravimetric analysis of fluid content of surgical gauze and sponges, and the measured volume of suctioned fluids. Each of these methods introduces some error into the calculation of EBL. Numerous studies have found substantial inaccuracy in the visual estimation of blood loss and poor inter-individual reliability. This is true whenever estimation of puddled blood is necessary, including child birth,[3–13] skin grafting,[14] trauma,[15,16] and epistaxis therapy.[17] Sponge weight is a more objective measurement, but is also subject to inaccuracy in measurement. The presence of other fluids, including irrigation and urine, will contribute to wet weight, overestimating blood loss, while evaporative fluid loss leads to underestimation of blood loss and is affected by surgical duration, room temperature, and humidity. Other fluids besides blood may be suctioned from the surgical field and the contribution of irrigation fluids or urine to suctioned fluids must be accurately deducted.

EBL may overestimate blood loss at very low volumes, but underestimates blood loss when volumes are high.[18] EBL has been found to vary from actual blood loss by 26% after major orthopedic procedures[19] and as much as 49% after delivery.[20]

Table 40.1 The calculation of anticipated postoperative hematocrit or hemoglobin

Average blood volume	
Adult women	60–65 ml/kg
Adult men	70–75 ml/kg
Infant	80 ml/kg
Full-term neonates	85–90 ml/kg
Premature infants	95–120 ml/kg

Estimated blood volume (EBV) = Weight (kg) × Average blood volume (ml/kg)
Estimated postoperative hematocrit* = Hct_{POST} = $Hct_{PRE} - \left(\frac{Hct_{PRE} \times EBL}{EBV}\right)$
*Hemoglobin may be substituted for hematocrit.

A significant discrepancy of the anticipated hemoglobin or hematocrit from measured values could be due to an inaccurate EBL. Anticipated hemoglobin in the *euvolemic* patient after appropriate volume resuscitation may be calculated by the formula in Table 40.1.

Dilutional anemia: Measured hemoglobin and hematocrit will reflect red blood cell loss, but also the degree of intravascular volume re-expansion. In the extreme form, rapid blood loss without volume replacement reduces circulatory volume but does not immediately alter hemoglobin or hematocrit. Too little volume replacement with crystalloids (under-resuscitation) results in an artifactually high hemoglobin/hematocrit measurement. Too much volume replacement with crystalloids (over-resuscitation) may result in an artifactually low measurement. Some degree of dilutional anemia is common in the early postoperative setting. Other indicators of hypervolemia may or may not be present.

Occult hemorrhage: Ongoing hemorrhage may be recognized in the postoperative setting by sanguineous seepage on to surgical dressings and output into surgical drains or chest tube. Unanticipated severe postoperative anemia should cause clinical suspicion for occult sources of bleeding. Occult hematoma formation can occur anywhere, including the limbs, thoracic, and retroperitoneal space where a significant proportion of the circulatory blood volume may be lost without clinical notice. Occult hemorrhage may be related to the surgical procedure or trauma, or may be related to other procedures or coincidental to the surgery. These later causes are often easily overlooked. Central line placement or regional anesthetic should raise concern for occult bleeding remote from the surgical site. If a hemothorax has occurred, a chest X-ray may show a large one-sided effusion. Retroperitoneal hematomas can be more challenging to diagnose because the most common signs of retroperitoneal hematomas are non-specific (hypotension and tachycardia). More specific findings in retroperitoneal hematomas are bruising and pain that occur in the peri-umbilical region (Cullen's sign) or in the flank (Grey Turner's sign). Abdominal, flank, groin, or lumbar radicular pain may be present. Fatal occult hemorrhage has been reported from lumbar sympathetic block with a 26-gauge needle,[21] so seemingly innocuous clinical interventions can have profound effects if recognition of occult hemorrhage is delayed.

Hemolysis: Although rare, hemolysis is an etiology of disproportionate postoperative anemia. Hemolysis is the premature destruction of erythrocytes. Hemolysis is most frequently a consequence of transfusion reaction, but may occur in surgical patients in the absence of blood transfusion. If hemolysis is suspected, the diagnosis can be confirmed by an abnormal blood smear demonstrating fragment red blood cells (schistocytes), elevated or normal reticulocyte count, elevated bilirubin, elevated lactate dehydrogenase, and a low haptoglobin.

Drug-induced hemolytic anemia can occur by autoimmune or non-autoimmune mechanisms. Over 125 medications have been identified in causing autoimmune hemolytic anemia.[22] The most commonly implicated medications that are frequently administered in the perioperative period are procainamide and antibiotics (especially penicillins and cephalosporins), but perioperative polypharmacy creates some small degree of risk in all surgical patients for this rare clinical phenomenon. Drug-induced non-immune hemolytic anemia is more common and can occur in predisposed individuals with enzymatic deficiencies. The most common is glucose-6-phosphate dehydrogenase (G6PD) deficiency. The highest prevalence of G6PD deficiency is among persons of African, Asian, or Mediterranean descent. Hemolysis is triggered by oxidative stress, including surgery itself and some medications. Methylene blue, sulfa drugs, and nitrofurantoin are unsafe for all patients with G6PD deficiency, but a larger number of medications may also cause hemolysis in individuals with severely deficient enzymatic activity (including diphenhydramine, prilocaine, acetaminophen, aspirin, procainamide).[23] Hemolysis can occur within hours of the exposure but usually is most apparent 24 to 72 hours after the oxidative stress.

Immune and non-immune etiologies of hemolysis can be differentiated with a direct Coombs' test or direct antiglobulin test (DAT). The DAT is positive in immune-mediated hemolysis. In non-immune-mediated hemolysis, the DAT is negative. The assay test that is performed to confirm a diagnosis of G6PD can be falsely negative during an active hemolytic episode. If G6PD deficiency is suspected, the offending agent should be discontinued, supplemental oxygen should be provided, and the patient referred to outpatient hematology and tested no sooner than 2 to 3 weeks after the hemolytic episode.

Other surgical patients may be at increased risk for hemolysis owing to underlying red blood cell defects. The most clinically common are sickle cell disease and hereditary spherocytosis. Sickle cell disease is an inherited mutation in the β-globin gene causing erythrocytes to form an abnormal sickle or crescent shape. The incidence is about 1 in every 500 African Americans. Red blood cell sickling can occur at any time, but is exacerbated when oxygen concentration in tissues is low. Maintenance of adequate oxygenation, hydration, normothermia, and analgesia are the fundamentals in preventing pain and hemolysis in a sickle cell patient. Hereditary spherocytosis is an inherited disease where the membrane of the erythrocyte is altered to be spherical instead of the normal discoid shape. The disease is encountered worldwide, but is most prevalent in people of northern European descent where it is found in about 0.02% to 0.03% of the population.[24] Affected patients may be completely asymptomatic, severely anemic, or somewhere between these extremes. Anemia is exacerbated during times of stress and viral infections. Findings to support the diagnosis of hereditary spherocytosis include: spherocytes on blood smear, small mean corpuscular volume (MCV), raised mean corpuscular hemoglobin concentration (MCHC), increased reticulocyte count, increased bilirubin, and splenomegaly.

Hemolysis may also be caused by direct red blood cell trauma in unique clinical circumstances. Mechanical valves, particularly ball-valves in the mitral position, and ventricular assist devices may cause hemolysis by this mechanism.

Anemia of chronic disease (AOCD): AOCD may be seen with certain chronic infections, malignancies, and autoimmune disorders. The disruptive effect of interleukin-6

(IL-6) upon iron metabolism has been identified as contributing to the development of anemia. Laboratory testing reveals below-normal hemoglobin, hematocrit, serum iron, serum transferrin, and transferrin saturation, but normal MCV.

A similar pattern of laboratory results consistent with AOCD is seen in patients with postoperative anemia, but the pattern is not observed clinically after hemorrhage unrelated to surgery. The acute effects of IL-6 and other inflammatory mediators released during surgical trespass may contribute to postoperative anemia.[25,26] Although postoperative anemia would seem to be merely a matter of surgical blood loss, postoperative anemia will develop after procedures without significant blood loss. Anemia was observed to develop and persist at 1 month after bunionectomy among patients with an average intraoperative blood loss of 4 ml.[25] Moreover, the development of postoperative anemia without significant blood loss appears to be independent of the type of anesthesia administered.[26,27]

The acute inflammatory state caused by surgical manipulation of tissue may produce anemia similar to that produced by chronic inflammation. This may exacerbate anemia in patients with surgical blood loss by impairing the compensatory reticulocytosis to replace lost red blood cells.

Management: Reduced red blood cell mass may be treated by replacing cells (transfusion) or supporting the ability of the body to produce new cells. The potential benefit of transfusion must be weighed against the potential risks including transfusion reaction, transmission of infectious disease, transfusion-related acute lung injury, and immunosuppression.

In a retrospective study of 125 women undergoing surgery but refusing blood transfusion owing to religious objections, increased mortality was seen with postoperative hemoglobin less than 8 g/dl, with a sharply increased mortality below 6 g/dl.[28] Significant comorbidity (cardiac, renal, hepatic) was a very poor prognostic sign in conjunction with severe postoperative anemia. The American Society of Anesthesiologists Task Force on Perioperative Blood Transfusion recommends that red blood cells should usually be administered to healthy adults if the hemoglobin is less than 6 g/dl and are not indicated if the hemoglobin concentration is more than 10 g/dl. For wide and clinically significant hemoglobin range of 6–10 g/dl, transfusion should be based on potential or ongoing bleeding, intravascular volume status, and risk factors for complications of inadequate oxygenation or poor organ perfusion.[29] The ultimate goal for treatment of anemia is to provide adequate oxygenation to vital organs, reduce cardiac and cerebral hypoxic damage while protecting the patient from potential harm from transfusions. No single transfusion trigger based upon hemoglobin or hematocrit values achieves this goal for all patients.

Nutritional supplementation

Iron, vitamin B12, and folate are necessary for reticulocytosis. Oral iron supplementation is favored by many orthopedic surgeons, although the medical literature does not show clear benefit of this practice in the therapy of postoperative anemia.[30,31] Parenteral iron supplementation as monotherapy[32,33] or in combination with erythropoietin has yielded similarly disappointing results.[34,35] This may in part be attributable to the interference with iron utilization created by postoperative inflammatory mediators. Anemia after bariatric surgery may offer a unique clinical challenge owing to the multiple disruptions in nutrient absorption from gastric resection.[36] Preliminary data suggest there may be

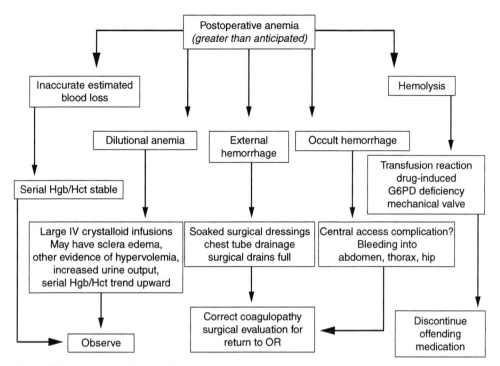

Figure 40.2 Approach to disproportionate postoperative anemia.

some benefit to parenteral iron supplementation after total gastrectomy for gastric carcinoma patients.[37] It is not yet determined whether this benefit extends to bariatric surgery patient populations as well.

An algorithmic approach to the evaluation of postoperative anemia which is out of proportion to surgical blood loss may be employed (Figure 40.2) to guide management.

References

1. J.P. Wallis, A.W. Wells, S. Whitehead, N. Brewster. Recovery from postoperative anaemia. *Transfus Med* 2005; 15:413–418.

2. A. Shander, K. Knight, R. Thurer, J. Adamson, R. Spence. Prevalence and outcomes of anemia in surgery: a systematic review of the literature. *Am J Med* 2004; 116 (7 Suppl 1):58–69.

3. H.A. Brant. Precise estimation of postpartum haemorrhage: difficulties and importance. *Br J Med* 1967; 1:398–400.

4. P.G. Higgins. Measuring nurses' accuracy of estimating blood loss. *J Adv Nurs* 1982; 7:157–162.

5. S.J. Duthie, D. Ven, G.L. Yung, *et al.* Discrepancy between laboratory determination and visual estimation of blood loss during normal delivery. *Eur J Obstet Gynecol Reprod Biol* 1991; 38:119–124.

6. S.J. Duthie, A. Ghosh, A. Ng, P.C. Ho. Intraoperative blood loss during elective lower segment caesarean section. *Br J Obstet Gynaecol* 1992; 99:364–367.

7. K. Razvi, S. Chua, S. Arulkumaran, S.S. Ratnam. A comparison between visual estimation and laboratory determination of blood loss during the third stage of labour. *Aust N Z J Obstet Gynaecol* 1996; 36:152–154.

8. W. Prasertcharoensuk, U. Swadpanich, P. Lumbiganon. Accuracy of the blood loss estimation in the third stage of labor. *Int J Gynaecol Obstet* 2000; 71:69–70.

9. P. Glover. Blood loss at delivery: how accurate is your estimation? *Aust J Midwifery* 2003; 16:21–24.

10. J.A. Kavle, S.S. Khalfan, R.J. Stoltzfus, *et al.* Measurement of blood loss at childbirth and postpartum. *Int J Gynaecol Obstet* 2006; 95:24–28.

11. C. Larsson, S. Saltvedt, I. Wilkund, S. Pahlen, E. Andolf. Estimation of blood loss after cesarean section and vaginal delivery has low validity with a tendency to exaggeration. *Acta Obstet Gynecol Scand* 2006; 85:1448–1452.

12. S.S. Buckland, C.S.E. Homer. Estimating blood loss after birth: using simulated clinical examples. *Women Birth* 2007; 20:85–88.

13. I. Stafford, G.A. Dildy, S.L. Clark, M.A. Belfort. Visually estimated and calculated blood loss in vaginal and cesarean delivery. *Am J Obstet Gynecol* 2008; 199:519.e1–519.e7.

14. P.G. Budny, P.J. Regan, A.H.N. Roberts. The estimation of blood loss during burns surgery. *Burns* 1993; 19:134–137.

15. G. Tall, D. Wise, P. Grove, C. Wilkinson. The accuracy of external blood loss estimation by ambulance and hospital personnel. *Emerg Med* 2003; 15:318–321.

16. K. Patton, D.L. Funk, M. McErlean, J.M. Bartfield. Accuracy of estimation of external blood loss by EMS personnel. *J Trauma* 2001; 50:914–916.

17. H.L. Beer, S. Duvvi, C.J. Webb, S. Tandon. Blood loss estimation in epistaxis scenarios. *J Laryngol Otol* 2005; 119:16–18.

18. G.A. Dildy, A.R. Paine, N.C. George, C. Velasc. Estimating blood loss: can teaching significantly improve visual estimation? *Obstet Gynecol* 2004; 104:601–606.

19. K.R. Sehat, R.L. Evans, J.H. Newman. Hidden blood loss following hip and knee arthroplasty. *J Bone Joint Surg Br* 2004; 86:561–565.

20. S. Maslovitz, G. Barkai, J.B. Lessing, A. Ziv, A. Many. Improved accuracy of postpartum blood loss estimation as assessed by simulation. *Acta Obstet Gynecol Scand* 2008; 87:929–934.

21. C. Maier, M. Gleim, T. Weiss, *et al.* Severe bleeding following lumbar sympathetic blockade in two patients under medication with irreversible platelet aggregation inhibitors. *Anesthesiology* 2002; 97:740–743.

22. G. Garratty. Immune hemolytic anemia associated with drug therapy. *Blood Rev* 2010; 24:143–150.

23. A.R. Elyassi, H.H. Rowshan. Perioperative management of the glucose-6-phosphate dehydrogenase deficient patient: a review of literature. *Anesth Prog* 2009; 56:86–91.

24. S.W. Eber, A. Pekrun, A. Neufeldt, W. Schröter. Prevalence of increased osmotic fragility of erythrocytes in German blood donors: screening using a modified glycerol lysis test. *Ann Hematol* 1992; 64:88–94.

25. D.H. Biesma, A. van de Wiel, Y. Benguin, R. Kraaijenhagen, J.J.M. Marx. Postoperative erythropoiesis is limited by the inflammatory effect of surgery on iron metabolism. *Eur J Clin Invest* 1995; 25:383–389.

26. C.E. van Iperen, R.J. Kraaijenhagen, D.H. Biesma, *et al.* Iron metabolism and erythropoiesis after surgery. *Br J Surg* 1998; 85:41–45.

27. H. Böhrer, M. Quintel, M.V. Fischer. Clinical evaluation of electrostimulation anesthesia for hysterectomy. *Acta Anaesthesiol Scand* 1991; 35:529–534.

28. J.L. Carson, R.K. Spence, R.M. Poses, G. Bonavita. Severity of anaemia and operative mortality and morbidity. *Lancet* 1988; 1:727–729.

29. Practice guidelines for perioperative blood transfusion and adjuvant therapies: an updated report by the American Society of Anesthesiologists Task Force on Perioperative Blood Transfusion and Adjuvant Therapies. *Anesthesiology* 2006; 105:198–208.

30. K.K.W. Lau, M.M. Utukuri, M. Ramachandran, D.H. Jones. Iron

supplementation for postoperative anaemia following major paediatric orthopaedic surgery. *Ann R Coll Surg Engl* 2007; 89:44–46.

31. M.J. Parker. Iron supplementation for anemia after hip fracture surgery: a randomized trial of 300 patients. *J Bone Joint Surg Am* 2010; 92:265–269.

32. J. Berniere, J.P. Dehuliu, O. Gail, I. Murat. Intravenous iron in the treatment of postoperative anemia in the surgery of the spine in infants and adolescents. *Rev Chir Orthop Reparatrice Appar Mot* 1998; 84:319–322.

33. M. Munoz, E. Naveira, J. Seara, *et al.* Role of parenteral iron in transfusion requirements after total knee replacement: a pilot study. *Transfus Med* 2006; 16:137–142.

34. S.N. Madi-Jebara, G.S. Sleilaty, P.E. Achouh, *et al.* Postoperative

intravenous iron used alone or in combination with low-dose erythropoietin is not effective for the correction of anemia after cardiac surgery. *J Cardiothorac Vasc Anesth* 2004; 18:59–63.

35. K. Karkouti, S.A. McCluskey, M. Ghannam, *et al.* Intravenous iron and recombinant erythropoietin for the treatment of postoperative anemia. *Can J Anaesth* 2006; 53:11–19.

36. A. von Drygalski, D.A. Andris. Anemia after bariatric surgery: more than just iron deficiency. *Nutr Clin Pract* 2009; 24:217–226.

37. O. Jeong, Y.K. Park. Effect of intravenous iron supplementation for acute postoperative anemia in patients undergoing gastrectomy for gastric carcinoma: a pilot study. *Ann Surg Oncol* 2014; 21:547–552.

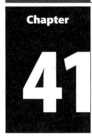

Chapter

41

Hemorrhage

Jeremy L. Hensley and Stephen O. Bader

- Acute hemorrhage may not immediately affect measured hemoglobin levels.
- Blood component therapy should be tailored to restore both oxygen carrying capacity and hemostasis.
- Hemostasis may be promoted by replacing depleted coagulation factors and platelets or by the administration of antifibrinolytic agents.

Postoperative bleeding is a common problem, representing 2.6% of all postoperative complications in one survey.[1] Bleeding may be observable, but often it is occult and may not be identified until sufficient intravascular volume-depletion has developed to cause hypotension. Since postoperative hypotension occurs frequently owing to diverse etiologies, clinical recognition of hemorrhage may be delayed. Diagnosis is made more difficult by the fact that hypovolemia from hemorrhage can be obscured by residual anesthetic effects and physiological changes associated with the surgical procedure. In the Post-Anesthesia Care Unit (PACU), clinicians should remain vigilant to the possibility of ongoing blood loss as a cause of postoperative hypovolemia. Frequently, it is necessary to institute therapy for hypotension before hemorrhage has been identified as the cause. Preparations for return to operating room should begin as soon as hemorrhage is suspected, since the availability of the proper personnel and operating room may require a significant time to coordinate.

Perioperative hemorrhage is the most common reason for blood transfusion.[2] Everyone involved in perioperative care of the surgical patient must be aware of the indications and complications of transfusion therapy.

Presentation and diagnosis

Occult hemorrhage typically presents as unexplained hypotension. Occasionally, anemia discovered incidentally on postoperative laboratory evaluation without associated hypotension will trigger further investigation for blood loss. Other more obvious signs of ongoing bleeding, such as bloody dressings or increased output from surgical drains, can be quickly identified, while laboratory and radiological assessments are made to confirm ongoing blood loss.

With acute blood loss in otherwise healthy patients, signs and symptoms may not appear until significant blood loss has occurred. Hypotension may not occur until >40%

Post-Anesthesia Care: Symptoms, Diagnosis, and Management, ed. James W. Heitz. Published by Cambridge University Press. © Cambridge University Press 2016.

of the blood volume has been lost in young patients without cardiovascular disease.[3] In patients with significant co-existing disease, or of advanced age, much smaller amounts of blood loss can result in hypotension. Other signs of hypovolemia and inadequate perfusion include reduced urine output, narrow pulse pressure, cool or mottled extremities, and poor capillary refill. These signs may precede hypotension and should not be ignored.

Intravascular hypovolemia may be due to inadequate fluid replacement because of evaporation, urine output, and edema formation intraoperatively, or the result of previous hemorrhage. If continued bleeding is suspected, the cause should be sought immediately. Postural hypotension and tachycardia usually precede frank hypotension, but may not be apparent in the supine patient after surgery. As blood loss increases, signs of decreased end-organ perfusion and hypovolemic shock may become apparent. These may include confusion, dyspnea, palor, diaphoresis, hypotension, and tachycardia. Typical physiological changes during recovery from anesthesia and anticholinergic or anti-adrenergic medications may obscure this clinical picture.

In evaluating hypovolemia in the PACU, anemia may not always be evident. Acute bleeding will not be reflected by a decreased hematocrit, if the intravascular volume loss has not been replaced. Once adequate resuscitation has been achieved using intravenous (IV) fluids, the hematocrit will reflect blood loss. Occasionally, overzealous fluid administration intraoperatively results in dilutional anemia that does not indicate blood loss. Serial measurement of hematocrit or hemoglobin concentration should be obtained, to follow the trend rather than the absolute value in determining whether bleeding is ongoing.

The causes of postoperative hemorrhage can broadly be broken down into technical (i.e. surgical) or non-technical (coagulopathy). Evaluation for both should take place simultaneously. Some estimate that early postoperative hemorrhage is due to inadequate surgical hemostasis in 75 to 90% of cases.[4] This is the so-called "silk deficiency." If bleeding from the surgical site is suspected, a thorough physical exam is warranted. Dressings should be examined for bleeding, and may require removal to inspect the wounds. If surgical drains are present, the output should be noted serially. If the patient has undergone an abdominal procedure, the abdomen may be distended or firm in cases of ongoing hemorrhage. The retroperitoneal space can accumulate a significant volume of blood, and signs such as Grey Turner's sign (flank ecchymosis) should be sought. The thighs can also hide a significant volume of lost blood before this becomes visually apparent. Furthermore, patients who have undergone orthopedic procedures may have splints/wraps that obscure inspection. If extremity hemorrhage is suspected, dressings should be removed for investigation as a limb-threatening compartment syndrome may develop.

A chest X-ray is sensitive for diagnosing hemothorax following thoracic or upper abdominal surgery or central venous access placement. CT scan should be considered in evaluating possible hemorrhage after abdominal and pelvic surgery, where plain X-ray films may not reveal even large collections of blood, especially if the bleeding is retroperitoneal. Angiography can be particularly useful for diagnosis of acute bleeding, as endovascular intervention can be performed immediately once the source is found. Bedside abdominal ultrasound has been validated to detect hemorrhage after trauma in the Emergency Department,[5] but does not yet have demonstrated efficacy in detecting postoperative hemorrhage.

Rarely, emergent interventions may be required in the PACU for hemorrhage unrelated to hypovolemia. Airway obstruction from hematoma following thyroid or anterior cervical spine surgery may require immediate opening of the incision to allow decompression of the airway obstructing hematoma. This responsibility may fall on PACU personnel if the surgeon is not immediately available. However, in less severe cases, the management may consist of a controlled return to the operating room for surgical exploration. The most important intervention to be made for bleeding is volume replacement with IV fluids and blood transfusion to maintain organ perfusion, while attempting to correct the underlying cause of bleeding.

Common medical causes of early postoperative bleeding include dilutional coagulopathy, inherited or acquired platelet disorders, hyperfibrinolysis, and inherited coagulation disorders. Dilutional thrombocytopenia is common after surgery owing to fluid resuscitation and blood transfusion. After transfusion of one blood volume, only 35% to 40% of platelets remain in circulation.[4] It should be noted that fibrinogen is also sensitive to hemodilution, and hypofibrinogenemia should always be considered as a medical cause for postoperative bleeding.[6] Loss of plasma coagulation factors can result in impaired thrombin generation, reflected by prolonged coagulation times.

Hyperfibrinolysis can be the result of large areas of tissue injury from trauma or extensive surgery, with resultant massive activation of the coagulation system.

The injured tissues release tissue factor, resulting in intravascular activation of coagulation and formation of thrombin and subsequent fibrin clots.[7] Fibrinolysis, which is feedback activated by thrombin generation, can become so avid as to cause premature breakdown of formed clot, resulting in further bleeding. Thus, massive clotting can result in massive fibrinolysis. Consequently, coagulation factors, platelets, and fibrinogen are further consumed, promoting further blood loss.

Assessment of platelet count, prothrombin time (PT), partial thromboplastin time (PTT) or activated partial thromboplastin time (aPTT), and fibrinogen concentration should be performed to detect coagulopathy when ongoing hemorrhage occurs. If the PT or PTT are prolonged more than 1.5 times normal values, the platelet count is less than 75K, or the fibrinogen is below 150 mg/dl, transfusion therapy should be considered to correct coagulopathy. Viscoelastic tests of coagulation, such as thromboelastography (TEG) and rotational thromboelastometry (ROTEM), can be used in the diagnosis of coagulopathy, when available, and can be particularly useful for identifying hyperfibrinolysis.[8,9]

Hypothermia is also common in the postoperative setting and contributes to thrombocytopenia through platelet sequestration in liver and spleen.[7] In addition, platelet surface molecules are altered, leading to impaired functioning of platelets that remain in circulation. A vicious cycle may result in which hypothermia causes more bleeding, which causes more hypothermia as room temperature fluids are administered during volume resuscitation. Rewarming of the patient causes desequestration of platelets and improved bleeding time. Plasma coagulation proteins are also sensitive to the effects of hypothermia. At 33 °C, the clotting deficiency seen is equivalent to a factor IX deficiency at 33% of its normal level.[10]

Metabolic derangements during surgery may also result in coagulation disturbance. Hypotension and hypoperfusion of end organs during surgery may result in lactic acidosis, which can impair the enzymatic processes of the coagulation cascade. There is a strong correlation between the duration of hypotension and coagulation abnormalities. One study demonstrated that shock-induced acidosis lasting greater than 150 minutes resulted in an increase in aPTT and decreased factor V activity.[11]

Blood component transfusion

Blood component transfusion has essentially replaced fresh whole blood (FWB) transfusion in the United States, with the exception of military use of FWB in austere settings. FWB may be the ideal transfusion product for traumatic or postoperative bleeding, but comes with significant safety and convenience concerns compared with blood component therapy.[12] Blood components available for transfusion include red blood cells (RBCs), fresh frozen plasma (FFP), platelets, and cryoprecipitate.

Units of whole blood are collected from volunteers and are treated with additive solutions to keep the blood product fluid and prolong storage. The separation of plasma and cellular components is accomplished by centrifugation. There are several commercial additives available. Common to these solutions is citrate, which binds to calcium ions in the collected blood, effectively anticoagulating the product, as calcium is then unavailable as a cofactor to the proteins of the coagulation system. Adenosine, phosphate, and dextrose are added to provide substrates for anaerobic metabolism, ATP synthesis, and buffering. The administration of blood products to the patient always includes the administration of the additive solution as well. Citrate toxicity can result when blood components are given rapidly, manifested by acute hypocalcemia.[13]

Hypothermia from rapid administration of cold blood products can worsen hemostasis further and has other adverse consequences for the patient. Therefore, when FFP and RBCs are transfused quickly (less than 1 hour per unit) in the PACU, a fluid warming system should be used. Slow infusions of blood products over several hours generally do not require fluid warming unless the patient is already hypothermic.

Red blood cells: In the United States, about 12 million units of RBCs are transfused annually.[2] The best indication for RBC transfusion is to improve oxygen carrying capacity. Blood transfusion is not indicated for purely intravascular volume expansion. Controversy surrounds the application of specific transfusion "triggers." Medical judgment continues to play a key role in the decision to initiate transfusion despite a hemoglobin concentration above or below a recommended threshold.

The beneficial effects of red cell transfusion are most evident in acute hypovolemia due to bleeding. The administration of red cells in response to acute blood loss provides needed intravascular volume and increases the oxygen carrying capacity. The use of volume replacement with crystalloid or colloid solutions in acute bleeding results in the anemia usually associated with blood loss.

Recommendations for specific hemoglobin and hematocrit values necessitating transfusion were developed during the NIH Health Consensus Conference.[14] These recommendations have changed little over the past 20 years. The authors recommended that acutely anemic patients with hematocrit values less than 21% will likely require RBC transfusion in the perioperative period. However, chronically anemic patients may safely tolerate lower values. Patient co-morbidities must be considered: many disease states, such as coronary artery disease, may require higher values owing to increased oxygen requirement. Clinical judgment plays a key role in these decisions.

The American Society of Anesthesiologists Practice Guidelines offered these recommendations in 2006[2]:

1. Transfusion is rarely indicated with hemoglobin values greater than 10 g/dl and almost always indicated if it is less than 6 g/dl, especially when acute.

2. Deciding whether or not to transfuse patients between these values should take patient risk into consideration.
3. The use of any specific transfusion "trigger" that does not take the patient's physiology into account is not recommended.
4. When appropriate, preoperative autologous blood donation, intraoperative and postoperative blood recovery, acute normovolemic hemodilution, and measures to decrease blood loss may be beneficial.
5. The indications for transfusing autologous blood may be more liberal than for allogenic blood because of decreased risk.

Ideally, all RBCs will be cross-matched before transfusion, reducing the risk of hemolytic transfusion reaction. In cases where time will not allow for cross-matching to be performed, type specific or type O uncrossed RBCs can be administered. Rh factor negative females of child-bearing potential should not receive Rh positive cells owing to the risk of developing antibodies that could cause fetal hydrops in a subsequent pregnancy. All others can receive either Rh positive or negative cells without consequence.

"Packed" RBCs have a high hematocrit of 70% to 80%, which varies by choice of processing and additive solutions. Transfusion of a single unit of RBCs can be expected to raise the hematocrit by about 3% in an average adult patient. Since volume is drawn into the intravascular space, packed RBC transfusion will result in volume expansion two to three times the actual volume infused. Most blood banks pass RBCs through white blood cell (WBC) filters in a process known as "leukoreduction." Leukoreduced RBCs may have a lower rate of febrile transfusion reactions and transmission of Cytomegalovirus and Epstein–Barr virus when compared with non-leukoreduced cells. Red cell irradiation is generally reserved for the very immunosuppressed patient at risk for graft-versus-host disease after blood transfusion as irradiation eliminates donor T-lymphocyte cells from the unit.[15]

Although RBC transfusion is performed to increase oxygen carrying capacity, stored RBCs may not initially deliver oxygen to the tissues as effectively as the patient's native cells. This so-called "storage lesion" of red cells becomes most apparent around 2 weeks of storage, and worsens as the stored unit approaches the expiration date.[16] Stored red cells may have less deformable cell membranes that impair microvascular blood flow and are more susceptible to aggregation. They have reduced intracellular levels of nitric oxide, ATP, and 2,3-diphosphoglycerate (2,3-DPG) levels, resulting in an inability to unload oxygen bound to hemoglobin and decreased tissue delivery.

In addition to impaired oxygen delivery, stored RBCs contain free hemoglobin, lysed cell membranes, and other immunomodulatory bioactive substances that may be responsible for increased morbidity and mortality in transfusion recipients. Transfusion-related acute lung injury (TRALI) is a well-recognized complication of red cell transfusion, but may be an under-appreciated complication in mild cases. The incidence of TRALI varies by type of transfusion, number of units, patient factors, and length of storage but ranges from 0.05% to 2.4%.[17] Units of red cells contain high levels of lactate due to anaerobic metabolism by the cells during storage, and can have very low pH (<7.0) when administered.[18] Cell lysis during storage also results in release of intracellular potassium, and rapid administration of red cells can result in hyperkalemia, of particular concern in patients with renal dysfunction. Transfusion of RBCs may also cause a higher rate of acute kidney injury and has been associated with an increase in mortality after surgery or trauma and in the critically ill.[19]

Platelets: Transfusion of platelets is frequent in the perioperative setting, with over 7 million units transfused annually in the United States. Platelets may be transfused for either absolute thrombocytopenia with a blood count less than 50,000/ml or for platelet dysfunction with normal platelet counts. Platelets should rarely be transfused if the count is above 100,000/ml. The latter indication is frequently associated with bleeding in patients who received preoperative antiplatelet therapy. Aspirin ingestion is associated with a qualitative but not quantitative decrease in platelet function. In most cases, aspirin therapy does not cause coagulopathy significant enough to warrant platelet transfusion. Other, more potent oral antiplatelet agents such as clopidogrel, ticlopidine, prasugrel, and ticagrelor are associated with a very high risk of bleeding in the perioperative period. These medications will generally be discontinued before surgery, except in the case of patients with recent drug-eluting coronary stents, as they have a high risk of acute stent thrombosis after discontinuation of antiplatelet therapy.

If a patient appears to have postoperative bleeding secondary to medication-induced platelet dysfunction, platelet transfusion is reasonable, despite normal platelet counts.[2] There are several commercially available platelet function analyzers, but there has been very little consensus on the value of these devices to guide transfusion. Platelet dysfunction can be identified using elastomeric coagulation tests, by reduced clot strength (reduced maximum amplitude (MA) on TEG, or maximum clot firmness (MCF) on ROTEM) despite normal traditional coagulation assays and platelet counts.

Platelets are prepared either from donated units of whole blood, or by donor plasmapheresis. In the case of platelets derived from whole blood units, they are separated by centrifugation and stored as single units, which are usually pooled with 4–6 other units of platelets at the time of transfusion. A unit contains approximately 5 million platelets/ml in 50 to 70 ml of plasma, and when a pool of 4–6 units is transfused to an average adult, the platelet count will rise by approximately 50,000/ml. Plasmapheresis-derived platelets are gathered from a single donor, and provide approximately the same effective dose of platelets as 4 to 6 pooled "random" units.[15]

Platelets are stored on rockers in citrated plasma for up to 5 days at 22 °C, leaving them more susceptible to bacterial contamination than other components that are stored at cooler temperatures. Platelet function is affected by cold storage, and if not kept in constant motion on rocker plates, they will clump and result in a lower delivered dose of platelets to the patient. Platelets are also associated with hypotension on administration, febrile transfusion reactions, and acute lung injury at the highest rate of all blood components.

Fresh frozen plasma: The most frequent indication for FFP in the PACU is to replace coagulant proteins that have been consumed or diluted by replacement fluid and RBC administration during hemorrhage. FFP administration also provides intravascular volume expansion, but FFP should not be transfused for this purpose solely. FFP use in fixed ratios with RBCs has been advocated for massive bleeding where greater than 0.5 to 1 blood volume is replaced, to reduce the incidence of coagulopathy of trauma.[20] Frequently, the PT is used to guide FFP therapy in the bleeding patient, with a recommended goal of maintaining the international normalized ratio (INR) less than 1.5. Correction of prolonged PT in the absence of hemorrhage is rarely clinically indicated.

After collection of whole blood from a donor, centrifugation results in cell-free plasma. This plasma is quickly cooled, frozen, and stored at less than –18 °C until it is needed. Frozen storage protects coagulation proteins from degradation. Even when frozen within 6 hours of collection, labile coagulation proteins V and VIII will degrade by about 30%.

Once thawed, FFP retains the majority of its coagulant protein activity, and can be stored for up to 24 hours refrigerated. Once at room temperature, thawed FFP must be administered immediately, to reduce loss of coagulant protein activity.

FFP is supplied in volumes of 200 to 250 ml, with each ml containing about 1 international unit of each plasma coagulation protein. In order to raise plasma coagulation factor activity by the minimum recommended level of 30%, 10 to 15 ml per kg body weight should be administered. For an average-sized adult considered to have depletion of plasma coagulation factors, a minimum of 4 units FFP should be transfused as rapidly as possible.[21] For many patients, even a 15 ml/kg dose may not be adequate, and larger doses should be considered.[22]

Patients on preoperative warfarin are at an increased risk for postoperative bleeding. In situations where the surgical procedure can be delayed, reversal of warfarin anticoagulation with either vitamin K-administration or simply discontinuing warfarin for several days is advisable. In situations where the surgical procedure must be performed more urgently, FFP transfusion is frequently used to reverse the effects of warfarin, by replacing the vitamin K-dependent factors whose synthesis is inhibited by warfarin. Complete return to normal laboratory values is frequently difficult acutely.

FFP is not cross-matched but should be ABO compatible with the recipient, since ABO incompatibility can result in hemolytic transfusion reactions. Transfusion of FFP is associated with many of the same transfusion-associated complications as RBCs, and is more commonly associated with acute lung injury than is transfusion of other blood components. The actual incidence of TRALI is unknown, but it appears to be more common than previously recognized.[23] Owing to the large amount of citrate in a unit of FFP, it is the most frequent component to cause citrate toxicity when rapidly administered.

Cryoprecipitate: Cryoprecipitate is prepared from plasma by a process of freezing and then thawing to refrigeration temperature of 4 °C. The cold-insoluble proteins that precipitate in this process are stored in a small volume of plasma, and delivered as a unit of cryoprecipitate. The unit is rich in factors VIII, XIII, von Willebrand factor, and fibrinogen. Historically, this product was used for the treatment of hemophilia A, but has been replaced by modern plasma-derived or recombinant factor VIII and IX concentrates. Cryoprecipitate is indicated for the treatment of bleeding associated with von Willebrand's disease that is not responsive to desmopressin therapy. In cases of postoperative bleeding with low plasma fibrinogen levels, a unit of cryoprecipitate contains about 150 to 250 mg of fibrinogen. This works out to each unit per 10 kg body weight can be expected to raise plasma concentration by approximately 50 mg/dl. For the average adult patient, 5 to 10 units cryoprecipitate is a typical initial dose. Traditionally, fibrinogen concentrations were considered acceptable above 80 to 100 mg/dl.[2] However, in the bleeding patient, it may be advantageous to maintain levels greater than 150 mg/dl.[6]

Hemostatic agents

Other intravascular hemostatic agents can be used to treat coagulopathy. In the case of a known congenital coagulation defect such as hemophilia, specific plasma-derived or recombinant factor replacement should be performed, usually with the aid of hematological consultation. Specific replacements for fibrinogen, factor VII, VIII, IX, XIII, and prothrombin complex concentrates containing factor II, IX, and X are available.

In cases of coagulopathy that is unresponsive to transfusion therapy, recombinant factor VIIa can be used as a hemostatic agent. Recombinant factor VIIa is currently approved by the US Food and Drug Administration in the treatment of hemophilia, but it has received widespread "off-label" use in the treatment of acquired coagulopathic states. It has been studied for use in intracranial hemorrhage,[24] trauma,[25] and cardiac surgery.[26] While generally found to be effective in reducing coagulopathic bleeding, factor VIIa therapy comes with an increased risk of thrombotic complications, which include lethal myocardial infarctions and stroke, confining its use to only the most extreme cases of coagulopathy.[27]

Desmopressin, also known as DDAVP, is a synthetic analog of arginine vasopressin, and has procoagulant as well as antidiuretic hormone effects. It has been used prophylactically in the treatment of patients with von Willebrand's disease to transiently increase circulating levels of von Willebrand factor. It also raises plasma levels of factor VIII and improves platelet adhesion. It can be of benefit in other coagulopathies. It may be reasonable to use this agent in disease states associated with platelet dysfunction, such as uremia, or after cardiac surgery.[28]

Antifibrinolytic drugs aminocaproic acid and tranexamic acid can be used to inhibit fibrinolysis in patients with bleeding secondary to excessive fibrinolysis. These drugs competitively antagonize plasmin by mimicking lysine residues on fibrin polymers. They have been used prophylactically in trauma, orthopedic, cardiac, and other surgery to reduce blood loss and blood transfusion. Their use in postoperative coagulopathy has not been as well studied. Viscoelastic coagulation studies will reveal hyperfibrinolysis by showing short lysis times. When a hyperfibrinolytic state has been diagnosed by TEG or ROTEM, intervention with antifibrinolytics may be appropriate.

Hemorrhage is a common postoperative complication that can often be difficult to diagnose in the PACU. Transfusion of blood products should be goal-directed to restore circulating blood volume, oxygen carrying capacity, and hemostasis. Coagulopathic conditions should be identified and treated promptly with appropriate blood components or hemostatic agents.

References

1. R. Hines, P.G. Barash, G. Watrous, T. O'Connor. Complications occurring in the postanesthesia care unit; a survey. *Anesth Analg* 1992; 74: 503–509.

2. ASA Task Force. Practice guidelines for perioperative blood transfusion and adjuvant therapies: an updated report by the American Society of Anesthesiologists Task Force on Perioperative Blood Transfusion and Adjuvant Therapies. *Anesthesiology* 2006; 105: 198–208.

3. T.F. Dagi. The management of postoperative bleeding. *Surg Clin N Am* 2005; 85: 1191–1213.

4. M. Marietta, L. Facchini, P. Pedrazzi, S. Busani, G. Torelli. Pathophysiology of bleeding in surgery. *Transplant Proc* 2006; 38: 812–814.

5. M.O. Dolich, M.G. McKenney, J.E. Varela, *et al.* 2,576 ultrasounds for blunt abdominal trauma. *J Trauma Acute Care Surg* 2001; 50: 108–112.

6. J.H. Levy, F. Szlam, K.A. Tanaka, R.M. Sniecisnki. Fibrinogen and hemostasis: a primary hemostatic target for the management of acquired bleeding. *Anesth Analg* 2012; 114: 261–274.

7. M. Lynn, I. Jeroukhimov, Y. Klein, U. Martinowitz. Updates in the management of severe coagulopathy in trauma patients. *Intensive Care Med* 2002; 28: S241–S247.

8. M. Brenni, M. Worn, M. Bruesch, D.R. Spahn, M.T. Ganter. Successful

rotational thromboelastometry-guided treatment of traumatic haemorrhage, hyperfibrinolysis and coagulopathy. *Acta Anaesthesiol Scand* 2010; 54: 111–117.

9. S. Ogawa, F. Szlam, E.P. Chen, *et al.* A comparative evaluation of rotation thromboelastometry and standard coagulation tests in hemodilution-induced coagulation changes after cardiac surgery. *Transfusion* 2011; 52: 14–22.

10. T.D. Johnston, Y. Chen, R.L. Reed. Functional equivalence of hypothermia to specific clotting factor deficiencies. *J Trauma* 1994; 37: 413–417.

11. H. Harke, S. Rahman. Haemostatic disorders in massive transfusion. *Bibl Haematol* 1980; 46: 179–188.

12. T.B. Repine, J.G. Perkins, D.S. Kauvar, *et al.* The use of fresh whole blood in massive transfusion. *J Trauma Acute Care Surg* 2006; 60: S59–S69.

13. W.H. Dzik, S.A. Kirkley. Citrate toxicity during massive blood transfusion. *Transfus Med Rev* 1988; 2: 76–94.

14. Perioperative red cell transfusion. *NIH Consensus Development Conference: Consensus Statement* 1988; 7: 27–29.

15. R.C. Arya, G.S. Wander, P. Gupta. Blood component therapy: which, when and how much. *J Anaesthesiol Clin Pharm* 2011; 27: 278–284.

16. C. Koch, L. Li, D.I. Sessler, *et al.* Duration of red-cell storage and complications after cardiac surgery. *N Engl J Med* 2008; 358: 1229–1239.

17. A.P.J. Vlaar, J.M. Binnekade, D. Prins, *et al.* The incidence, risk factors, and outcome of transfusion-related acute lung injury in a cohort of cardiac surgery patients: a prospective nested case-control study. *Blood* 2011; 117: 4218–4225.

18. E. Bennett-Guerrero, T.H. Veldman, A. Doctor, *et al.* Evolution of adverse changes in stored RBCs. *Proc Natl Acad Sci U S A* 2007; 104: 17063–17068.

19. W.P. Robinson, J. Ahn, A. Stifler, *et al.* Blood transfusion is an independent predictor of increased mortality in nonoperatively managed blunt hepatic and splenic injuries. *J Trauma Acute Care Surg* 2005; 58: 437–445.

20. J.B. Holcomb, C.E. Wade, J.E. Michalek, *et al.* Increased plasma and platelet to red blood cell ratios improves outcome in 466 massively transfused civilian trauma patients. *Ann Surg* 2008; 248: 447–458.

21. E.S. Cooper, A.W. Bracey, A.E. Horvath, *et al.* Practice parameters for the use of fresh frozen plasma, cryoprecipitate, and platelets. *JAMA* 1994; 271: 777–781.

22. P. Chowdhury, A.G. Saayman, U. Paulus, G.P. Findlay, P.W. Collins. Efficacy of standard dose and 30 ml/kg fresh frozen plasma in correcting laboratory parameters of haemostasis in critically ill patients. *Br J Haematol* 2004; 125: 69–73.

23. P.E. Marik, H.L. Corwin. Acute lung injury following blood transfusion: expanding the definition. *Crit Care Med* 2008; 36: 3080–3084.

24. S.A. Mayer, N.C. Brun, K. Begtrup, *et al.* Efficacy and safety of recombinant activated factor VII for acute intracerebral hemorrhage. *N Engl J Med* 2008; 358: 2127–2137.

25. K.D. Boffard, B. Riou, B. Warren, *et al.* Recombinant factor VIIa as adjunctive therapy for bleeding control in severely injured trauma patients: two parallel randomized, placebo-controlled, double-blind clinical trials. *J Trauma* 2005; 59: 8–15.

26. K. Karkouti, W.S. Beattie, D.N. Wijeysundara, *et al.* Recombinant factor VIIa for intractable blood loss after cardiac surgery: a propensity score–matched case-control analysis. *Transfusion* 2004; 45: 26–34.

27. M. Levi, J.H. Levy, H.F. Anderson, D. Truloff. Safety of recombinant activated factor VII in randomized clinical trials. *New Engl J Med* 2010; 363: 1791–1800.

28. J.E. Kaufmann, U.M. Vischer. Cellular mechanisms of the hemostatic effects of desmopressin (DDAVP). *J Thromb Haemost* 2003; 1: 682–689.

Chapter 42

Intraoperative awareness

Michelle Beam and James W. Heitz

- Intraoperative awareness occurs in low frequency in modern anesthetic care.
- Only one-third of patients experiencing intraoperative awareness will report it in the Post-Anesthesia Care Unit (PACU).
- Differentiating awareness from intraoperative dreaming may be challenging for some patients.
- Patients suffering intraoperative awareness should be offered psychological counseling to prevent sequelae.

Intraoperative awareness is an infrequent complication of general anesthesia, but can have distressing consequences when it occurs. Depending upon how it is defined and measured, intraoperative awareness has an incidence of 0.13%[1,2] to 1%.[3,4] A more recent audit in the UK found a much lower incidence of 1 in 15,000 general anesthetics.[5] By definition, intraoperative awareness must include both awareness and explicit recall of the events occurring while anesthetized. Studies utilizing an isolated forearm technique (a tourniquet is applied to the arm prior to dosing of a neuromuscular blocker, sparing that limb from paralysis) demonstrate that a subset of patients receiving general anesthesia will follow simple verbal commands while anesthetized, but typically have no explicit recall of the event.[6] Awareness without explicit memory formation appears to occur at a higher frequency than does intraoperative awareness, but the clinical significance of this, if any, is unknown.

Memory of awareness may be a source of psychological trauma to the patient. Patients may report anxiety, fear, or sleep disturbances. A higher than expected frequency of post-traumatic stress disorder (PTSD) has been observed among patients after episodes of intraoperative awareness.[7,8] In a recent prospective study examining the incidence of PTSD among patients with intraoperative awareness compared with match control surgical patients without intraoperative awareness, an elevated incidence of PTSD was noted among both the intraoperative awareness group and the control group as compared with the general population.[9] PTSD may be an under-recognized consequence of the psychological trauma associated with surgery and not specific to intraoperative awareness.

Intraoperative awareness can range from recall of conversations to recall of portions of the procedure or pain. The Michigan Awareness Classification Instrument was designed to facilitate classification of intraoperative awareness.[10] Under this classification system,

Post-Anesthesia Care: Symptoms, Diagnosis, and Management, ed. James W. Heitz. Published by Cambridge University Press. © Cambridge University Press 2016.

Class 0 = no awareness, Class 1 = isolated auditory perceptions, Class 2 = tactile percep-tions, Class 3 = pain, Class 4 = awareness of paralysis, and Class 5 = pain and paralysis. Most intraoperative awareness is Class 1 with comments about body habitus forming the most common content of conversation recall. Class 3 or greater intraoperative awareness is very rare and often associated with equipment malfunction that interferes with delivery of the anesthesia (e.g. empty anesthesia vaporizer).

In determining that intraoperative awareness has occurred, it is important to exclude other things that might be mistaken as intraoperative awareness. Dreaming with general anesthesia occurs with 27% of propofol-based and 28% of desflurane-based anesthetics.[11] Dreaming with anesthesia is common and is not awareness. Recall of any portion of a procedure in which conscious sedation or regional anesthesia, including spinal or epidural anesthesia, is administered is not intraoperative awareness. Some recall during sedation is anticipated. Recall of events in the operating room either before or after the anesthetic is sometimes mistakenly attributed to intraoperative awareness.

Despite advancements in the pharmacology of general anesthesia and the technology that monitors the anesthetized patient, true intraoperative awareness cannot always be anticipated or detected. Adequacy of anesthesia has traditionally been assessed by monitoring hemodynamics monitoring for tachycardia or hypertension, but awareness may occur without hemodynamic signs. More recently, monitors that evaluate processed electroencephalogram information have been increasingly utilized as part of the monitoring during anesthesia. Current commercially available monitors include: BIS™ (Bispectral Index, Coviden, Mansfield, MA), Narcotrend™ (Monitor Technik, Bad Bramstedt, Germany), Entropy™ (GE Healthcare Technologies, Waukesha WI), SedLine™ (Masimo, Irvine, CA), SNAP II™ (Everest Biomedical Instruments, Chesterfield, MO), and Cerebral State Monitor™ (Danmeter A/S, Odense, Denmark). The choice of a par-ticular brand of monitor is usually one of institutional preference, and no single device has demonstrated clear superiority over others. While these devices can provide valuable information to aid in the dosing of anesthesia, intraoperative awareness continues to occur despite their use.[7] For the Bispectral Index and the Narcotrend monitors, readings consistent with possible awareness have a positive predictive value less than 20% for responsiveness.[12,13] Referring to these devices as "awareness monitors" is a too frequently used misnomer.

Risk factors associated with awareness include female gender, young age, obstetrical and cardiac procedures, "light" anesthesia, and a prior episode of awareness.[14] A prior history of intraoperative awareness increases the risk of an individual patient experiencing intraoperative awareness in a subsequent surgery by five fold compared with a patient without prior intraoperative awareness.[15]

Approximately 35% of patients reporting an experience of intraoperative awareness do so in the PACU. Half of patients will eventually report the experience to a healthcare provider, but for the other half it is necessary to actively question the patient to elicit the history.[14] The best results for eliciting intraoperative awareness are obtained by a standard-ized interview. The Brice Interview as modified by Sandin is frequently used in screening for intraoperative awareness and comprises five questions:[16,17]

1. *What was the last thing you remember before going to sleep?*
2. *What is the first thing you remember after waking up?*
3. *Do you remember anything between going to sleep and waking up?*

4. *Did you dream during your procedure?*
5. *What was the worst thing about your operation?*

Patients who spontaneously report intraoperative awareness or are identified on post-operative visits using the Modified Brice Interview should receive follow-up care.

Management: When a patient reports possible intraoperative awareness, the anesthesiologist who administered the anesthetic should be notified (see Figure 42.1).[18,19] Patients may not report awareness for several days or longer after the surgery, so the anesthesiologist may not be cognizant unless contacted. The patient should be interviewed by that anesthesiologist or his/her surrogate with knowledge about intraoperative awareness. Different portions of the brain have different sensitivities to anesthetics, so a partially anesthetized brain may form incomplete and inaccurate memories regarding the event. Determining whether or not awareness occurred is not necessarily straightforward, since reports of the experience of intraoperative awareness often contain elements of hallucination or confabulation. Inconsistencies in the memory do not exclude the possibility of elements of true recall.

It is important that healthcare providers refer the patient back to the anesthesiologist for evaluation. Dismissing reports of awareness as merely dreaming because of disprovable elements may contribute to preventable psychological stress and harm. It is equally important to refrain from offering opinions that someone must have done something wrong for this to have occurred. A low incidence of awareness under general anesthesia is unavoidable with current medications and technology. Moreover, intraoperative conditions may arise that increase the risk for intraoperative awareness. If cardiac instability or hemorrhage occurs during surgery, compromising the ability of the patient to tolerate general anesthesia, an anesthesiologist may choose to reduce the anesthesia during resuscitation and risk awareness rather than allowing hypotension to persist, risking death. The anesthesiologist who provided the anesthetic is in the best position to perform the evaluation of the patient reporting intraoperative awareness.

In managing a case of suspected awareness, the American Society of Anesthesiologists (ASA) Task Force on Intraoperative Awareness recommends that patients reporting possible intraoperative awareness be interviewed to obtain a detailed account of the patient's experience and an explanation offered to the patient as to reasons why this may have occurred. Patients should be offered counseling and psychological support, and if awareness is suspected, an occurrence report should be generated for quality management.[20] The Joint Commission, which offers accreditation for healthcare organizations in the United States, offers the same recommendations as the ASA. Additionally, the Joint Commission suggests that an apology be offered to the patient if awareness has occurred and that the patient be reassured that their account is believed by the physician. The Joint Commission recommends that each Anesthesiology Department maintain a policy on intraoperative awareness and that all members of the perioperative team including surgeons, nurses, and other key personnel be educated about intraoperative awareness and how to manage it.[21] The Anesthesiology Department should also establish a relationship with specific counselors and psychiatric support teams that are experienced in cases of awareness.

Although apologies to patients over undesirable clinical outcomes have been demonstrated to reduce subsequent litigation, many physicians are still reluctant to offer apologies. Many fear that apologies may be construed as admission of malpractice and could be introduced as evidence of guilt during subsequent civil litigation. Previously, spontaneous apologies have been admissible as evidence in civil litigation as an exception to the hearsay

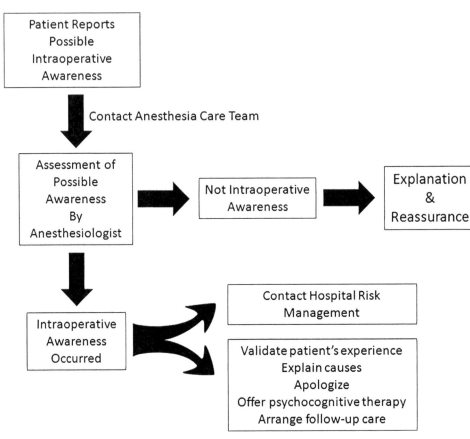

Figure 42.1 Postoperative management of intraoperative awareness.

rule. Recognizing that this has an inhibiting effect of disclosure of adverse healthcare events, many states now shield healthcare providers with the creation of "apology laws." The first apology law was enacted in Massachusetts in 1986 and states:

> "Statements, writings or benevolent gestures expressing sympathy or a general sense of benevolence relating to the pain, suffering or death of a person involved in an accident and made to such person or to the family of such person shall be inadmissible as evidence of an admission of liability in a civil action."[22]

Most states have now created their own apology laws. An apology does not need to acknowledge error if none has occurred. An effective apology may merely be an empathetic acknowledgement of the patient's distress. Statements such as "I'm sorry this happened to you" may suffice. However, some studies have shown that apologies that go beyond mere expressions of sympathy and accept responsibility for the outcome may have a greater effect in reducing litigation.[23]

Psychological support and counseling is prudent for the intraoperative awareness patient and should be offered to all patients troubled by the experience. Individuals experiencing Michigan Awareness Class 3 or greater should be particularly encouraged to enroll in counseling and offered appropriate follow-up care.

References

1. R.H. Sandin, G. Enlund, P. Samuelsson, C. Lennmarken. Awareness during anaesthesia: a prospective case study. *Lancet* 2000; 355:707–711.

2. P.S. Sebel, T.A. Bowdle, M.M. Ghoneim, *et al.* The incidence of awareness during anesthesia: a multicenter United States study. *Anesth Analg* 2004; 99:833–839.

3. C.L. Errando, J.C. Sigl, M. Robles, *et al.* Awareness with recall during general anaesthesia: a prospective observational evaluation of 4001 patients. *Br J Anaesth* 2008; 101:178–185.

4. L. Xu, A.S. Wu, Y. Yue. The incidence of intraoperative awareness during general anesthesia in China: a multicenter observational study. *Acta Anaesthesiol Scand* 2009; 53:873–882.

5. J. Pandit, T. Cook, W. Jonker, E. O'Sullivan. A national survey of anaesthetists (NAP 5 baseline) to estimate an annual incidence of accidental awareness during general anaesthesia in the UK. *Br J Anaesth* 2013; 110:501–509

6. R.D. Sanders, G. Tononi, S. Laureys, J.W. Sleigh. Unresponsiveness ≠ unconsciousness. *Anesthesiology* 2012; 116:946–959.

7. R.R. Bruchas, C.D. Kent, H.D. Wilson, K.B. Domino. Anesthesia awareness: narrative review of psychological sequelae, treatment, and incidence. *J Clin Psychol Med Settings* 2011; 18:257–267.

8. K. Leslie, M.T.V. Chan, P.S. Myles, A. Forbes, T.J. McCulloch. Posttraumatic stress disorder in aware patients from the b-aware trial. *Anesth Analg* 2010; 110:823–828.

9. E.L. Whitlock, T.L. Rodebaugh, A.L. Hasset, *et al.* Psychological sequalae of surgery in a prospective cohort of patients from three intraoperative awareness prevention trials. *Anesth Analg* 2015; 120:87–95.

10. G.A. Mashour, R.K. Esaki, K.K. Tremper, *et al.* A novel classification instrument for intraoperative awareness events. *Anesth Analg* 2010; 100:813–815.

11. K. Leslie, J. Sleigh, M.J. Paech, *et al.* Dreaming and electroencephalographic changes during anesthesia maintained with propofol or desflurane. *Anesthesiology* 2009; 111:547–555.

12. I.F. Russell. The Narcotrend 'depth of anaesthesia' monitor cannot reliably detect consciousness during general anaesthesia: an investigation using the isolated forearm technique. *Br J Anaesth* 2006; 96:346–352.

13. I.F. Russell. The ability of bispectral index to detect intraoperative wakefulness during total intravenous anesthesia compared with the isolated forearm technique. *Anaesthesia* 2013; 68:502–511.

14. M.M. Ghoneim, R.J. Block, M. Haffarman, J. Matthews. Awareness during anesthesia: risk factors, causes and sequel. A review of reported cases in the literature. *Anesth Analg* 2009; 108:527–535.

15. A. Arake, S. Gradwhol, A. Ben-Abdallah, *et al.* Increased risk of intraoperative awareness in patients with a history of awareness. *Anesthesiology* 2013; 119:1275–1283.

16. D.D. Brice, R.R. Hetherington, J.E. Utting. A simple study of awareness and dreaming during anaesthesia. *Br J Anaesth* 1970; 42:535–542.

17. O. Nordström, A.M. Engström, S. Persson, R. Sandin. Incidence of awareness in total i.v. anaesthesia based on propofol, alfentanil and neuromuscular blockade. *Acta Anaesthesiol Scand* 2008; 41:978–984.

18. F. Guerra. Awareness during anaesthesia. *Can Anaesth Soc J* 1980; 27:178.

19. G.A. Mashour, L.Y. Wang, R.K. Esaki, N.N. Naughton. Operating room desensitization as a novel treatment for post-traumatic stress disorder after intraoperative awareness. *Anesthesiology* 2008; 109:927–929.

20. J.L. Apfelbaum, J.F. Arens, D.J. Cole, *et al.* Practice advisory for intraoperative awareness and brain function monitoring. *Anesthesiology* 2006; 104:847–864.

21. Joint Commission Sentinel Alert Issue 32 October 6, 2004. Preventing,

and managing the impact of, anesthesia awareness. http://www.jointcommission.org/assets/1/18/SEA_32.PDF. Accessed 12/1/2104.

22. M. Wei. Doctors, apologies, and the law: an analysis and critique of apology laws. *J Health Law* 2007; 40:107–159.

23. J.K. Robbennolt. Apologies and settlement. *Court Rev* 2009; 45:90–97.

Chapter

43

Special considerations for mechanical ventilation

Yousef Hamdeh, Zara Y. Mergan, and James W. Heitz

- Many of the reasons for mechanical ventilation of the surgical patient are unique to the postoperative setting.
- The benefit of sedation in the PACU is dependent upon the reason for mechanical ventilation.
- Mechanical ventilation needs to be considered in the differential diagnosis of postoperative hypotension.

The indications for mechanical ventilation in the Post-Anesthesia Care Unit (PACU) and early postoperative period are different than those in the intensive care unit (ICU). In medical patients, mechanical ventilation is most typically instituted to correct underlying hypoxia or severe acid–base disturbance due to pathology. In surgical patients, if mechanical ventilation is necessary in the early postoperative period it is often due to iatrogenic reasons, which are rapidly reversible, including residual neuromuscular blockade, negative pressure pulmonary edema, hypothermia, and delayed emergence from general anesthesia. The therapeutic objective is to provide supportive ventilation until reversible factors thwarting safe tracheal extubation have resolved. Extubation criteria in the perioperative period are therefore unique. The decision of whether or not to provide sedation during mechanical ventilation in the early postoperative period is dependent upon the reason for mechanical ventilation.

Residual neuromuscular blockade

There are two pharmacological subtypes of neuromuscular blockers: depolarizing and non-depolarizing. Succinylcholine (suxamethonium) is a nicotinic acetylcholine receptor agonist that produces depolarizing blockade, but is rapidly metabolized by pseudocholinesterase. In individuals with normal activity of pseudocholinesterase, the duration of action of succinylcholine is limited to 3 to 5 minutes. The rapid onset and rapid offset are the major clinical advantages of the medication and the reason it is in clinical use. However, in individuals with pseudocholinesterase deficiency, the duration of neuromuscular blockade is extended. Deficiencies of pseudocholinesterase may be quantitative or qualitative, and inherited or acquired.

Pseudocholinesterase has no identified biological function besides the metabolism of a few pharmaceuticals, so individuals with an inherited lack of normal enzymatic function

Post-Anesthesia Care: Symptoms, Diagnosis, and Management, ed. James W. Heitz. Published by Cambridge University Press. © Cambridge University Press 2016.

are phenotypically normal and often cannot be identified preoperatively. After exposure to succinylcholine, paralysis is prolonged. Over 65 genetic mutations have been identified as producing abnormal or deficient pseudocholinesterase.[1] Depending upon the mutation and whether the individual is homozygous or heterozygous for the gene encoding for the defective enzyme, the duration of action of succinylcholine may be extended by several minutes to several hours. The most severe inherited enzymatic deficiency is the silent variant. The incidence of the homozygous silent variant mutation is estimated to be between 1 in 40,000[2] and 1 in 100,000[3] among individuals of European descent and produces clinical paralysis of 4 to 8 hours after exposure to succinylcholine.[2] Among the ethnic Vysya of India the incidence climbs to 1 in 24.[3] It is not possible to acutely identify the cause of prolonged paralysis from succinylcholine, so affected patients need to be monitored for return of neuromuscular function. Analysis of pseudocholinesterase activity is best deferred until the interfering effect of succinylcholine has dissipated.[2] Many of the variants of abnormal pseudocholinesterase produce paralysis of 1 to 2 hours' duration when challenged with succinylcholine, so if more than 2 hours has elapsed since administration the individual likely possesses a severe mutation. Acquired deficiencies in serum pseudocholinesterase may be observed in liver disease, renal insufficiency, malnutrition, pregnancy, malignancy, and leprosy,[3] although the increased duration of action of succinylcholine is rarely clinically significant with these disorders. Deficient pseudocholinesterase activity may also be acquired from the concurrent administration of other pharmaceuticals. The most clinically significant is administration of competitive cholinesterase inhibitors including neostigmine, physostigmine, or pyridostigmine. These medications are typically administered at the conclusion of surgery for reversal of non-depolarizing neuromuscular blockade. If succinylcholine is administered as part of emergency airway management of failed extubation, prolonged paralysis may result. A number of other medications also prolong the action of succinylcholine through pseudocholinesterase inhibition, but the effects are generally short-lived and rarely of clinical significance (Table 43.1).

Non-depolarizing neuromuscular blocker duration of action is variable and dependent upon the particular pharmaceutical administered. Typically, spontaneous recovery from an

Table 43.1 Factors influencing neuromuscular blockade duration

	Depolarizing	Non-depolarizing
Pharmacological	Echothiophate eyedrops, phenelzine, pancuronium, oral contraceptives, metoclopramide, donepezil	Antibiotics (gentamicin, tobramycin) local anesthetics, inhalational agents, magnesium, lithium, calcium entry blockers, antiarrhythmics, diuretics
Pathophysiological	Liver disease, renal insufficiency, malnutrition, malignancy, burns, leprosy	Acidosis, hypothermia, hypokalemia, hypocalcemia, hypernatremia, diseases of neuromuscular junction, hepatic or renal disease (hepatic or renal excretion medications)
Physiological	Pregnancy	Elderly

intubating dose of a non-depolarizer occurs within 2 hours. There are many factors that can affect the duration of non-depolarizing neuromuscular blockade, including interference from other pharmaceuticals, hepatic or renal insufficiency, electrolyte disturbances, hypothermia, acidosis, and pre-existing pathology at the neuromuscular junction.

Recovery from neuromuscular blockade is evaluated by utilizing a twitch monitor to determine a train-of-four (TOF) ratio. The TOF ratio is defined as four successive electrical stimulations each occurring every half second. The response to the fourth stimulus is compared with the response to the first stimulus. A ratio of 0.9 signifies that pharyngeal function has been restored; if pharyngeal function is not restored there may be an increased risk of upper airway obstruction upon extubation. Of note, diaphragmatic function returns before pharyngeal function does. Therefore, adequate tidal volumes during spontaneous ventilation are not sufficient for extubation. At the end of an anesthetic the trachea is extubated, but only when the effects of the neuromuscular blockade have been terminated. The termination of neuromuscular blockade is facilitated by spontaneous recovery (metabolism by the body) or by pharmacological antagonism (reversal). Reversal is achieved by using an cholin esterase inhibitor such as neostigmine. Residual neuromuscular blockade is a common complication in the PACU with approximately 40% of patients exhibiting TOF ratios <0.9.[4]

Management: Significant residual neuromuscular blockade may require intubation and mechanical ventilation, both to ensure adequacy of oxygenation and ventilation, and for airway protection.[5] When a patient presents to the PACU intubated with residual neuromuscular blockade, assess TOF ratio and evaluate need for sedation. Clinically weak patients requiring mechanical ventilation should be sedated. Neuromuscular blockade is terrifying for the awake patient, and anxiolysis and amnesia should be supplied. Once the TOF ratio is >0.9 one can assume that pharyngeal tone has been restored and extubation can be performed.[6] If TOF monitoring is not available, assessment of adequate clinical strength for extubation may be achieved with a 5 second head lift.[7]

Negative pressure pulmonary edema

Negative pressure pulmonary edema is a type of non-cardiogenic pulmonary edema. Any type of airway obstruction can lead to negative pressure pulmonary edema, but the most common cause of precipitating obstruction is laryngospasm.[8] The underlying cause of the pulmonary edema is thought to be the creation of a large pressure gradient across the pulmonary capillary wall. The creation of a large negative intrathoracic pressure against an obstruction draws fluid from the interstitial space/capillaries and into the alveoli.[9] The process is also mediated by a disruption of the alveolar capillary membrane secondary to this large negative pressure. This phenomenon is observed in 1 of every 1,000 general surgeries.[10]

Management: This will lead to pulmonary edema and potentially hypoxia. Intubation and mechanical ventilation is reserved for only the most severely affected individuals and is rarely necessary. Management is supportive care. The pathophysiology is a transudative process, not volume overload, so the role of diuretics in management is controversial.[11] Some advocate diuresis for affected patients, but the evidence of benefit is anecdotal and limited to case reports. Spontaneous recovery is also common. Severely affected patients requiring mechanical ventilation will most likely require only short-term support and may benefit from brief sedation.

Hypothermia

Hypothermia in the PACU is frequently observed. Most anesthetics agents promote vaso-dilation, which in turn will lead to an increase in heat loss and subsequently hypothermia. Mild hypothermia is defined as a core temperature between 33.0 °C and 36.4 °C. It can affect coagulation, electrolytes, acid–base status, and the renal, neurological, cardiac, and respiratory systems.[12] The respiratory rate and tidal volume will decrease with decreasing temperature, leading to hypoventilation and hypoxemia. This in turn may necessitate mechanical ventilation and a secure airway.

Management: The best treatment of hypothermia is prevention, but if inadvertent hypothermia has developed, active rewarming with forced air devices is indicated. Extubation is generally deferred until the patient is sufficiently rewarmed. Sedation during mechanical ventilation is warranted.

Prolonged sedation

The differential diagnosis of delayed emergence from anesthesia is robust, but is sometimes attributable to individual variability of drug metabolism and prolonged sedation. Short periods of mechanical ventilation in the PACU may be necessary for some patients.

Management: Extubation in the PACU is possible for most patients with prolonged sedation. Sedation during mechanical ventilation is generally avoided, since once consciousness is restored, most patients may be successfully extubated.

Upper airway edema and pulmonary edema

Surgical patients requiring endotracheal intubation owing to upper airway edema from surgical manipulation or cardiogenic pulmonary edema from volume overload typically require mechanical ventilation for a longer duration than allows for extubation in the PACU. If extubation is not planned, sedation is clinically prudent.

Sedation and mechanical ventilation in the PACU

Traditionally, patients requiring mechanical ventilation are sedated to minimize agitation and anxiety. Multiple studies have demonstrated the negative consequences of prolonged, deep sedation, and the benefits of maintaining lighter sedation levels in adult ICU patients.[13] Deep sedation was found to be an independent negative predictor of the time to extubation, hospital death, and 180-day mortality.[14] There is no analogous data for outcome of sedation provided for short-term mechanical ventilation in the PACU, and it is impossible to make meaningful extrapolation from studies of ICU patients. However, in the PACU, it seems clinically reasonable to provide sedation with attention to the underlying reason for mechanical ventilation. For ICU patients, the specific etiology of the need for mechanical ventilation is often trivial to the decision to provide sedation. For surgical patients receiving mechanical ventilation in the PACU, it is important that sedation be short-acting to allow for timely extubation of patients requiring only short-term mechanical ventilation. Virtually all patients with residual neuromuscular blockade should be sedated, but sedation should be used much more judiciously in individuals with prolonged sedation.

Extubation in the PACU

Extubation in the PACU is very different than extubation in the ICU. Extubation criteria exist for patients in the ICU which take into account spontaneous breathing trials, assessment of negative inspiratory force, and arterial blood gas analysis among many other criteria. Mechanically ventilated patients in the PACU usually do not have the same pathologies as patients in the ICU. For this reason extubation criteria based in the ICU setting are non-applicable, but we can apply some of the same principles to the PACU. Prior to extubation, the patient should be able to maintain oxygen saturation while receiving a FiO_2 <50%, possess the ability to generate adequate tidal volumes, and display hemodynamic stability. Application of clinical judgment that is used in the operating room setting for extubation is appropriate for extubation in the PACU.

Hypotension during mechanical ventilation

Hypotension is common in the perioperative period and may be exacerbated by positive pressure ventilation. The positive intrathoracic pressure generated by mechanical ventilation during inspiration decreases cardiac preload and decreases cardiac output. Excessively high intrathoracic pressure may be clinically recognized as hypotension. Common triggers of increased intrathoracic pressure in the mechanically ventilated PACU patient include bronchospasm, auto-PEEP (positive end expiratory pressure), pneumothorax, and patient–ventilator asynchrony (bucking).

Bronchospasm

Perioperative bronchospasm usually presents during the induction of anesthesia but can arise at any stage of anesthesia. Of note, 20% of perioperative bronchospasm happens during the emergence from anesthesia.[15] It occurs most commonly in patients with a history of reactive airway disease and patients who are smokers. Triggers include environmental, pharmacological, and mechanical such as the endotracheal tube, laryngoscopy, or airway suctioning.[16] One should suspect bronchospasm in a mechanically ventilated patient in the PACU if their work of breathing or airway peak pressures have increased, or hypoxia or hypotension develops. The diagnosis is a clinical one and is based on physical examination. Upon auscultation of the chest one may hear wheezing or even absent breath sounds. A rise in peak pressure usually accompanies bronchospasm. Treatment includes an increase in the FiO_2, inhaled beta-2 agonism, systemic steroids, manual bag ventilation to assess compliance, and potentially epinephrine if the bronchospasm is associated with cardiovascular collapse.[15]

Auto-PEEP

PEEP is pressure in the alveoli at the end of exhalation that is greater than atmospheric pressure.[17] Normally, passive exhalation occurs; the lungs empty via elastic recoil and alveolar pressure equals atmospheric pressure. Auto-PEEP or breath stacking is unwanted PEEP at the end of exhalation. Patients who are at risk for auto-PEEP are those with obstructive lung diseases such as asthma and chronic obstructive pulmonary disease. These patients usually require a longer time for expiration secondary to their disease process. However, it can happen in those with healthy lungs, which is the more common case in the PACU, if the respiratory rate is too high or expiratory time is too low or with any process that decreases the amount of time for exhalation. This will lead to the creation of positive airway pressure at the end of exhalation. Auto-PEEP can increase work of breathing; to overcome the positive pressure in the alveoli, the diaphragm now has to generate more negative pressure. A decrease in arterial oxygen tension occurs because of an uneven distribution of inspired gas leading to worsening gas exchange.[18] Auto-PEEP can also cause a decrease in cardiac output.[19] Auto-PEEP can be suspected if exhalation continues until the next breath begins.[18] Once detected, it can be treated by disconnecting the circuit and allowing the patient to exhale passively. It can be prevented by decreasing the respiratory rate and/or changing the inspiratory:expiratory ratio, which would give the patient more time to exhale.

Tension pneumothorax

Tension pneumothorax can develop precipitously in the mechanically ventilated patient. Classic signs include deviation of the trachea, decreased or asymmetrical chest expansion, decreased breath sounds, increased percussion note, and possibly distended neck veins. It is important to note that the hypovolemic surgical patient may not display distended neck veins and that classic signs of tension pneumothorax may be absent, complicating diagnosis. Tension pneumothorax in the PACU may first be recognized by mild hypotension,[20] profound hypotension,[21] or hypoxia.[22] It is important that tension pneumothorax be rapidly excluded as causing hypotension in the mechanically ventilated surgical patient after surgery.

References

1. L.R. Mikami, S. Wieseler, R.L. Souza, et al. Five new naturally occurring mutations of the BCHE gene and frequencies of 12 butyryl cholinesterase alleles in a Brazilian population. Pharmacogenet Genomics 2008; 18(3):213–218.

2. J.D. Whittington, H.D. Pham, M. Procter, D.G. Grenache, R. Mao. A patient with prolonged paralysis. Clin Chem 2012; 58(3):496–501.

3. I. Manoharan, S. Wieseler, P.G. Layer, O. Lockridge, R. Boopathy. Naturally occurring mutation Leu307Pro of human butyrylcholinesterase in the Vysya community of India. Pharmacogenet Genomics 2006; 16(7):461–468.

4. G.S. Murphy, S.J. Brull. Residual neuromuscular block: lessons unlearned. Part I: definitions, incidence, and adverse physiologic effects of residual neuromuscular block. Anesth Analg 2010; 111(1):120–128.

5. D.R. Bevan. Neuromuscular blockade. Inadvertent extubation of the partially paralyzed patient. Anesthesiol Clin North America 2001; 19(4):913–922.

6. L.I. Eriksson, E. Sundman, R. Olsson, et al. Functional assessment of the pharynx at rest and during swallowing in partially paralyzed humans: simultaneous videomanometry and mechanomyography of awake human volunteers. Anesthesiology 1997; 87(5):1035–1043.

7. J.B. Brand, D.J. Cullen, N.E. Wilson, H.H. Ali. Spontaneous recovery from nondepolarizing neuromuscular blockade: correlation between clinical and evoked responses. Anesth Analg 1977; 56(1):55–58.

8. M. Lemyze, J. Mallat. Understanding negative pressure pulmonary edema. Intensive Care Med 2014; 40(8):1140–1143.

9. D.J. Krodel, E.A. Bittner, R.E. Abdulnour, R.H. Brown, M. Eikermann. Negative pressure pulmonary edema following bronchospasm. Chest 2011; 140(5):1351–1354.

10. K. Deepika, C.A. Kenaan, A.M. Barrocas, J.J. Fonseca, G.B. Bikazi. Negative

pressure pulmonary edema after acute upper airway obstruction. *J Clin Anesth* 1997; 9(5):403–438.

11. S.J. Singh Bajwa, A. Kulshrestha. Diagnosis, prevention and management of postoperative pulmonary edema. *Ann Med Health Sci Res* 2012; 2(2):180–185.

12. D.I. Sessler. Complications and treatment of mild hypothermia. *Anesthesiology* 2001; 95(2):531–543.

13. J. Barr, G.L. Fraser, K. Puntillo, *et al.* Clinical practice guidelines for the management of pain, agitation, and delirium in adult patients in the intensive care unit. *Crit Care Med* 2013; 41(1):263–306.

14. Y. Shehabi, R. Bellomo, M.C. Reade, *et al.* for the Sedation Practice in Intensive Care Evaluation (SPICE) Study Investigators; ANZICS Clinical Trials Group. Early intensive care sedation predicts long-term mortality in ventilated critically ill patients. *Am J Respir Crit Care Med* 2012; 186(8):724–731.

15. P. Dewachter, C. Mouton-Faivre, C.W. Emala, S. Beloucif. Case scenario: bronchospasm during anesthetic induction. *Anesthesiology* 2011; 114(4):1200–1210.

16. B.D. Woods, R.N. Sladen. Perioperative considerations for the patient with asthma. *Br J Anaesth* 2009; 103(Suppl 1):57–65.

17. M.M. Mughal, D.A. Culver, O.A. Minai, A.C. Arroliga. Auto-positive end-expiratory pressure: mechanisms and treatment. *Cleve Clin J Med* 2005; 72(9):801–809.

18. R. Brandoles, C. Broseghini, G. Polese, *et al.* Effects of intrinsic PEEP on pulmonary gas exchange in mechanically ventilated patients. *Eur Respir J* 1993; 6(3):358–363.

19. T. Luecke, P. Pelosi. Clinical review: positive end-expiratory pressure and cardiac output. *Crit Care* 2005; 9(6):607–621.

20. J. Du, J. Zuo. Unexpected tension pneumothorax occurring in an elderly patient in the post anesthesia care unit. *Pak J Med Sci* 2011; 27(4):906–908.

21. A.C. Mega, J.M. Encinas, N.P. Blanco, T.M. Martins. Tension pneumothorax in post-anesthetic care unit: case report. *Rev Bras Anestesiol* 2004; 54(5):681–686.

22. S.J. Lee, D.-J. Lee, M.-C. Kim, U.-J. Im. Pneumothorax in a post-anesthetic care unit after right thyroidectomy with left neck dissection: a case report. *Korean J Anesthesiol* 2010; 59(6):429–432.

Chapter

44

Special considerations for the pediatric patient

Peter Jonathan Gambino, Allan F. Simpao, and Zvi Grunwald

- A multimodal approach to pain control allows the clinicians to treat the pain at multiple points in the process of pain generation.
- Postoperative nausea and vomiting (PONV) may be due to multiple factors that are similar for adult and pediatric patients.
- A clinician's initial assessment of hydration status should focus on estimating capillary refill time, skin turgor, and respiratory patterns.

Pediatric patients in the Post-Anesthesia Care Unit (PACU) require vigilant attention after they receive anesthesia. One-to-one nursing, special vital sign monitoring, and the ability to evaluate patients quickly and accurately are some of the requirements of a pediatric PACU. The evaluation and treatment of a pediatric patient may require the clinician to utilize alternative methods than those used for an adult patient. For example, a child undergoing bilateral myringotomy tube placement may not have an intravenous (IV) catheter present to administer anti-emetic and pain medications.

The goal of managing a pediatric patient is to transition patients safely from anesthesia to discharge from the PACU. In addition to stable vital signs and adequate oxygenation and ventilation, three important patient factors to assess are adequate pain control, hydration status, and the degree of nausea and vomiting.

Assessments

Assessments of pediatric patients in the PACU should always begin with ensuring a patent airway, as well as assessing breathing and circulation (ABCs). Table 44.1 lists the normal, age-specific values for respiratory rate, heart rate, and blood pressure in awake pediatric patients.

Pain in pediatric patients

All patients, from neonates to adults, can perceive pain. Therefore, it is imperative to accurately assess and treat pain with standardized methods in a patient of any age. Adequate pain control in children is complicated by their inability to communicate the type, intensity, and location of their pain. Many patients are pre-verbal or possess mental challenges that make communication difficult. However, many tools are available to evaluate a child at any

Post-Anesthesia Care: Symptoms, Diagnosis, and Management, ed. James W. Heitz. Published by Cambridge University Press. © Cambridge University Press 2016.

Table 44.1 Age-specific vital sign norms

Age	Respiratory rate (breaths/min)	Heart rate (beats/min)	Systolic blood pressure (mmHg)	Diastolic blood pressure (mmHg)
0–3 months	35–55	100–150	65–85	45–55
3–6 months	30–45	90–120	70–90	50–65
6–12 months	25–40	80–120	80–100	55–65
1–3 years	24–30	70–110	90–105	55–70
3–6 years	20–25	65–110	95–110	60–75
6–12 years	14–22	60–95	100–120	60–75
12+ years	12–18	55–85	110–135	65–85

Source: R. Kliegman et al. (editions), Nelson Textbook of Pediatrics 19th edition. Philadelphia, PA: Saunders, 2011.

Table 44.2 CRIES neonatal post operative pain management

	0	1	2
Crying	No	High pitched	Inconsolable
O_2 required to maintain SpO_2 >95%	No	FiO_2 21–30%	FiO_2 greater than 30%
Vital signs	HR and BP less than or equal to preoperative values	HR and BP up to 20% greater than preoperative	HR and BP over 20% greater than preoperative
Expressions	None	Grimace	Grimace/grunt
Sleeplessness	No	Wakes at frequent intervals	Constantly awake

HR, heart rate; BP, blood pressure.

age or development stage. They are categorized as being either observational or self-reported. Self-reported pain levels become relevant by the age of 5 to 6 years.[1]

Neonate pain assessment involves monitoring vital signs and observing the child. The CRIES (Crying, Requires O_2 for SpO_2 >95%, Increased vital signs, Expression, Sleepless) neonatal post operative pain measurement score shown in Table 44.2 was developed at the University of Missouri, Columbia.[2] Assessment should be carried out after every pain intervention. A CRIES score of zero represents no pain, while a score of 10 signifies maximal pain.

Several tools can be used to evaluate pain in patients aged 1 year old to pre-verbal. Commonly used scales include The Children's Hospital of Eastern Ontario Pain Scale (CHEOPS), Toddler–Preschooler Postoperative Pain Scale (TPPPS), and the Fingers, Legs, Arms, Cry and Consolability (FLACC) scale,[3] which rely on vocal, facial, and bodily pain assessments. The FLACC scale (Table 44.3) is a measurement tool that assesses pain in

Table 44.3 The Fingers, Legs, Arms, Cry and Consolability (FLACC) scale

Criteria	0	1	2
Fingers	No particular expression, or smile	Occasional grimace or frown, withdrawn or uninterested	Frequent to constant quivering chin, clenched jaw
Legs	Normal position or relaxed	Uneasy, restless, tense	Kicking or legs drawn up
Arms	Lying quietly, normal position, moves easily	Squirming, shifting back and forth, tense	Arched, rigid, or jerking
Cry	No cry (awake or asleep)	Moans or whimpers, occasional complaints	Crying steadily, screams or sobs
Consolability	Content, relaxed	Reassured by occasional touching, hugging, or being talked to	Difficult to console or comfort

children between the ages of 2 months and 7 years. The scale is scored from zero (no pain) to 10 (severe pain). It does not rely on a child's ability to verbalize his or her degree of pain.

Assessing pain in the verbal child can be facilitated by tools that help the child convey their level of pain to the practitioner. Some tools available are the Oucher,[4] Faces pain scale, Numeric pain scale, and Visual Analog scale. These tools can help a clinician accurately evaluate pain in a pediatric patient.

Treatment of pain

The pain response is generated and transmitted via multiple mechanisms and pathways. A multimodal approach to pain control allows the clinicians to treat the pain at multiple points in the process of pain generation. Acetaminophen, non-steroidal anti-inflammatory drugs (NSAIDs), and opioids have all been shown to provide safe and effective analgesia in children.[5] Aspirin is not regularly used in the pediatric population because of its association with Reye syndrome.[6]

Medication administration may be complicated by the lack of IV access in some pediatric postoperative patients (e.g. myringotomy tubes). Oral, intramuscular, intraosseous, and rectal administration routes are options in patients without IV access. Dosing of medication is usually determined by weight in the pediatric population. In many instances, the dose of medication may differ from the adult dose. When using weight-based dosing, the dose should not exceed the recommended dose for adults.

Acetaminophen provides analgesia and antipyretic activity and is available in oral, IV, and rectal forms. The oral and IV dose is 15 mg/kg every 6 hours. The dose for rectal acetaminophen is 35 mg/kg every 6 hours. The maximum dose of the drug is the same for all routes of administration. The dose in neonates should not exceed 60 mg/kg/day. The dose in infants/children should not exceed 4 g/day.[7]

NSAIDs have been found to be effective in the treatment of pain in children after ambulatory surgery. They have a synergistic analgesic effect with opioids, while reducing the occurrence of opioid-related side effects.[8] Ibuprofen, naproxen, and ketorolac have all been studied in the pediatric population (Table 44.4).

Table 44.4 NSAIDs in the pediatric population

Drug	Dose	Interval	Max dose
Ibuprofen	6–10 mg/kg PO	4–6 hr	Lesser of 40 mg/kg day or 2.4 g
Naproxen	5–10 mg/kg PO	12 hr	20 mg/kg/day
Ketorolac*	0.5 mg/kg IV	6 hr	Lesser of 2 mg/kg/day or 120 mg

*Do not use for more than 5 days

Table 44.5 Opioid dosing in pediatrics

Drug	Age	Dose	Interval
Morphine			
Oral, immediate release	Infants/children	0.3 mg/kg	3–4 hr
Oral, extended release	Infants/children	0.25–0.5 mg/kg	8–12 hr
IV bolus	Preterm neonate	10–25 mcg/kg	2–4 hr
IV bolus	Full term neonate	25–50 mcg/kg	3–4 hr
IV bolus	Infants/children	50–100 mcg/kg	3 hr
Hydromorphone			
Oral	Infants/children	40–80 mcg/kg	4 hr
IV bolus	Infants/children	10–20 mcg/kg	3–4 hr
Fentanyl			
Intranasal	Infants/children	1–2 mcg/kg	Once
IV bolus	Infants/children	0.5–1 mcg/kg	1–2 hr
Nalbuphine			
IV bolus	Preterm neonate	10–25 mcg/kg	2–4 hr
IV bolus	Full term neonate	25–50 mcg/kg	2–4 hr
IV bolus	Infants/children	50–100 mcg/kg	2–4 hr

Source: J.B. Rose. Pediatric analgesia pharmacology. In: Ronald S Litman, *Pediatric Anesthesia: The Requisites in Anesthesiology*. Philadelphia, PA: Mosby, 2004.[8]
Preterm: newborn <37 weeks' gestation
Full term: newborn >37 weeks' gestation
Infant: >3 months of age

Opioids are used commonly to control moderate to severe pain in pediatric patients. The dosing is based upon the child's weight. The side effects are similar to those seen in adults. Nausea, vomiting, pruritus, sedation, respiratory depression, and constipation are commonly seen. Table 44.5 shows some commonly used opioids and their doses. If an opioid overdose is suspected, naloxone can be administered to reverse the opioid effect; however, one must take into account the patient's clinical presentation and the implications of opioid receptor antagonism in a postoperative patient (Table 44.6).

Table 44.6 Naloxone dosing

Age	Dose	Interval
Less than 1 mo	0.1 mg/kg IV	2–3 min prn
1 mo to 5 yr and less than 20 kg	0.1 mg/kg IV	2–3 min prn
Greater than 5 yr and greater than 20 kg	2 mg IV	2–3 min prn

Hydration status in the pediatric patient

Hydration status can affect a pediatric patient's suitability for discharge from the PACU and the hospital. Many centers do not require that the patient be able to consume liquids and urinate. Therefore, it is necessary to have the ability to assess hydration status and treat a patient prior to discharge.

A clinician's initial assessment should focus on estimating capillary refill time, skin turgor, and respiratory patterns. Additional signs of dehydration are sunken eyes, dry mucous membranes, sunken fontanelles, and overall poor appearance. The exact degree of dehydration is difficult to determine because of the imprecision and inaccuracy of available tests.[9]

Assessment of capillary refill time determines the body's ability to perfuse end organs. Patient's age and temperature should be considered when testing an individual. Compress a patient's fingernail to remove blood from the capillaries. Release pressure and note the time until color is restored in the fingernail. Normal capillary refill time in an infant is 2 seconds.

Skin turgor is a late sign of dehydration. It occurs with a loss of 5% of bodily fluids. Edema makes it difficult to assess skin turgor in a patient. A clinician should pinch the skin on the back of the hand, upper arm, or abdomen till it tents. Once pressure is released, the skin should return to normal within one second.

An abnormal breathing pattern is a hallmark of dehydration in children. Moderate to severe dehydration is categorized by rapid and deep breathing patterns.

Nausea and vomiting in the pediatric patient

Nausea and vomiting is a common cause of unanticipated hospital admissions. Postoperative nausea and vomiting (PONV) may be due to multiple factors that are similar between adult and pediatric patients. Both the location of the surgical site and the use of inhalation anesthetics can increase the risk of PONV – particularly laparoscopic (especially gynecological), strabismus, middle ear, orchiopexy, stomach, duodenal, gall bladder, and extracorporeal shock wave lithotripsy. Patient factors include age (peaks between 11 and 14 years), female sex, obesity, anxiety/stress, history of PONV, and full stomach. Postoperative causes of nausea and vomiting include oral intake, motion, and postoperative narcotics.

Because the biochemical pathways contributing to PONV involve multiple receptor types (e.g. serotonin, dopamine), treatment of PONV should utilize a multimodal approach. When one agent fails to relieve nausea and vomiting, the patient should be given a medication from a different drug class. Many of the drugs available for adults have been studied in children (Table 44.7); however, drug dosing differs between adults and children. Pediatric dosing is weight-based.

Table 44.7 Anti-emetic medication doses in pediatric patients

Drug	Dose	Age/weight range	Max dose	Side effects
Serotonin antagonists				
Ondansetron	0.1 mg/kg IV	1 mo to 12 yr and <40 kg	4 mg/dose	QT prolongation
Steroid				
Dexamethasone	0.5–1 mg/kg IV	None	10–20 mg	Insomnia, hyperactivity

Postoperative complications

Stridor is a postoperative complication that must be addressed immediately. A clinician should be concerned for impending airway obstruction and respiratory failure. The management of the patient depends upon the cause of the obstruction. If the surgery involved the upper airway, the surgical service should be consulted immediately.

Laryngospasm is an obstruction of the airway at the level of the vocal cords that presents with stridor and is commonly seen when a patient is in stage 2 of anesthesia. Stage 2 is the "excitement stage," where contact with the vocal cords can elicit muscular spasms. Children who have an upper airway infection or who are regularly exposed to tobacco smoke are at increased risk of laryngospasm. Pediatric patients are at increased risk for laryngospasms when they are extubated in deeper stages of anesthesia and then brought to the PACU to emerge from anesthesia. These "deep extubation" patients should receive one-to-one nurse monitoring to identify laryngospasm at its onset. A mask, an oxygen supply, and oral airways should be available at the bedside for any child emerging from anesthesia.[10]

Treatment of laryngospasm involves establishing a patent upper airway (e.g. chin lift and jaw thrust maneuvers, oral and/or nasal airways), delivery of 100% FiO_2, and the application of continuous positive airway pressure. Muscle relaxant administration and tracheal intubation should be considered immediately. The laryngospasm may also be broken by increasing anesthetic depth via IV medications, such as propofol (2.5 mg/kg). However, one should weigh the risk of administering medications that affect cardiac function in a patient with worsening hypoxemia and possible bradycardia.

Post-intubation croup is inspiratory stridor associated with retraction of accessory muscles of respiration for at least 30 minutes that is severe enough to require treatment with humidified O_2 or racemic epinephrine. Studies have placed the incidence rate of post-intubation croup at 0.1%.[11] The cause of the obstruction is usually edema in the subglottic region. Symptoms often resolve with humidified O_2 and rarely require racemic epinephrine. Overnight admission and observation should be considered for patients with additional episodes of post-intubation croup. While several studies have shown a benefit to steroid administration in post-intubation croup, their use remains controversial.[12]

Emergence delirium has been described as a "mental disturbance during the recovery of general anesthesia consisting of hallucination, delusions, and general confusion manifested by moaning, restlessness, involuntary physical activity, and thrashing about in bed."[13] Emergence delirium can range from 25% to 80% of patients depending on the criteria used to define it.[14] Emergence delirium occurs within 30 minutes of emergence from volatile anesthesia, is self-limiting with variable duration, and disrupts the PACU environment.

Assessment of the patient should include a review of the anesthetic and surgical course, as well as a focused history and physical exam. Common causes of distress should be addressed prior to a diagnosis of emergence delirium, such as pain, anxiety, hypoxia, hypercarbia, full bladder, hypovolemia, and cerebral irritation. A diagnosis of emergence delirium should be made only after other life-threatening causes have been excluded.

Management involves preventing children from harming themselves and reducing their agitation. While soft restraints can protect children and preserve their IV access, most small children can be kept safe by being held by nursing staff or parents. Stimulation should be minimized; lights should be lowered, while the child should be swaddled and encouraged to sleep. The child's parents should not only be allowed at bedside to help reduce the child's anxiety, but also be informed of the transient nature of this condition to relieve their anxiety. Vital signs should be monitored and adequate oxygenation and blood pressure maintained.

Pharmaceutical management of emergence delirium is directed at calming the child and encouraging the patient to sleep. Propofol (0.5 mg/kg IV) or midazolam (0.02 mg/kg IV) can accomplish these objectives. The use of benzodiazepines in children has been associated with a paradoxical reaction causing an increase in agitation. If a paradoxical reaction is suspected, flumazenil 0.01 mg/kg IV (maximum dose 0.2 mg) at 1–2-minute intervals to maximum dose of 1 mg can be used to reverse the effects of the benzodiazepines. Opioid use in treating emergence delirium (e.g. morphine 0.05 mg/kg) is aimed at sedating the child and allowing him or her to sleep through the delirium.[10]

Discharge

There are many criteria that can be used to determine if a pediatric patient is ready for discharge from the PACU. There have been attempts to establish specific criteria for discharge, such as the Steward Post-anesthetic Recovery Score. There is still debate on how well the criteria established in these studies correlate to other variables.[15] Discharge criteria are institution-dependent. The clinician should establish and utilize PACU discharge criteria that best fit his or her institution and patient population.

References

1. Z.N. Kain, D.V. Cicchetti, B.C. McClain. Measurement of pain in children: state-of-the-art considerations. *Anesthesiology* 2002; 96:523–526.

2. L.S. Krechel, J. Bildner. CRIES: a new neonatal postoperative pain measurement score. Initial testing of validity and reliability. *Paediatr Anaesth* 1995; 5:53–61.

3. S.I. Merkel. T. Voepel-Lewis, J.R. Shaveevitz, S. Malviva. The FLACC: a behavioral scale for scoring postoperative pain in young children. *Pediatr Nurs* 1997; 23:293–297.

4. Pain Associates in Nursing. OUCHER Pain Scale. www.oucher.org. Accessed October 4, 2012.

5. M. Yaster. Multimodal analgesia in children. *Eur J Anaesthesiol* 2010; 27:851–857.

6. E.D. Belay, J.S. Bresse, R.C. Holman, *et al.* Reye's syndrome in the United States from 1981 through 1997. *N Engl J Med* 1999; 340:1377–1382.

7. C.B. Berde, N.F. Sethna. Analgesics for the treatment of pain in children. *N Engl J Med* 2002; 347:1094–1103.

8. J.B. Rose. Pediatric analgesia pharmacology. In: Ronald S Litman, *Pediatric Anesthesia: The Requisites in Anesthesiology*. Philadelphia, PA: Mosby, 2004 pp. 196–205.

9. M.J. Stiener, D. Dewalt, J. Byerly. Is this child dehydrated? *JAMA* 2004; 291:2746–2754.

10. L.J. Mason. Problems and pitfalls of pediatric anesthesia. http://www.iars.org/assets/1/7/2008_IARS_Review_Course_Lectures.pdf/. Accessed August 17, 2015.

11. R. Litman, T.P. Keon. Postintubation croup in children. *Anesthesiology* 1991; 75:1122–1123.

12. M. Ausejo, A. Saenz, B. Pham, D. Moher, T. Chalmers. The effectiveness of glucocorticoids in treating croup: meta-analysis. *Br Med J* 1999; 319:595–600.

13. T. Wilson, S. Graves. Pediatric considerations in a general post anesthesia care unit. *Perianesth Nurs* 1990; 5:16–24.

14. N. Sikich, J. Lerman. Development and psychometric evaluation of the Pediatric Anesthesia Emergence Delirium Scale. *Anesthesiology* 2004; 100:1138–1145.

15. R. Litman. Postoperative considerations. In: Ronald S Litman, *Pediatric Anesthesia: The Requisites in Anesthesiology*. Philadelphia, PA: Mosby, 2004 pp.185–190.

Special considerations for the pregnant patient after non-obstetric surgery

Suzanne Huffnagle and H. Jane Huffnagle

- Knowledge of the physiological changes that occur during pregnancy is important for proper postoperative care of the pregnant patient.
- Treat maternal hypotension aggressively using fluids, phenylephrine, and ephedrine when appropriate.
- Most opioids and anti-emetics are safe for use in pregnancy.
- Utilize continuous electronic fetal heart rate and contraction monitoring for 24 hours in the postoperative period if the fetus is considered viable.
- Pregnancy is a hypercoagulable state, and thromboembolism prophylaxis is vital.

Taking care of the post-surgical pregnant patient in the Post-Anesthesia Care Unit (PACU) can be a challenging experience. It may be appropriate for some pregnant patients having surgical procedures to recover in the labor and delivery suite. The decision is usually made by the obstetrician. This chapter will focus on the pregnant patient going to the general PACU.

It is essential to have knowledge of the physiological changes that occur in pregnant patients, making them different from the general population. In addition, the development of preterm labor and fetal heart rate abnormalities must be promptly recognized and treated. Good communication between several services including surgery, anesthesiology, and obstetrics is imperative. We will discuss some of the most important physiological changes occurring in pregnancy which may impact PACU care, some of the most common surgical procedures performed on pregnant patients, what medications are safe to give in the PACU, and some guidelines for discharge of the pregnant patient after non-obstetric surgery.

Physiological changes in pregnancy that impact PACU stay

In the PACU, it is important to be aware of several physiological changes that occur in pregnant patients. Pregnant patients have decreased functional residual capacity beginning about the fifth month of pregnancy, which further decreases in the supine position.[1] Periods of hypoventilation or apnea in the postoperative period, as well as higher oxygen consumption during pregnancy, result in more rapid maternal hypoxemia than in the

Post-Anesthesia Care: Symptoms, Diagnosis, and Management, ed. James W. Heitz. Published by Cambridge University Press. © Cambridge University Press 2016.

non-pregnant counterpart.[2] Supplemental oxygen in the PACU minimizes maternal hypoxemia and may increase oxygen delivery to the fetus.

Supine hypotension syndrome, characterized by maternal hypotension, tachycardia (or bradycardia), diaphoresis, nausea, vomiting, and mental status changes can occur from aortocaval compression by the gravid uterus when a parturient lies supine. This decrease in venous return of blood to the heart reduces the maternal cardiac output and may result in impairment of uteroplacental blood flow. Placing a wedge under the parturient's right hip, to displace the gravid uterus away from the abdominal vessels, can improve maternal venous return, cardiac output, and blood pressure.

Approximately 30% to 50% of pregnant women experience gastroesophageal reflux during pregnancy.[3] Aspiration during an episode of reflux in a sedated postoperative pregnant patient is of concern. Raising the head of the bed may help minimize reflux, but postoperative nausea and vomiting (PONV) is still a potential problem. We will discuss medications to treat PONV which are safe in pregnancy later in this chapter. Pregnant patients experience vascular engorgement of the airway and friable mucous membranes, and may have a higher incidence of airway obstruction, making airway management more difficult in the event of over-sedation in the PACU.[4]

Postoperative pain control is important to alleviate excess catecholamine outflow in the pregnant patient, thus minimizing the development of preterm labor. Decreased protein binding associated with low albumin concentrations may result in a larger fraction of unbound drug, with the potential for greater drug toxicity during pregnancy. Since most opioid analgesics are at least moderately protein-bound, the pregnant patient may be more sensitive to the analgesic and respiratory depressant effects of these drugs.[5]

Lastly, pregnancy induces a hypercoagulable state, predisposing a parturient to thromboembolism, so pneumatic compression devices placed in the operating room should be maintained in the PACU.[6] Early mobilization in the event of a prolonged PACU stay (no post operative beds available) is imperative.

Surgical procedures performed on pregnant patients

About 0.3% to 2.2% of pregnant women will undergo a surgical procedure each year, requiring approximately 115,000 anesthetics.[7] Surgery may be necessary in any stage of pregnancy, but the second trimester is the optimal time as it avoids the period of organogenesis, and the risk of developing preterm labor is lowest. Laparoscopic surgery for gynecological indications is the most common first trimester procedure, whereas appendectomy is the most common procedure during the remainder of pregnancy. Indications for pregnancy-related surgery include cervical incompetence and ovarian cysts. Non-pregnancy-related surgery includes appendectomy, cholecystectomy, trauma-related procedures, craniotomy, electroconvulsive shock therapy, cardiac surgery, ureterolithotomy, and surgeries for malignancy. Unfortunately, many of these procedures require general anesthesia. Patients undergoing neurosurgical and cardiac procedures frequently recover in the intensive care unit, so our discussion will focus on the other common surgical situations where pregnant patients will recover in the PACU.

Specific postoperative considerations after regional anesthesia

Cervical cerclage placement, ovarian cystectomy, and urological procedures during pregnancy can often be performed utilizing regional anesthesia. These postoperative pregnant patients enter the recovery room awake, relatively pain free, and able to maintain a patent airway. Postoperative pain and nausea/vomiting may accompany regression of the block and will be discussed later. Postdural puncture headache presenting in the PACU is very rare, as the headache usually presents on the first or second day after the dural puncture.[8] When these patients are hemodynamically stable, and their nausea, vomiting, and pain are adequately treated, one study suggests that a two segment regression of sensory block may be adequate for discharge from the PACU.[9] Since two segment regression of sensory block occurs early and progresses in a linear fashion, patients do not need to remain in PACU until the block completely recedes.[9] In the rare event that the patient experiences severe back pain, a significant delay in normal recovery of the block, or deterioration of lower extremity or bladder function, emergent imaging of the spine is warranted to rule out epidural or spinal hematoma.[10] Monitoring of the fetus and other considerations will be discussed later.

Postoperative considerations for the fetus

Most anesthetics for surgery during pregnancy involve general anesthesia. These patients enter the PACU sedated and may be in some discomfort. Not only does one have to assess the mother, but one must consider the fetus as well. We will discuss some guidelines for monitoring the fetus, and concerns about medications to treat nausea, vomiting, and pain that are safe in pregnant patients. We will also touch on some strategies for prevention of thromboembolism.

The American College of Obstetricians and Gynecologists Committee on Obstetric Practice has several *guidelines* for monitoring the fetus in the perioperative period when a pregnant patient must have surgery.[11] Because of the difficulty of conducting large-scale randomized clinical trials in this population, there are no data to allow for specific recommendations. Some of these guidelines are as follows:

1. If possible, non-urgent surgery should be performed in the second trimester when preterm contractions and spontaneous abortion are least likely.
2. Surgery should be done at an institution with neonatal and pediatric services.
3. An obstetric care provider with cesarean delivery privileges should be readily available.
4. A qualified individual should be readily available to interpret the fetal heart rate pattern.
5. If the fetus is considered previable (<24 weeks), it is generally sufficient to ascertain the fetal heart rate by Doppler before and after the procedure.
6. At a minimum, if the fetus is considered to be viable (around 24 weeks or over),[12] simultaneous electronic fetal heart rate and contraction monitoring should be performed before and after the procedure to assess fetal well-being and the absence of contractions.

These guidelines are purposely vague to allow for individual decisions based upon the surgical situation, the patient's condition, available resources, and the obstetrician's input. We recommend continuous electronic fetal heart rate and contraction monitoring for 24 hours in the postoperative period if the fetus is considered viable and the abdomen is accessible (personal communication with our obstetricians). A qualified individual (obstetrical nurse) should be available to interpret the fetal heart rate patterns during fetal heart rate monitoring. This does not mean that the parturient must remain in the PACU during the entire monitoring period. Transfer to a maternal observation or labor and delivery unit for the remainder of monitoring after initial recovery from anesthesia is acceptable.

Table 45.1 FDA Classification of Fetal Harm Risk from Drugs

Category A	Human studies: controlled studies show no risk to fetus in any trimester, fetal harm is remote. Example: water
Category B	Human studies: no risk to fetus in any trimester Animal studies: show adverse effect
Category C	Human studies: no controlled studies done, no data available Animal studies: adverse effects (teratogenic, embryocidal). Only give if benefits outweigh risks
Category D	Human studies: positive evidence of fetal risk, use if life-threatening disease where no safer drug exists. Example: diazepam
Category X	Human studies: teratogenicity to fetus Animal studies: teratogenicity in animals. Contraindicated in pregnancy. Example: thalidomide

(Briggs GG, Freeman RK, Yaffe SJ. *Drugs in Pregnancy and Lactation*. 8th edition. Philadelphia: Lippincott Williams & Wilkins 2008)

If a non-reassuring fetal heart rate pattern or preterm maternal contractions develops, timely communication with appropriate personnel is important to ensure the best fetal outcome. Adequate hydration, placing oxygen on the mother, treating maternal hypotension, and maintaining left uterine displacement, are easy steps to temporize these conditions until the obstetrical team can make more definitive plans.

Treatment of hypotension, hypertension, nausea, vomiting, and maternal pain may require giving medications to the mother. What medications are safe for the developing fetus? In 1979 the US Food and Drug Administration (FDA) introduced a classification system of drug risk to the fetus which includes Category A (safest), B, C, D, and X (known danger).[13] This classification system is based on review of the literature and helps physicians weigh risks and benefits when giving drugs during pregnancy (Table 45.1).

Maternal hypotension from any cause can jeopardize uteroplacental perfusion and cause fetal asphyxia. It is initially treated with fluids (crystalloid, colloid, blood products) when appropriate; phenylephrine and ephedrine are the two most common vasopressors used in pregnancy. Randomized controlled trials comparing ephedrine with phenylephrine for the treatment of maternal hypotension have shown there is no difference between them in efficacy, nor incidence of true fetal acidosis, although maternal bradycardia was more common with phenylephrine.[14] One should attempt to keep maternal blood pressure within 20% of the preoperative baseline.

Maternal hypertension in the PACU is usually from inadequately treated pain, but may also be from sympathetic overactivity, which could compromise uteroplacental perfusion. Most antihypertensive medications can be used safely in the PACU while monitoring the fetal heart rate, with the exception of esmolol and angiotensin-converting enzyme (ACE) inhibitors. Esmolol may cause a prolonged fetal heart rate bradycardia and a reduction in fetal PaO_2;[15] ACE inhibitors are teratogenic (Table 45.2).

Opioid analgesics commonly used in the PACU lack teratogenic effects in clinical doses; however, they do decrease FHR variability.[7] Most are considered Category C drugs when used during pregnancy (Table 45.2). Occasionally, anxiolytics are needed in the PACU. Benzodiazepines are Category D because of an association with first trimester use and an

Table 45.2 Fetal risk classification of drugs used in the PACU

Drug category	Drug	FDA risk category
IV opioids	Fentanyl	C
	Morphine	C
	Hydromorphone	C
	Meperidine	C
Benzodiazepines	Midazolam	D
	Diazepam	D
	Lorazepam	D
Anti-emetics	Ondansetron	B
	Droperidol	C
	Metoclopramide	B
	H$_2$ blockers	B
	Promethazine	C
	Hydroxyzine	C
Anti hypertensives	Labetalol	C
	Nifedipine	C
	Alpha methyldopa	B
	ACE inhibitors	D
	Angiotensin receptor blockers (ARBs)	D
	Magnesium	A
Vasopressors	Ephedrine	C
	Phenylephrine	C
	Epinephrine	C
Other pain relievers	NSAIDs	D
	Tramadol	C
	Aspirin	D (3rd trimester)
	Acetaminophen	B
Antithrombotics	Heparin	C
	Enoxaparin	B
Glucocorticoids	Dexamethasone	C

(Briggs GG, Freeman RK, Yaffe SJ. *Drugs in Pregnancy and Lactation*. 8th edition. Philadelphia: Lippincott Williams & Wilkins 2008)

increased incidence of cleft lip and palate, neural tube defects, intestinal atresia, and limb defects.[16] Although the consensus among teratologists is that benzodiazepines are not proven human teratogens, the package insert for these drugs warns of these risks. Of bigger concern is over-sedating the postoperative pregnant patient. Adequate supervision and monitoring in the PACU are essential to minimize the incidence of airway obstruction, apnea, and aspiration which can result in maternal death.[17]

Aspirin causes permanent inhibition of prostaglandin synthetase in platelets and may increase the risk of bleeding after certain surgical procedures. Acetaminophen does not, and both are considered safe for use during pregnancy. Although non-steroidal anti-inflammatory drugs (NSAIDs) do not cause teratogenicity, they can cause constriction of the fetal ductus arteriosus if used after 32 weeks' gestation.[18]

Postoperative nausea and vomiting in the pregnant patient can lead to dehydration, which may precipitate the development of preterm labor. Most agents used to treat nausea and vomiting in the PACU are Category B or C in pregnancy (Table 45.2). These include H_2-receptor antagonists, metoclopramide, promethazine, droperidol, and ondansetron.[18] Glucocorticoids are used to hasten fetal lung maturity in threatened preterm deliveries, so one can infer that a dose of dexamethasone in the PACU to alleviate PONV would not be harmful.

Since pregnancy is a hypercoagulable state, postoperative thromboembolism prophylaxis should be continued in the postoperative period. Early mobilization for a pregnant patient in the PACU may not be feasible during continuous fetal heart rate monitoring, but one should get the parturient out of bed as soon as possible if the PACU stay will be lengthy. Other methods of prophylaxis include continuing the use of intraoperatively placed pneumatic compression devices or anti-embolic compression stockings, and continuing any preoperative anticoagulation measures when appropriate. Low molecular weight heparin and unfractionated heparin are safe in pregnancy and may be given in the PACU under the direction of the surgeon or obstetrician.[18] If the parturient has received regional anesthesia, one should follow the guidelines recommended by the American Society of Regional Anesthesiologists when beginning postoperative anticoagulation.[19]

References

1. R. Geiser. Physiologic changes of pregnancy, Chapter 2 in *Obstetric Anesthesia Principles and Practices*. Chestnut DH. 4th edition. Philadelphia: Mosby Elsevier. 2009; p. 28.

2. G.W. Archer Jr., G.F. Marx. Arterial oxygen tension during apnoea in parturient women. *Br J Anaesth* 1974; 46:358–360.

3. R.E. Richter. Review article: the management of heartburn in pregnancy. *Aliment Pharmacol Ther* 2005; 22:749–757.

4. S. Pilkington, F. Carli, M.J. Dakin, et al. Increase in Mallampati score during pregnancy. *Br J Anaesth* 1995; 74:638–642.

5. M.J. Wunsch, V. Shanard, S.H. Schnoll. Treatment of pain in pregnancy. *Clin J Pain* 2003; 19:148–155.

6. A.J. Duhl, M.J. Paidas, S.H. Ural, et al. Antithrombotic therapy and pregnancy: consensus report and recommendations for prevention and treatment of venous thromboembolism and adverse pregnancy outcomes. *Am J Obstet Gynecol* 2007; 197:457.e1–457.e21.

7. M. Van de Velde. Nonobstetric surgery during pregnancy, Chapter 17 in *Obstetric Anesthesia Principles and Practices*. Chestnut DH. 4th edition. Philadelphia: Mosby Elsevier. 2009; pp. 337–358.

8. Headache Classification Committee of the International Headache Society. *Cephalalgia* 2004; 24:1–60.

9. S.E. Cohen, C.L. Hamilton, E.T. Riley, et al. Obstetric postanesthesia care unit stays: reevaluation of discharge criteria after regional anesthesia. *Anesthesiology* 1998; 89:1559–1565.

10. F. Reynolds. Neurologic complications of pregnancy and neuraxial anesthesia, Chapter 32 in *Obstetric Anesthesia Principles and Practices*. Chestnut DH. 4th edition. Philadelphia: Mosby Elsevier. 2009; pp. 701–726.

11. American College of Obstetricians and Gynecologists Committee Opinion Number 474: nonobstetric surgery during pregnancy. *Obstet Gynecol* 2011; 117:420–421.

12. L.P. Halamek. Prenatal consultation at the limits of viability. *NeoReviews* 2003; 4:e153–e156.

13. G.G. Briggs, R.K. Freeman, S.J. Yaffe. *Drugs in Pregnancy and Lactation*. 8th edition. Philadelphia: Lippincott, Williams & Wilkins, 2008.

14. A. Lee, W.D. Ngan Kee, T. Gin. A quantitative, systematic review of randomized controlled trials of ephedrine versus phenylephrine for the management of hypotension during spinal anesthesia for cesarean delivery. *Anesth Analg* 2002; 94:920–926.

15. J.C. Eisenach, M. Castro. Maternally administered esmolol produces beta-adrenergic blockade and hypoxemia in sheep. *Anesthesiology* 1989; 71:718–722.

16. D. Kjae, E. Horvath-Puhó, J. Christersen, *et al.* Use of phenytoin, phenobarbital, or diazepam during pregnancy and risk of congenital abnormalities: a case-time-control study. *Pharmacoepidemiol Drug Saf* 2007; 16:181–188.

17. J. Mhyre, M.N. Riesner, L.S. Polley. A series of anesthesia related maternal deaths in Michigan 1985–2003. *Anesthesiology* 2007; 106:1096–1104.

18. J. Yankowitz. Nonanesthetic drugs during pregnancy and lactation, Chapter 14 in *Obstetric Anesthesia Principles and Practices*. Chestnut DH. 4th edition. Philadelphia: Mosby Elsevier. 2009; pp. 285–303.

19. T.T. Horlocker, D.J. Wedel, J.C. Rowlingson, *et al.* Regional anesthesia in the patient receiving antithrombotic or thrombolytic therapy: American Society of Regional Anesthesia and Pain Medicine evidence-based guidelines (3rd edition). *Reg Anesth Pain Med* 2010; 35:64–101.

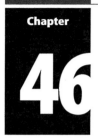

Chapter

Special considerations for the cardiac patient with implanted devices

46

Ryan P. Maxwell and Jordan E. Goldhammer

- Patients with implantable cardiac devices present a special challenge when presenting for non-cardiac surgery.
- A working knowledge of these devices is necessary for safe care of the cardiac patient after non-cardiac surgery.

Left ventricular assist device

Over the 2-year period of 2009–2011, implantation of left ventricular assist devices (LVADs) in the United States increased ten-fold when selected for destination therapy.[1] LVADs can be utilized in three clinical scenarios: (1) acute ventricular failure as a bridge to recovery; (2) chronic ventricular failure as a bridge to heart transplant; or (3) permanent implantation in those not suitable for heart transplantation. All LVADs fall into one of two physiological categories: pulsatile or non-pulsatile devices. Non-pulsatile, or continuous-flow, LVADs are smaller in size, operate silently, and have proven more durable when compared with pulsatile flow LVADs.[2] In patients selected for destination therapy, the continuous-flow Heartmate II device has demonstrated improved patient survival when compared with the pulsatile LVAD Heartmate XVE (58% vs. 24%, 2-year survival).[3] Thus, continuous-flow LVADs are more common and practitioners in the Post-Anesthesia Care Unit (PACU) setting are likely to encounter a continuous-flow VAD.

The VAD is implanted during a surgical procedure utilizing cardiopulmonary bypass. The left ventricle is emptied by a cannula located at the apex. This cannula delivers blood into a sub-diaphragmatic pre-peritoneal or intra abdominal pump. The rotary pump is capable of generating flow, a surrogate of cardiac output, of up to 10 l/min. Blood is returned from the device to the ascending aorta. LVADs are sensitive to changes in both preload (volume status) and afterload (systemic vascular resistance). LVAD patients will either have a weak or non-palpable pulse. The failing left ventricle cannot generate sufficient intrinsic contractile strength to create pulsatile flow beyond the continuous flow of the device.

Vital sign monitoring: The non-pulsatile flow of an LVAD can create difficulty in measuring basic vital signs in the PACU. Pulse oximetry estimates the percentage of oxygenated hemoglobin in arterial blood based upon characteristic light absorption of oxygenated and deoxygenated hemoglobin. Arterial saturation is differentiated from the

Post-Anesthesia Care: Symptoms, Diagnosis, and Management, ed. James W. Heitz. Published by Cambridge University Press. © Cambridge University Press 2016.

"background" oxygen saturation of venous blood by detecting arterial pulsations. In the absence of pulsatile flow, standard pulse oximetry will be unreliable. In this situation it is best to confirm clinical signs of tissue oxygenation such as mental status, capillary refill, and skin pallor. If concern exists regarding a patient's oxygenation, arterial blood gas analysis is indicated. In addition to pulse oximetry, automatic non-invasive blood pressure cuffs require pulsatility to generate accurate blood pressure measurements. A trial of a non-invasive cuff is warranted, however, as a mean blood pressure may be detected in those with weak pulsatility. In the absence of pulsatility, an alternative method for blood pressure measurement involves using a manual blood pressure cuff and an audible Doppler. The Doppler probe is placed over a distal artery as the manual cuff is slowly deflated. The blood pressure cuff reading when audible flow is heard by Doppler should be considered in the range of the patient's mean blood pressure.[2] In the absence of consistent blood pressure monitoring, mental status, urine output, and tissue oxygenation should be monitored as clinical signs of normotension. If concern exists regarding the patient's blood pressure, an arterial line should be considered. The use of ultrasound or Doppler can be of assistance in cannulating an artery with little or no palpable pulse.

LVAD console: A mechanical circulation coordinator or nurse who is familiar with the patient's assist device settings will accompany the majority of patients with a VAD. Should a specialized nurse not be available, standard VAD systems include a monitor that displays the pump speed (RPM), power (watts), flow (l/min), and pulsatility index (PI). The pump is run in a fixed speed mode in the range of 8,000 to 10,000 revolutions per minute (RPM).[4] The fixed speed is determined shortly after device placement and is based upon both optimal emptying of the left ventricle and right ventricular function. The pump power is a direct measurement of power output and self-adjusts to maintain pump speed based upon changes in afterload and viscosity. When evaluating the patient's VAD settings, a continual increase in power, or an absolute power value greater than 10–12 watts may indicate the presence of a thrombus inside the LVAD.[4] PI represents the contribution of the native left ventricle to cardiac output.[4] The PI ranges from 1 to 10 and is averaged every 15 seconds. The higher the PI, the more the left ventricle is contributing to flow through the VAD. A progressively lower PI often represents a decrease in left ventricular preload as the native heart can no longer augment flow through the LVAD.

Hypotension: LVAD patients are sensitive to changes in preload owing to the fixed cardiac output generated by the device. PI can be used as a surrogate for preload; however, it will not differentiate true hypovolemia from decreased device inflow secondary to right ventricular failure. The evaluation of severe hypotension in the PACU should include an emergent transthoracic or transesophageal echocardiogram to determine right ventricular function, volume status, and inflow or outflow problems intrinsic to the device.[5] Treatment should be tailored based on the echocardiographic findings with volume resuscitation for hypovolemia and inotropic therapy for progressive right ventricular failure.

Suction event: A significant drop in left ventricular preload can result in suction of the ventricular wall, most often the intraventricular septum, into the inflow cannula, as the pump continues to rotate at a set speed. A suction event will often trigger ventricular arrhythmias and can result in profound hypotension and circulatory collapse. Treatment of a suction event includes immediate restoration of left ventricular preload and treatment of malignant arrhythmias to restore biventricular function. Suction events are sensed by the LVAD system when there is an acute and severe decrease in the PI.[4] In this instance, the LVAD will automatically drop its speed to a previously set low limit to temporize the problem and minimize suction forces against the ventricular wall. This temporary decrease in RPM allows the clinician a window to restore circulating volume and maintain normal device function. After the suction event has resolved, the LVAD will slowly increase its speed, in 100 RPM intervals, until it reaches the standard RPM setting.

Other concerns for LVAD patients: Careful consideration of the LVAD patient's anticoagulation status is important in their PACU management. VAD patients are anticoagulated with a regimen consisting of antiplatelet agents and warfarin. Some centers use a target INR (international normalized ratio) of 2.0 to 3.0 whereas others use 1.5 to 2.5.[2] The antiplatelet agent also varies, but may include aspirin 81 mg daily with or without dipyridamole 75 mg. Although the etiology is not yet completely understood, many continuous-flow LVAD patients demonstrate reduced levels of von Willebrand factor, which may further increase their bleeding diathesis.[6]

Right ventricular output is not supported by an LVAD, and rhythms such as sustained ventricular tachycardia and ventricular fibrillation can quickly lead to hemodynamic compromise. A patient with an LVAD can safely receive cardioversion or defibrillation. Caution is advised in performing chest compressions on a VAD patient owing to the risk of dislodging or damaging the inflow and outflow grafts. In a situation where augmented circulation is necessary, abdominal compressions may be performed.[4] VADs contain ferromagnetic components, and these patients should not be subjected to an MRI.

Intra-aortic balloon pump

The intra-aortic balloon pump (IABP) is a mechanical assist device typically utilized for patients in cardiogenic shock. The PACU provider may encounter an IABP in patients following cardiac surgery, interventional cardiac catheterization, or non-cardiac surgery patients who have experienced a perioperative myocardial infarction.

The IABP is an inflatable balloon placed percutaneously into the femoral artery and advanced into the descending thoracic aorta. Proper localization of the balloon is at the proximal descending thoracic aorta, 1 to 2 cm distal to the aortic arch. Echocardiography, fluoroscopy, or chest X-ray is utilized to ensure proper positioning.

The goal of the device is two-fold: (1) improve systemic blood flow by afterload reduction; and (2) improve coronary artery perfusion during ventricular diastole, therefore improving myocardial oxygen supply and demand dynamics. The IABP inflates during diastole, thereby increasing aortic diastolic pressure, and driving blood flow into the coronary arteries, improving myocardial perfusion. Rapid, pre-systolic balloon deflation enhances ventricular ejection by reducing left ventricular afterload and wall tension, and improving myocardial energy balance up to 15%.[7]

IABP management: Several key points are important for the PACU provider managing an IABP. The device is set to synchronize with either an arterial waveform tracing or ECG. Balloon inflation occurs at the start of diastole, identified by the device console as either the T wave on ECG tracing, indicating ventricular repolarization, or the dicrotic notch on the arterial waveform, signifying aortic valve closure. Deflation occurs at the onset of the next ventricular contraction, as the arterial pressure tracing reaches its nadir, or the R wave on ECG. Most modern IABP devices have a sensor on the tip of the balloon capable of measuring a direct arterial waveform; therefore, a dedicated arterial catheter is not always necessary. If triggering IABP function based upon ECG, additional leads must be connected to the IABP console.

Improperly timed device inflation can cause significant hemodynamic compromise and increased myocardial work. If this situation is identified in the PACU, expert consultation should be sought. The pumping frequency of the IABP is indicated as a ratio of balloon pump beats to native cardiac beats, with 1:1 being the maximum pump benefit. As the pump frequency ratio is dropped from 1:1 to 1:2 to 1:4 or less, the inotropic requirements of the patient will often increase.[8] Anticoagulation with heparin is used to prevent thrombus formation during IABP therapy. Target activated partial thromboplastin time (aPTT) is 1.5 to 2 times the normal value.[8] The IABP must never be turned off completely owing to the risk of thrombus formation.[7]

Hypotension: Patients in cardiogenic shock require careful monitoring and hemodynamic fluctuations are to be expected; however, special considerations must be investigated in a patient with an IABP who experiences sudden, severe hemodynamic deterioration. Improper device timing may cause hemodynamic compromise and increased myocardial work, as the native ventricle will have difficulty ejecting against an increased afterload caused by the inflated balloon. Bedside echocardiography or fluoroscopy can be utilized to determine balloon desynchronization, and expert consultation should be sought if this scenario is considered. Complete device failure may occur secondary to power failure or an interruption of ECG or arterial waveform monitoring. ECG and/or arterial monitoring should be immediately re-established and power failure corrected. The IABP console has a battery pack for patient transport; however, when stationary, the device should remain attached to a standard electric power source. Finally, device migration can cause hemodynamic compromise if the balloon migrates into the aortic arch. IABP inflation in the arch may impair perfusion of the great vessels and coronary arteries by direct vascular occlusion from the balloon. If malpositioning is suspected, a portable chest X-ray in the PACU can confirm location of the proximal tip of the balloon.

Other considerations: Major contraindications to placement of an IABP include: pre-existing aortic regurgitation, which will worsen during diastolic balloon inflation; severe vascular disease, owing to risk of balloon inflation dislodging atherosclerotic plaque; or sepsis, which will risk bacterial contamination of the implantable device.

Chest compressions can be safely performed in patients with an IABP; however, in this situation, the device should be turned off to ensure that incorrect device timing will not impede blood flow.

Once the IABP is removed, it is important to closely monitor the ipsilateral lower extremity for signs of vascular compromise. The most common complications associated with IABP are vascular in nature, with a reported incidence of 6% to 33%.[9]

Pacemakers

There are approximately 225,000 new pacemakers implanted annually in the United States and nearly 3 million patients are currently living with a pacemaker.[10] Indications for permanent pacemaker insertion include symptomatic brady-arrhythmias, Mobitz type II or greater heart block, sinoatrial node dysfunction, ventricular tachycardia, certain supraventricular tachycardias, cardiomyopathies, and long QT syndrome.[11] In the perioperative and PACU setting, attention must be paid to the patient's native or underlying cardiac rhythm, current medications, and pacemaker settings.

Pacemaker function: Pacemakers are coded by five letters that describe their function. The first letter refers to the chamber paced, second to the chamber sensed, and third to the sensed event. The last two letters refer to the device's programmability and the anti-tachycardia function. In the first two letter positions, "A" indicates atria, "V" indicates ventricle, and "D" indicates dual, implying both the atria and ventricle are paced or sensed. "O" indicates that nothing is sensed. For the third letter position, "I" represents an inhibition, "T" represents a trigger, and "D" indicates dual, when both triggering and inhibition occur, such as the atrium is triggered and the ventricle is inhibited. "O" in this position represents no sensed event. In the fourth position an "R" indicates a change in rate associated with exercise. "O" in this position represents no programmed rate response. A letter in the fifth position indicates anti-bradycardia and anti-tachycardia pacing capabilities. "P" in this letter position indicates anti-tachycardia pacing, "S" indicates shock, "D" represents dual anti-tachycardia pacing and shocking functions. "O" signifies no anti-tachycardia pacing or shocking functions are present.[12]

Special considerations for perioperative management include pacemaker reprogramming or placing the device in an asynchronous mode. In general, these changes are made to avoid intermittent inhibition via electromagnetic interference caused by electrosurgical cautery, or inappropriate delivery of a defibrillation or cardioversion shock. Communication of perioperative device manipulation between the intraoperative and PACU provider is paramount. If a pacemaker has been reprogrammed, or a magnet placed to convert to an asynchronous mode, device interrogation in the PACU may be necessary to restore preoperative pacemaker settings and ensure device integrity.

Magnet application to pacemaker: Most current pacemakers respond to magnet application in a single or dual chamber asynchronous pacing mode. This asynchronous mode is device-specific for each manufacturer. Medtronic pacemakers will pace at 85 beats/min (bpm) in AOO or DOO mode. Guidant pacemakers will pace at a rate of 100 bpm, and St. Jude devices will pace at 98.6 bpm.[12] Additionally, magnet application will disable intrinsic cardioversion and defibrillation capabilities. External cardioversion and defibrillation equipment must be immediately available. Oftentimes defibrillation pads are placed on the patient intraoperatively and should remain on the patient in the PACU until device interrogation is complete and normal function is restored.

Generator malfunction: In the event of generator failure, immediate expert consultation should be sought. As a temporizing measure, a magnet may be placed over the malfunctioning device to initiate an asynchronous mode and disable cardioversion and defibrillation therapy. Alternative modalities for temporary pacing should be utilized, such as transcutaneous, transesophageal, or transvenous pacing.[12,13] A pacing pulmonary artery catheter can also be considered. Intravenous chronotropic drugs such as isoproterenol, ephedrine, or epinephrine should be available.

External cardioversion or defibrillation: External shock will cause temporary inhibition of an implanted device and occasionally permanent malfunction. Special consideration of the proximity of the external paddles to the pulse generator should be taken to avoid pulse generator damage. It is recommended by device manufacturers to utilize an anterior–posterior configuration with the paddles or pads at least 10 cm from the pulse generator. Additionally, it is advised to use the lowest amount of energy possible for external cardioversion or defibrillation. All devices should be interrogated by a cardiologist following defibrillation from an external power source for signs of malfunction or pacemaker failure, as reprogramming or even replacement of the device may be necessary.[14]

References

1. G.C. Stewart, L.W. Stevenson. Controversies in cardiovascular medicine: keeping left ventricular device acceleration on track. *Circulation* 2011; 123:1559–1568.

2. M.S. Slaughter, F.D. Pagani, J.G. Rogers, *et al.* Clinical management of continuous-flow left ventricular assist devices in advanced heart failure. *J Heart Lung Transplant* 2010; 29:S1–S39.

3. M.S. Slaughter, J.G. Rogers, C.A. Milano, *et al.* Advanced heart failure treated with continuous-flow left ventricular assist device. *N Engl J Med* 2009; 361:2241–2251.

4. *Heartmate II LVAS Left Ventricular Assist System Operating Manual.* Pleasanton, CA: Thoratec, 2010. pp. 1–263.

5. J.D. Estep, R.F. Stainback, S.H. Little, G. Torre, W.A. Zoghbi. The role of echocardiography and other imaging modalities in patients with left ventricular assist devices *JACC Cardiovasc Imaging* 2010; 3:1049–1064.

6. S. Crow, D. Chen, C. Milano, *et al.* Acquired von Willebrand syndrome in continuous-flow ventricular assist device recipients. *Ann Thorac Surg* 2010; 90:1263–1269.

7. J. Kaplan, D.L. Reich, J.S. Savino. *Kaplan's Cardiac Anesthesia.* 6th edition. 2011. pp. 1034–1039.

8. J. Ferguson, M. Cohen, R.J. Freedman Jr., *et al.* The current practice of intra-aortic balloon counterpulsation: results from the Benchmark Registry. *J Am Coll Cardiol* 2001; 38:1456–1462.

9. U. Melhorn, A. Kröner, E.R. de Vivi. 30 years of clinical intra-aortic balloon pumping: facts and figures. *Thorac Cardiovasc Surg* 1999; 47:298–303.

10. A.J. Greenspon, J.D. Patel, E. Lau, *et al.* Trends in permanent pacemaker implantation in the United States from 1993 to 2009. Increasing complexity of patients and procedures. *J Am Coll Cardiol* 2012; 60:1540–1545.

11. C.M. Tracy, A.E. Epstein, D. Darbar *et al.* 2012 ACCF/AHA/HRS focused update of the 2008 Guidelines for Device-Based Therapy of Cardiac Rhythm Abnormalities: a report of the American College of Cardiology Foundation/American Heart Association Task Force on Practice Guidelines. *J Am Coll Cardiol* 2012; 60:1297–1313.

12. J. Kaplan, *et al. Kaplan's Cardiac Anesthesia.* 5th edition. 2006. pp. 790–806.

13. K.R. Stone, C.A. McPherson. Assessment and management of patients with pacemakers and implantable cardioverter defibrillators. *Crit Care Med* 2004; 32: S155–S165.

14. J.L. Appfelbaum, P. Belott, R.T. Connis, *et al.* for the American Society of Anesthesiologists Committee on Standards and Practice Parameters. American Society of Anesthesiology practice advisory for the perioperative management of patients with rhythm management devices: pacemakers and implantable cardioverter-defibrillators. *Anesthesiology* 2011; 114:247–261.

Chapter

Special considerations
for the morbidly obese patient

47

Emily J. MacKay and Michele Mele

- Obesity is associated with multiple co-morbidities, affecting cardiopulmonary, endocrine, gastrointestinal, and vascular systems.
- Obesity in combination with perioperative opioid administration predisposes to pulmonary complications in the Post-Anesthesia Care Unit (PACU) such as obesity hypoventilation, hypoxia, hypercarbia, and apnea.
- Obesity may complicate airway management.
- Opioid-sparing multimodal analgesia is recommended for obese surgical patients.

The prevalence of obesity is increasing to epidemic proportions. It currently affects 1.7 billion people worldwide[1] and 78 million (34.9%) in the United States.[2] Overweight is defined as having a body mass index (BMI) 25.0–29.9 kg/m^2; obese, BMI 30.0–34.9 kg/m^2; and morbidly obese, BMI>35.0 kg/m^2.[1] Obesity is the second leading cause of death in the United States with "poor diet and physical inactivity" contributing to 400,000 deaths, 16.6% of all deaths in the United States (2000).[3] As obesity becomes an ever more frequent co-morbidity among surgical patients, an understanding of the physiological implications of obesity is crucial for anticipating and minimizing perioperative complications (Figure 47.1).

Obesity affects every organ system. Cardiovascular diseases include coronary artery disease, sudden cardiac death, obesity-related cardiomyopathy, hypertension, hyperlipidemia, and right-sided heart failure (cor pulmonale).[4,5] Pulmonary diseases include restrictive lung disease, obstructive sleep apnea (OSA), obesity hypoventilation syndrome (OHS)[5] and decreased residual lung volume.[4] Gastrointestinal diseases include hiatal hernia[4,5] and gastro esophageal reflux (GERD).[5] The most common endocrine disease is diabetes mellitus type II (DMII).[4] Musculoskeletal diseases include osteoarthritis of the weight-bearing joints and chronic back pain.[4,5] (See Table 47.1.) An increased incidence of postoperative complications detectable among obese surgical patients compared with lean controls includes myocardial infarction, peripheral nerve injury, wound infection, and urinary tract infection.[5] An increased incidence of difficult airway management in the perioperative period is controversial, with conflicting data in the medical literature.[5,6]

Post-Anesthesia Care: Symptoms, Diagnosis, and Management, ed. James W. Heitz. Published by Cambridge University Press. © Cambridge University Press 2016.

Table 47.1 Co-morbidities associated with obesity associated with postoperative complications

Organ system	Disease	Potential postoperative complications
Cardiovascular	• Coronary artery disease • Sudden cardiac death • Cardiomyopathy • Hypertension • Hyperlipidemia • Cor pulmonale	• Myocardial infarction • Arrhythmia • Hypertension • Urgency/Emergency
Pulmonary	• Restrictive lung disease • OSA • OHS • Decreased residual lung volume	• Hypoxemia • Hypercapnia • Apnea
Gastrointestinal	• GERD • Hiatal hernia	• If emergent intubation required: aspiration risk
Endocrine	• DMII	• Hyperosmolar hyperglycemic non-ketotic coma • Hypoglycemia • "Silent" myocardial infarction
Musculoskeletal	• High body mass index	• If emergent intubation needed: potential difficult airway

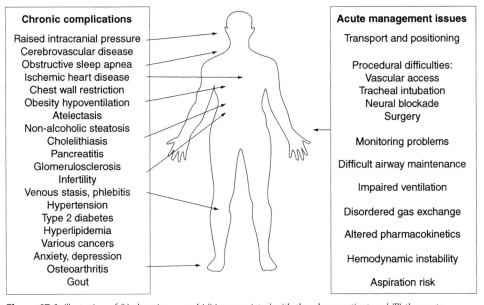

Chronic complications	Acute management issues
Raised intracranial pressure Cerebrovascular disease Obstructive sleep apnea Ischemic heart disease Chest wall restriction Obesity hypoventilation Atelectasis Non-alcoholic steatosis Cholelithiasis Pancreatitis Glomerulosclerosis Infertility Venous stasis, phlebitis Hypertension Type 2 diabetes Hyperlipidemia Various cancers Anxiety, depression Osteoarthritis Gout	Transport and positioning Procedural difficulties: Vascular access Tracheal intubation Neural blockade Surgery Monitoring problems Difficult airway maintenance Impaired ventilation Disordered gas exchange Altered pharmacokinetics Hemodynamic instability Aspiration risk

Figure 47.1 Illustration of (L) chronic co-morbidities associated with the obese patient and (R) the acute perioperative concerns important to the anesthetic management of the obese patient.
Adapted from: A. Malhotra, D. Hillman. *Thorax* 2008; **63:**925–931.[9] *Used with permission.*

Pulmonary complications

Obstructive sleep apnea: The prevalence of OSA is 5% among morbidly obese patients.[7] The incidence of OSA is 12 to 30-fold higher than in the general population.[8] OSA is defined as frequent episodes of apnea or hypopnea during sleep (apnea being greater than 10 seconds of cessation of airflow despite continuous effort against a closed glottis).[9] OSA may be associated with daytime somnolence and snoring, but definitive diagnosis can only be made by an overnight sleep study.[9] The morbidly obese patient is at risk for OSA owing to the anatomical and physiological changes associated with obesity: BMI >30 kg/m^2, collar size >16.5 inches, and increased soft tissue surrounding the trachea.[8] OSA causes physiological changes such as hypoxemia and hypercapnia as well as pulmonary and systemic vasoconstriction leading to subsequent development of pulmonary and systemic hypertension.[5] The presence of OSA for patients undergoing total hip and knee arthroplasty increases the incidence of airway and pulmonary complications requiring Intensive Care Unit (ICU) admission and the length of inpatient hospitalization.[10]

Obesity hypoventilation syndrome: OHS is similar to but distinct from OSA. While the OSA patient is only hypercapneic while asleep, the OHS patient is hypercapneic at rest and while awake. OHS is defined as episodes of apnea without respiratory effort or "central apnea."[5] The pathogenesis of obesity hypoventilation remains unclear but it is accepted that these patients have a decrease in central nervous system control of respiratory drive from hypercapnia and have an increasing reliance on hypoxemia as respiratory drive.[5,11] The hallmark used to differentiate OHS from OSA is the *lack* of respiratory effort against a closed glottis seen during periods of apnea in the OSA patient. The patient with OHS will desaturate, become hypoxic, and will have no physiological respiratory drive to mitigate the effect. A severe form of OHS is "Pickwickian syndrome," characterized by obesity, hypersomnolence, hypoxia, hypercapnia, right ventricular failure, and polycythemia.[5,12]

The obese patient has impaired gas exchange secondary to mass loading on the thorax and abdomen. Implications of the excess mass means a significant reduction in functional residual capacity (FRC), expiratory reserve volume (ERV), and total lung capacity (TLC).[5] FRC decreases exponentially with increasing BMI. A decreased FRC leads to significant pulmonary complications such as ventilation–perfusion mismatch, right-to-left shunting, and arterial hypoxemia.[5] Anesthesia compounds the insufficiency. Data shows the FRC to be reduced by 20% in the non-anesthetized obese patient, and further reduced by 50% in the anesthetized patient.[13]

The obese patient is at risk for gas exchange abnormalities. The supine position of the obese patient under anesthesia leads to additional anatomical complications; increased work of breathing, increased carbon dioxide production, decreased compliance, and increased lung resistance.[5]

The post-anesthesia obese patient is potentially at risk for one or more of the above complications. Clinical guidelines have been developed for the obese patient with OSA:[5,13]

1. Identify OSA early;
2. Use continuous positive airway pressure (CPAP) postoperatively;
3. Anesthetic of choice is regional;
4. Judicious reversal of neuromuscular blockade;
5. Awake tracheal extubation following general anesthesia (if difficult airway);
6. Lateral positioning preferred over supine positioning, and extended and close monitoring in the postoperative period.[5,9]

Guidelines for the obese patient with OHS have not been developed, and the clinician must rely heavily on clinical judgment. Special attention to analgesia is prudent for patients with both obesity and OHS as increased sensitivity to opioid medications may have a profound impact upon ventilation.

After general anesthesia, to mitigate pulmonary complications in the morbidly obese patient, the following recommendations can be made:[4,5]

1. Always transport the patient sitting up at a 45-degree angle with oxygen.
2. Once in the PACU, respiratory rate and oxygen saturation should be monitored vigilantly, and opioid medication should be administered cautiously.[4,5]
3. Appropriate communication when transferring care to a PACU nurse or anesthesiologist should include documentation and communication of reversal of neuromuscular blockade; neostigmine/glycopyrrolate dosing and response.
4. Morbidly obese patients with significant co-morbid cardiopulmonary disease could potentially benefit from prolonged mechanical ventilation.[5]

Cardiovascular complications

Obesity is a risk factor for cardiovascular disease including ischemic heart disease, cardiac dysrhythmias, hypertension, hyperlipidemia, and obesity-induced cardiomyopathy (related to the interrelationship between OSA, with or without pulmonary and/or systemic hypertension). Pulmonary arterial hypertension from OSA may lead to right ventricular hypertrophy. Pulmonary venous hypertension and systemic hypertension may lead to left ventricular hypertrophy.[5,14] The risk of postoperative cardiac ischemia or myocardial infarction is increased in the obese patient.[6]

There is significant interrelationship of cardiovascular disease and pulmonary disease. Therefore, the clinician should have an elevated index of suspicion of myocardial ischemia in the obese patient with or without OSA, OHS, or parenchymal lung disease. An effort to reduce myocardial demand by decreasing heart rate, avoiding tachycardia, and decreasing systemic hypertension will aid in reducing the morbidly obese patient's risk of an ischemic event following anesthesia.

Endocrine complications

Obesity itself is a risk factor for DMII. One study reported the incidence of diabetes at 20% in the morbidly obese.[15] Postoperative management of the diabetic patient begins with a full understanding of the extent of end-organ disease (cardiovascular, renal, nervous system, immune). Attentive postoperative care of the diabetic patient is important to avoid life-threatening complications including diabetic ketoacidosis (DKA) and hyperglycemic hyperosmolar non-ketotic (HHNK) state. In addition, diabetic patients are prone to subclinical coronary artery disease which may be associated with silent ischemia postoperatively owing to cardiac denervation. It is also well understood that diabetic patients have abnormal granulocyte function. Consequently, poorly controlled glucose levels will increase the risk of postoperative wound infection.[6] The management of perioperative and postoperative insulin requirements and level of ideal glucose control is a topic of great controversy. The catabolic effect of surgery may require administration of postoperative insulin.[5] Regular (short-acting) insulin is preferred because of its rapid onset and ease of titration with the rapidly changing metabolic requirements in the immediate postoperative period.

Intravenous is the ideal route of administration since the subcutaneous route has unpredictable absorption, especially in a hypothermic patient.

Thromboembolic disease

Obesity is considered one of the risk factors for development of deep vein thrombosis (DVT). In the obese patient, the risk of a DVT is twice that of a normal weight patient: 48% incidence in obese patients vs. 23% in normal weight patients in an orthopedic population studied.[10] Obese patients possess risk factors for acquiring a DVT and/or pulmonary embolism (PE) postoperatively: higher incidence of previous DVT/PE, poor ambulation, and inadequate lower extremity circulation (lymph edema, varices). The increased risk of DVT/PE may be due to increased pressure in the lower limbs, prolonged immobility, increased fibrinogen concentration (coagulation in the setting of endothelial injury), and decreased antithrombin III levels. While there is no universally accepted DVT/PE prophylaxis regimen, early ambulation, pneumatic compression devices, and subcutaneous heparin administration are the most commonly used and effective interventions in preventing the complication of thromboembolic disease. Judicious compliance with the prophylaxis regimen chosen, a high index of suspicion for DVT, and increased vigilance in the immediate postoperative period are critical in order to prevent this dangerous morbidity.

Difficult airway

Obese patients appear to be at increased risk of difficult mask ventilation and intubation, and hypoxemia during tracheal intubation, but the literature regarding airway management of the obese patient is conflicting.[5,6] Because of the potential for an airway emergency in the PACU, awareness of the high likelihood of a difficult airway in the obese patient is critical. Control of the airway is potentially hindered by reduced neck mobility and altered oropharyngeal anatomy.[16] Pharyngeal space is narrowed owing to soft tissues, and there is often a higher Mallampati airway evaluation score.[4] A morbidly obese patient should be considered a difficult airway until proven otherwise and treated accordingly throughout the perioperative period. Clinicians skilled in the management of the difficult airways and emergency airway equipment must be immediately available. A recent retrospective study concluded that more than half of hypoxic episodes occur more than 30 minutes after arrival to the PACU, so continuous attention to the special needs of the obese patient in the early postoperative period is required.[17]

Monitoring

Watchful and alert postoperative monitoring of the obese patient is critical. Basic PACU monitoring should include oxygen saturation, blood pressure, electrocardiogram (ECG), and respiratory rate. Because of the anatomical changes associated with obesity, postoperative monitoring of the obese patient can be challenging. Obesity can be associated with a wide variety of ECG changes including leftward shift in P wave, QRS, and T wave axes, and low voltage QRS. In addition, measuring blood pressure in the obese patient using non-invasive monitoring techniques can often be inaccurate. An inappropriately fitted blood pressure cuff owing to a conical-shaped upper arm is often the major limitation. Obtaining a more accurate blood pressure reading can be achieved by using a standard size cuff applied to the forearm 13 cm below the elbow.[18]

Patient positioning

There is limited literature to conclusively determine the ideal positioning of obese patients in the postoperative period. Improved Apnea Hypopnea Index Scores are seen when adult patients with OSA are in lateral or sitting positions. Current recommendations suggest the supine position should be avoided if there is clinical evidence of OSA.

Oxygenation

Supplemental oxygen should be administered to patients in the PACU until they are able to maintain their baseline oxygen saturation on room air. Patients with OSA who have been using CPAP devices prior to surgery should continue CPAP use in the immediate post-operative period unless contraindicated. Currently, there is insufficient literature to support instituting the use of CPAP in patients who were not using this modality prior to surgery.

Drug dosing

Drug dosing in the obese patient is the subject of conflicting data in the literature. Pharmacokinetic parameters such as volume of distribution (V_d), clearance (Cl), and protein binding may be different for certain drugs in the obese patient. The adult dosing recommendations from drug manufacturers are often weight-based. Because of this, how to scale drug dosing in the obese patient can be challenging. Most authors suggest administration of drugs commonly used by anesthesiologists (propofol, fentanyl, neuromuscular blockers, benzodiazepines) can be dosed either on ideal body weight or actual body weight. Dosing should be decreased in drugs that have a narrow therapeutic index (digoxin), as the risk of toxicity is increased in obese patients.[5,19] V_d is increased in obese patients for highly lipid-soluble drugs and will require increased dose (volatile anesthetics and benzodiazepines).[19] Interestingly, propofol, although highly lipid soluble, does not require an increased dose and can even be dosed effectively at ideal body weight.[5,8] Phase I elimination (oxidation, reduction, and hydrolysis) is unchanged in the obese. Phase II reactions are consistently increased in the obese patient because of increased plasma volume and subsequent increased glomerular filtration rate.[5,8]

Postoperative analgesia

The American Society of Anesthesiologists (ASA) Practice Guidelines recommend regional anesthesia as the anesthetic of choice for obese patients at risk for the aforementioned pulmonary complications.[20] Regional anesthesia greatly reduces the need for systemic opioids, reducing the risk of pulmonary suppression. If patient-controlled systemic opioids are required, background basal infusions should be avoided if possible. Multimodal pain control including non-steroidal anti-inflammatory drugs (NSAIDs), acetaminophen, and ketamine should be considered when acceptable, owing to their opioid-sparing effects.

PACU discharge criteria

Standardized outpatient discharge criteria can be followed for obese patients without a preoperative diagnosis of OSA.[20] However, for obese patients with known OSA it is recommended that in addition to standard outpatient discharge criteria, room air saturation should return to baseline with no episodes of hypoxemia or airway obstruction in the

PACU. ASA clinical practice guidelines recommend patients with OSA should be monitored for 3 hours longer than non-OSA patients before being discharged from the PACU.[20]

Postoperative care of the morbidly obese patient differs from the protocol for persons within a normal weight range. Best practice requires not only attention to the documented past medical conditions of the patient, but also awareness of the physiological and anatomical changes resulting from excess weight. Timely diagnosis and intervention is crucial in assuring optimum patient outcomes.

References

1. M. Deitel. Overweight and obesity worldwide now estimated to involve 1.7 billion people. *Obesity Surg* 2003; 13:329–330.

2. C.L. Ogden, M.D. Carroll, B.K. Kit, K.M. Flegal. Prevalence of childhood and adult obesity in the United States, 2011–2012. *JAMA* 2014; 311(8):806–814.

3. A.H. Mokdad, J.S. Marks, D.F. Stroup, J.L. Gerberding. Actual causes of death in the United States, 2000. *JAMA* 2004; 291(10):1238–1245.

4. J.P. Adams, P.G. Murphy. Obesity in anaesthesia and intensive care. *Br J Anaesth* 2000; 85:91–108.

5. O.A. Bamgbade, T.W. Rutter, O.O. Nafiu, P. Dorje. Postoperative complications in the obese and nonobese patients. *World J Surg* 2007; 31:556–560.

6. H.C. Hemmings, P.M. Hopkins, P.G. Murphy. Obesity. In *Foundations of Anaesthesia. Basic and Clinical Sciences.* London: Mosby. 2000:703–711.

7. T. Young, M. Palta, J. Dempsey, *et al.* The occurrence of sleep-disordered breathing among middle-aged adults. *N Engl J Med* 1993; 328:1230–1235.

8. J. Peiser, P. Lavie, A. Ovnat, I. Charuzi. Sleep apnea syndrome in the morbidly obese as an indication for weight reduction surgery. *Ann Surg* 1984; 199(1):112–115.

9. A. Malhotra, D. Hillman. Obesity and the lung: 3. Obesity, respiration, and intensive care. *Thorax* 2008; 63(10):925–931.

10. R.M. Gupta, J. Parvizi, A.D. Hanssen, P.C. Gay. Postoperative complications in patients with obstructive sleep apnea syndrome undergoing hip or knee replacement: a case-control study. *Mayo Clin Proc* 2001; 76(9):897–905.

11. C.W. Zwillich, F.D. Sutton, D.J. Pierson, *et al.* Decreased hypoxic ventilator drive in the obesity-hypoventilation syndrome. *Am J Med* 1975; 59(3):343–348.

12. C.S. Burwell, E.D. Robin, R.D. Whaley, *et al.* Extreme obesity associated with alveolar hypoventilation – A Pickwickian syndrome. *Am J Med* 1956; 21(5):811–818.

13. G. Damia, D. Mascheroni, M. Croci, L. Tarenzi. Perioperative changes in functional residual capacity in morbidly obese patients. *Br J Anaesth* 1988; 60(5):574–578.

14. K. Usui, J.D. Parker, G.E. Newton, *et al.* Adaptations to obstructive sleep apnea in dilated cardiomyopathy. *Am J Respir Crit Care Med* 2006; 173(100):1170–1175.

15. W.J. Pories, J.F. Caro, E.G. Flickinger, H.D. Meelheim, M.S. Swanson. The control of diabetes mellitus (NIDDM) in the morbidly obese with the Greenville gastric bypass. *Ann Surg* 1987; 206(3):316–323.

16. J.B. Brodsky, H.J. Lemmens, J.G. Brock-Utne, M. Vierra, L.J. Saidman. Morbid obesity and tracheal intubation. *Anesth Analg* 2002; 94(3):732–736.

17. R.H. Epstein, F. Dexter, M.G. Lopez, J.M. Ehrenfeld. Anesthesiologist staffing considerations consequent to the temporal distribution of hypoxemic episodes in the postanesthesia care unit. *Anesth Analg* 2014; 119(6):1322–1333.

18. S.A. Nasraway, T.M. Hudson-Jinks, R.M. Keller. Multidisciplinary care of the obese patient with chronic critical illness after surgery. *Crit Care Clin* 2002; 18(3):643–657.

19. L.E.D. Baerdemaeker, E.P. Mortier, M.M.R.F. Struys. Pharmacokinetics in obese patients. *Contin Educ Anaesth Crit Care Pain* 2004; 4(5):152–155.

20. Practice guidelines for the perioperative management of patients with obstructive sleep apnea: a report by the American Society of Anesthesiologists Task Force on Perioperative Management of Patients with Obstructive Sleep Apnea. *Anesthesiology* 2006; 104(5):1081–1093.

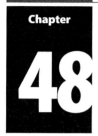

Chapter

48

Special considerations for the renal failure patient

Eric S. Schwenk

- High-risk patients and those undergoing high-risk surgery should be counseled on the possibility of postoperative renal failure as mortality rates are high.
- Renal failure may be classified as prerenal, intrinsic renal, and postrenal, and these categories can aid in diagnosis.
- Patients who have chronic renal failure on dialysis introduce special considerations, such as electrolyte disturbances, anemia, and excretion of drugs.

Acute kidney injury

Definition and epidemiology of AKI: Acute renal failure, or acute kidney injury (AKI), occurs in approximately 1% of surgical patients, although this number is substantially higher in high-risk populations.[1] The mortality rate for perioperative AKI may be as high as 50%,[2] making its diagnosis and treatment important for anyone involved in care of surgical patients in the Post-Anesthesia Care Unit (PACU). The definition of AKI is not uniform throughout the literature; however, the Acute Kidney Injury Network in 2007 defined AKI as an abrupt (within 48 hours) absolute increase in serum creatinine of greater than or equal to 0.3 mg/dl, a 50% or greater increase in serum creatinine, or oliguria of less than 0.5 ml/kg for more than 6 hours.[3] In the PACU environment, patients are typically discharged after a few hours at most, so the 6-hour definition may not apply in this specific patient population. Patients who are oliguric in the PACU for several hours, particularly those who have risk factors or those who underwent high-risk surgery, should be managed aggressively in an attempt to prevent worsening of their renal function.

Risk factors for perioperative AKI: Although there is not a consensus of what constitutes the risk factors for perioperative AKI, several have been suggested. One review of the literature found that preoperative increased serum creatinine, blood urea nitrogen (BUN), or renal dysfunction predicted postoperative renal failure the best of any factors studied, while advanced age, pre-existing congestive heart failure (CHF), bacterial endocarditis, decreased serum albumin, malignancy, gout, vascular disease, elevated serum bilirubin, and prior cardiac surgery were weakly associated with postoperative AKI.[4] The type of surgery also influences the risk, with cardiac, vascular

Post-Anesthesia Care: Symptoms, Diagnosis, and Management, ed. James W. Heitz. Published by Cambridge University Press. © Cambridge University Press 2016.

(especially abdominal aortic aneurysm repair), and liver transplantation having the highest incidence of postoperative AKI.[2]

Classification of AKI: AKI is traditionally divided into prerenal, intrinsic renal, and postrenal causes. In the PACU setting, postrenal causes usually involve obstruction of the ureters, bladder, or urethra, either mechanically or pharmacologically via decreased bladder tone. Certain surgical procedures, such as urological or gynecological, would obviously make a postrenal etiology more likely. Surgical injury to the genitourinary tract, renal stones, and benign prostatic hypertrophy are common mechanical causes, while bladder dysfunction can result from medications such as cholinergic antagonists or opioids. A bladder scan, which is a non-invasive method of detecting bladder volume, can suggest bladder dysfunction as the cause of postrenal failure. Alternatively, a Foley catheter or straight catheter may be placed (if it is not already in place) to look for the presence of retained urine. In patients with a Foley catheter already in place, the catheter should be checked for patency and flushed, if necessary, to ensure proper position. Postrenal causes can frequently be detected by one of these simple maneuvers, and in most cases a postrenal source of oliguria should be ruled out first because it is quick and easy to do so.

Prerenal causes, namely renal hypoperfusion, may represent 90% of perioperative AKI,[1] although it is not clear at what point prolonged hypoperfusion causes acute tubular necrosis (ATN), which may be the underlying pathology in many cases of perioperative AKI.[2] Prerenal AKI is due to decreased renal perfusion, usually through hypotension, hypovolemia, decreased cardiac output, renal artery stenosis, or sepsis. Oliguric patients in the PACU who experienced prolonged intraoperative hypotension or significant surgical blood loss should be aggressively managed with crystalloids, red blood cells, and, if needed, inotropes and vasopressors to maintain adequate renal perfusion and prevent the development of permanent kidney damage. Indeed, optimization of hemodynamics, especially blood pressure, in the perioperative period has been found to decrease both postoperative AKI and mortality.[5] Patients in the PACU commonly develop oliguria, and a simple initial therapy involves the administration of a fluid challenge. Unless an obvious source of renal insult exists (a large dose of a nephrotoxin or a urethral obstruction, for example), the practitioner is left with an uncertain etiology, and a fluid challenge offers little downside in the large majority of patients. An increase in urine production following fluid administration suggests hypovolemia as the problem, while a lack of a response may prompt one to consider other causes, such as cardiac failure, sepsis, or intrinsic renal pathology. A BUN:creatinine ratio >20 suggests a prerenal cause, as does a fractional excretion of sodium (FENa) of <1%.[6] Some patients may require multiple fluid boluses to establish urine output; however, be wary of the patient who does not respond after significant fluid administration as another cause may be likely.

The third type of renal failure seen in the PACU is that involving intrinsic renal injury. Common sources of such injury include medications (aminoglycosides, angiotensin-converting enzyme [ACE] inhibitors, vancomycin, non-steroidal anti-inflammatory drugs [NSAIDs], intravenous contrast dye), endotoxin, myoglobin, and prolonged ischemia.[1] AKI due to prerenal causes, such as hypotension, can progress to ATN if not corrected. If one suspects an intrinsic renal problem, consultation with a nephrologist is recommended, as prompt treatment is mandatory.

Chronic renal failure

Patients with chronic renal failure (CRF) frequently undergo surgical procedures, and as a result those involved in PACU care are faced with the challenge of caring for them. The following discussion will focus on patients with end stage renal disease (ESRD) on dialysis. Overall, the increase in mortality in patients with ESRD who undergo general surgery is greater than 4%, significantly higher than that of patients with normal renal function.[7,8] During the handoff from the intraoperative to the postoperative period, the timing of the last dialysis session and the frequency of dialysis should be mentioned. A CRF patient who was dialyzed several days ago can present very differently from one who received dialysis several hours prior to surgery. The patient's current weight and dry weight (if known) should be discussed, as this is often a good indicator of his or her fluid status. A plan for fluid management in the PACU should be made and the choice of fluid should also be determined, although the commonly held belief that lactated Ringer's solution (which contains a small amount of potassium) should be replaced with normal saline in ESRD patients is unfounded.[9]

Electrolyte abnormalities: Patients with ESRD exhibit multiple electrolyte abnormalities, the most important of which for the practitioner in the PACU is hyperkalemia. Patients with CRF are at greater risk for hyperkalemia due to both decreased excretion and increases from multiple sources, such as blood products, medications, and a shift of potassium from the intra- to the extracellular compartment that follows acidosis.[7] It is the most frequent cause of perioperative morbidity in patients with ESRD.[7] Of primary concern to those providing care in the PACU are possible electrocardiogram (ECG) changes that can occur with hyperkalemia. At potassium levels of 5.5 to 7.0 mmol/l, tall, peaked, narrow T waves are observed, along with fascicular block.[10] This can progress to ST segment depression and eventually sinus arrest. Any ESRD patient with these changes observed on the PACU monitor should have a 12-lead ECG performed and a serum.

The chronicity of the patient's hyperkalemia and his or her baseline potassium level can also play a role in guiding the decision to treat or not. A patient with baseline potassium of 5.0 mmol/l, for example, may tolerate the increase to 6.0 mmol/l better than a patient with baseline potassium of 4.0 mmol/l. Treatment of acute hyperkalemia in the PACU involves administering calcium carbonate or calcium gluconate to stabilize cardiac membranes and prevent lethal arrhythmias, followed by insulin with glucose to shift potassium from the extracellular compartment to the intracellular compartment. A recent review concluded that insulin, at a dose of 10 to 20 units, effectively decreases serum potassium levels 0.5 to 1.0 mmol/l faster than albuterol for a period of about 2 hours.[11] It must be given with glucose to prevent hypoglycemia.

Nebulized albuterol and other β_2 agonists are another effective treatment of hyperkalemia. However, they may take up to 30 minutes to take effect, making them less desirable in the PACU setting.[11]

Sodium bicarbonate, advocated by some for hyperkalemia treatment, has not been shown to be as effective as insulin and β_2 agonists for the acute setting.[11]

Postoperative bleeding and anemia: For multiple reasons, patients with CRF are more likely to bleed postoperatively than patients with normal renal function. First, CRF patients have a qualitative platelet dysfunction that impairs the platelet–platelet and platelet–vessel wall interactions, creating a propensity to bleed.[12] The dysfunction is not typically severe enough to cause spontaneous bleeding but with the insult of surgery can certainly make existing bleeding more significant. Second, CRF patients often have co-morbidities, such as atrial fibrillation, coronary artery disease, and valvular disorders, that require anticoagulation. A large, prospective cohort study found that the incidence of atrial fibrillation in patients with mild to moderate renal failure was 20%, which is three times the incidence in the general population, and 25% in those patients age 70 or greater.[13] Consequently, many CRF patients take warfarin, or various other medications that affect coagulation. One needs a high index of suspicion for bleeding in the PACU as a possible cause of postoperative hypotension in a patient with ESRD, especially in abdominal, thoracic, or orthopedic surgery where the bleeding may not be obvious.

ESRD patients on dialysis are frequently anemic because of the inability of the failing kidney to effectively produce erythropoietin. This decreases aerobic capacity and quality of life and could worsen myocardial dysfunction in certain patients.[14] As a result, surgical blood loss that would ordinarily not be problematic in normal patients can compromise oxygen delivery to the tissues or necessitate blood transfusion.

Renal excretion of drugs

Many frequently administered medications in the perioperative setting are primarily excreted by the kidneys. As one of the most commonly given analgesics in the perioperative period, morphine deserves special consideration. Morphine is a μ-opioid agonist used for moderate to severe pain with a slow onset, half-life of 2 hours, and duration of 4 to 5 hours.[15] It is metabolized by the liver into morphine-6-glucuronide and morphine-3-glucuronide, with the former possessing significant analgesic properties.[16] Because these metabolites are renally excreted, their levels can build up significantly in patients with CRF, potentially leading to prolonged respiratory depression and unwanted side effects, such as sedation, pruritus, and nausea and vomiting.[16,17] Other renally metabolized opioids to avoid in the PACU setting in ESRD patients include codeine[18] and meperidine.[19]

The aminosteroid neuromuscular blockers (NMBs) represent another class of commonly encountered medications that can be affected by CRF. Significant renal disease may delay clearance of vecuronium and rocuronium, two of the most commonly used NMBs.[20] Residual neuromuscular blockade should be considered in the differential diagnosis of any CRF patient in the PACU with respiratory distress, hypoxia, or weakness. In addition, anticholinesterase drugs, such as neostigmine and edrophonium, are also prolonged by renal failure, often as much as or more than the NMBs,[20] so prominent cholinergic effects may present, including bradycardia, bronchoconstriction, salivation, and increased gastrointestinal peristalsis.

References

1. P. Carmichael, A.R. Carmichael. Acute renal failure in the surgical setting. *ANZ J Surg* 2003; 73:144–153.

2. D.J. Jones, H.T. Lee. Perioperative renal protection. *Best Pract Res Clin Anaesthesiol* 2008; 22;193–208.

3. R.L. Mehta, J.A. Kellum, S.V. Shah, *et al.* Acute Kidney Injury Network: report of an initiative to improve outcomes in acute kidney injury. *Crit Care* 2007; 11:R31.

4. B.K. Novis, M.F. Roizen, S. Aronson, R.A. Thisted. Association of preoperative risk factors with postoperative acute renal failure. *Anesth Analg* 1994; 78:143–149.

5. N. Brienza, M.T. Giglio, M. Marucci, T. Fiore. Does perioperative hemodynamic optimization protect renal function in surgical patients? A meta-analytic study. *Crit Care Med* 2009; 37:2079–2090.

6. C.R. Parikh, S.G. Coca. Defining prerenal azotemia in clinical practice and research. *Nat Rev Nephrol* 2010; 6:641–642.

7. P.S. Kellerman. Perioperative care of the renal patient. *Arch Intern Med* 1994; 154:1674–1688.

8. A. Mathew, P.J. Devereaux, A. O'Hare, *et al.* Chronic kidney disease and postoperative mortality: a systematic review and meta-analysis. *Kidney Int* 2008; 73:1069–1081.

9. C.M.N. O'Malley, R.J. Frumento, M.A. Hardy, *et al.* A randomized, double-blind comparison of lactated Ringer's solution and 0.9% NaCl during renal transplantation. *Anesth Analg* 2005; 100:1518–1524.

10. N. El-Sherif, G. Turitto. Electrolyte disorders and arrythmogenesis. *Cardiol J* 2011; 18:233–245.

11. M.J. Elliott, P.E. Ronksley, C.M. Clase, S.B. Ahmed, B.R. Hemmelgarn. Management of patients with acute hyperkalemia. *CMAJ* 2010; 182:1631–1635.

12. M. Galbusera, G. Remuzzi, P. Boccardo. Treatment of bleeding in dialysis patients. *Semin Dial* 2009; 22:279–286.

13. E.Z. Soliman, R.J. Prineas, A.S. Go, *et al.* Chronic kidney disease and prevalent atrial fibrillation: The Chronic Renal Insufficiency Cohort (CRIC). *Am Heart J* 2010; 159:1102–1107.

14. D. Trainor, E. Borthwick, A. Ferguson. Perioperative management of the hemodialysis patient. *Semin Dial* 2011; 24:314–326.

15. S.M. Macres, P.G. Moore, S.M. Fishman. Acute pain management. In: Barash PG, Cullen BF, Stoelting RK, Cahalan MK, Stock MC, eds. *Clinical Anesthesia.* 6th edition. Philadelphia, PA: Wolters Kluwer; 2009: 1473–1504.

16. D. Paul, K.M. Standifer, C.E. Inturrisi, G.W. Pasternak. Pharmacological characterization of morphine-6β-glucuronide, a very potent morphine metabolite. *J Pharmacol Exp Ther* 1989; 251:477–483.

17. J.X. Mazoit, K. Butscher, K. Samii. Morphine in postoperative patients: pharmacokinetics and pharmacodynamics of metabolites. *Anesth Analg* 2007; 105:70–78.

18. M. Dean. Opioids in renal failure and dialysis patients. *J Pain Symptom Manage* 2004; 28:497–504.

19. H. Hassan, B. Bastani, M. Gellens. Successful treatment of normeperidine neurotoxicity by hemodialysis. *Am J Kidney Dis* 2000; 35:146–149.

20. S. Garwood. Renal disease. In: Hines RL, Marschall KE, eds. *Stoelting's Anesthesia and Co-Existing Disease.* 5th edition. Philadelphia, PA: Churchill Livingstone; 2008: 323–347.

Chapter 49

Special considerations for pain management

Benjamin Vaghari, Jaime Baratta, and Kishor Gandhi

- Multimodal analgesia is of key importance for the opioid-tolerant surgical patient.
- A high degree of suspicion for obstructive sleep apnea is necessary when designing an anesthetic regimen as many patients may be undiagnosed.
- Analgesics with renal clearance of metabolites must be used with caution in the presence of renal insufficiency.
- Pain assessment of the pediatric patient may be particularly challenging after surgery.

Managing the patient with pain in the Post-Anesthesia Care Unit (PACU) can be challenging. Even a sound understanding of the different modalities of pain management and methods for their most effective utilization may not be adequate to meet the demands of certain patient populations. These patient groups may require the clinician to make certain modifications to what would be an otherwise effective analgesic plan in the majority of patients. The following chapter will discuss some of these patient groups that can present a challenge even to a thoroughly prepared and experienced PACU clinician.

The opioid-tolerant patient

The combination of chronic pain and the liberal use of prescription drugs in the United States has resulted in an epidemic of opioid tolerance. Tolerance is further compounded by abuse and diversion of prescription drugs by patients. Opioid tolerance results when patients are chronically exposed to opioids and develop a reduced analgesic effect of these drugs. These patients will often require large amounts of pain medication compared with the opioid-naïve patient. Studies have shown that increasing opioids in such patients will lead to hyperalgesia and a further increase in opioid tolerance. Furthermore, dose escalation can result in increases in adverse events such as respiratory depression, sedation, urinary retention, ileus, nausea/vomiting, and pruritus.

The current understanding of opioid tolerance is that it occurs owing to desensitization of opioid receptors and second-messenger systems in the central nervous system (CNS).[1] A multimodal pain management technique involves utilization of pharmacological agents that target different receptors at the pain cascade. A multimodal technique allows for minimization of opioid use, thus decreasing peripheral and central sensitization.

Post-Anesthesia Care: Symptoms, Diagnosis, and Management, ed. James W. Heitz. Published by Cambridge University Press. © Cambridge University Press 2016.

The concept of multimodal therapy in opioid tolerance involves identification of patients prior to surgery. This can occur during their surgical or preoperative clinic visit where chronic opioid use can be identified by their medication profile. With proper communication between the surgeons and anesthesiologist, an analgesic strategy can be formed and implemented for the patient. As a first step, we recommend instructing patients to take their opioids on the morning of surgery.

An effective multimodal analgesic plan requires utilization of non-opioid analgesic techniques and medications. The optimal pain control strategy for opioid tolerance often involves utilization of regional anesthesia services. A continuous neuraxial or peripheral catheter can provide prolonged pain control for these patients. In addition to regional anesthesia, many medications such as acetaminophen, clonidine (α_2-agonist), celecoxib (COX-2 inhibitor), gabapentin/pregabalin (calcium channel), and ketamine (NMDA receptor antagonist) can be instituted prior to surgery for better control of postoperative pain. These agents serve to act peripherally and centrally to minimize primary sensitization if used prior to pain stimulus. All of these agents have also been found to have opioid-sparing effects in clinical trials.[2–4]

Once surgery is completed and patients arrive to the PACU, a proper signout to the PACU team is critical for vigilant continuity of care in opioid tolerance. Patients can be given boluses of hydromorphone (0.2 mg) titrated to comfort and respiratory rate. If an intravenous patient-controlled analgesia (PCA) will be utilized in the postoperative period, we suggest beginning a hydromorphone PCA in the PACU once comfort is achieved or when respiratory rate limits further bolus dosing. Additionally, postoperative ketamine infusions can be continued for up to 3 to 4 days depending on patient tolerance. Multimodal analgesic therapy agents (e.g. clonidine, acetaminophen, celecoxib, gabapentin, and pregabalin) should be continued during hospitalization to decrease reliance on opioids and facilitate patient discharge.

Obstructive sleep apnea

Obstructive sleep apnea (OSA), a syndrome in which an individual experiences recurrent subtotal or complete airway obstruction during sleep despite intact respiratory effort, is likely to be increasingly encountered given the rising rate of obesity. OSA must be carefully addressed as it poses significant challenges in pain management postoperatively. However, many patients will present lacking a clinical diagnosis of OSA; therefore, it is imperative to identify those at risk via a detailed history. Although obesity is common, it is not pathognomonic, while a history of loud snoring, daytime somnolence, witnessed apnea during sleep, neck circumference greater than 40 cm, body mass index (BMI) greater than 35, and concurrent hypertension should raise concern for OSA.

Most clinicians are well aware that opioids have significant respiratory depressant effects. Opioids have been shown to cause hypoxia and hypercapnia in healthy volunteers as well as obstructive apnea and hypoxia in the postoperative period in patients without OSA.[5] Hence, there are significant concerns regarding the consequences of opioid administration to patients with OSA. Minimizing opioids and other potential sedatives regardless of the route or technique of administration is recommended.[5]

In 2014, The American Society of Anesthesiologists (ASA)Task Force of Perioperative Management of Patients with Obstructive Sleep Apnea recommended utilizing a multimodal analgesic approach to minimize opioids and opioid side effects and incorporate regional anesthesia/analgesia whenever possible.[6] An effective multimodal approach would entail using regional anesthetic in conjunction with local anesthetic whenever possible, while incorporating non-opioid analgesics such as acetaminophen, non-steroidal anti-inflammatory drugs (NSAIDs), COX-2 inhibitors, anti-neuropathic agents, and ketamine in order to limit opioid-induced respiratory depression in patients with suspected OSA.[5] Despite a multimodal approach, unfortunately opioids often cannot be avoided in efforts to achieve pain control. While the ASA Task Force did not find data to suggest superiority of nursing-administered opioids or PCA, it is recommended that basal infusion be avoided and proper monitoring for respiratory depression continued in the PACU.[6] In addition, long-acting opioids (oral and parenteral) should be used with caution and neuraxial opioids should be avoided in patients with diagnosed or suspected OSA.

Chronic kidney and end stage renal disease

Pain management in the PACU of patients with either chronic kidney or end stage renal disease is becoming more and more common. Safe use of analgesics for these patients involves awareness of prolonged drug clearance and the ramifications of such alterations. Further, those with chronic kidney disease and those undergoing some form of dialysis should not be considered one patient population. While dosing for many medications needs to be adjusted for those with decreased glomerular filtration rates (GFR), certain medications, such as NSAIDs, may or may not need to have dosing alterations. In patients with severely reduced GFRs and those on dialysis with some residual kidney function (i.e. those patients that still make urine), high dose and/or prolonged NSAID use may reduce kidney function. However, for those patients receiving dialysis that have no residual kidney function, NSAID doses do not require decreased dosing as these patients no longer have functioning kidneys. A second scenario to consider when administering analgesics to patients on dialysis is whether the medication is dialyzable. As an example, propoxyphene is poorly dialyzable, and its metabolites are associated with respiratory depression, cardiac conduction disturbances, and hypoglycemia.[7,8] The unwanted side effects make propoxyphene a drug that should absolutely be avoided in patients with end stage renal disease.

There are a number of opioids that can be safely used in patients with reduced GFR in the PACU (Table 49.1). Fentanyl primarily undergoes hepatic elimination and has a long history of safe use in these patients. Sufentanil has also been used safely despite potential for poor clearance during dialysis. These medications are excellent for use in the PACU as they are both potent and fast-acting analgesic options. Hydromorphone is another good option, with the advantage of extended duration of action to that of fentanyl. However, hydromorphone has a metabolite hydromorphone-3-glucuronide which can accumulate in patients with renal failure causing a neuro-excitatory phenomenon. This side effect becomes more prevalent when multiple dosages are administered over an extended period of time, although this may be less of a concern in a PACU setting. For oral medications, tramadol, hydrocodone, and methadone can be used, although all require some dosage reductions depending on the GFR. Oxycodone, which has active metabolites, can be used in patients with chronic kidney disease with appropriate dosing changes but should be avoided in patients undergoing dialysis.

There are a few opioid analgesics that should be used cautiously or avoided altogether in patients with significantly reduced GFRs. Morphine, the most widely used opioid

Table 49.1 Commonly used opioids in the PACU in patients with chronic kidney disease and end stage renal disease

Opioid	Recommendation
Morphine	CRF – Careful use ESRD – Careful use or best to avoid
Fentanyl	Appears safe
Hydromorphone	CRF – Careful use ESRD – Careful use, may accumulate but dialyzable
Hydrocodone	Metabolized to hydromorphone, see previous
Oxycodone	CRF – Careful use ESRD – Best to avoid
Codeine	Avoid
Propoxyphene	Avoid

CKD, chronic kidney disease; ESRD, end stage renal disease.

medication in the world, has an active metabolite morphine-6-glucuronide which, while dialyzable, will accumulate in patients with reduced GFRs. This active metabolite can often cause over-sedation as it accumulates, making morphine an opiate to avoid if better alternatives are available. Opioid medications that should certainly be avoided are meperidine, codeine, and propoxyphene.[9] These three medications all have toxic metabolites that will accumulate in these patients.

Overall, many of the commonly used opioid medications can be used safely in patients with chronic kidney disease (CKD) or dialysis. The overall safety of these medications often rests with judicious use and monitoring by the administering clinicians.

Special considerations for the pediatric population

Postoperative pain management of the pediatric population can prove to be very challenging and is further complicated by the inability to adequately communicate in many of the patients. Still, it is imperative to achieve adequate analgesia in the pediatric population as inadequate analgesia may lead to hypersensitivity or altered development of neuroanatomy and subsequent psychological or behavioral problems.[10] As no single assessment tool exists, familiarity with developmental milestones, subjective pain assessment by the patient, and observational cues collected by parents and nursing staff as well as physical signs of pain must be used in order to properly quantify pain and guide treatment in pediatric patients.

Although PCA may be difficult to use for pediatric patients, it has been shown to be effective in children older than 5 years of age, but proper education of the parents and child is necessary.[11] In addition, non-opioids and regional analgesia should be included in a multimodal approach whenever possible. Regardless of technique, providers must be vigilant of pediatric dosing of each medication administered.

References

1. L.F. Chu, M.S. Angst, D. Clark. Opioid-induced hyperalgesia in humans: molecular mechanism and clinical considerations. *Clin J Pain* 2008; 24:479–496.

2. H. Clarke, S. Perieira, D. Kennedy, *et al.* Gabapentin decreases morphine consumption and improves functional recovery following total knee arthroplasty. *Pain Res Manag* 2009; 14:217–222.

3. A. Buvanendran, J.S. Kroin, C.J. Della Valley, *et al.* Perioperative oral pregabalin reduces chronic pain after total knee arthroplasty: a prospective, randomized controlled trial. *Anesth Analg* 2010; 110:199–207.

4. R.W. Loftus, M.P. Yeager, J.A. Clark, *et al.* Intraoperative ketamine reduces perioperative opiate consumption in opiate-dependent patients with chronic back pain undergoing back surgery. *Anesthesiology* 2010; 113:639–646.

5. K. Gandhi, J.W. Heitz, E.R. Viscusi. Challenges in acute pain management. *Anesthesiol Clin* 2011; 29:291–309.

6. ASA Task Force on Perioperative Management of Patients with Obstructive Sleep Apnea. Practice guidelines for the perioperative management of patients with obstructive sleep apnea: an updated report by the American Society of Anesthesiologists Task Force on Perioperative Management of Patients with Obstructive Sleep Apnea. *Anesthesiology* 2014; 120:268–286.

7. S.J. Mauer, C.L. Paxon, B. von Hartizsch, *et al.* Hemodialysis in an infant with propoxyphene intoxication. *Clin Pharmacol Ther* 1975; 17:88–92.

8. R.L. Barkin, S.J. Barkin, D.S. Barkin. Propoxyphene (dextropropoxyphene): a critical review of a weak opioid analgesic that should remain in antiquity. *Am J Ther* 2006; 13:534–542.

9. M. Dean. Opioids in renal failure and dialysis patients. *J Pain Symptom Manage* 2004; 28:497–504.

10. V.Y. Sohn, D. Zenger, S.R. Steele. Pain management in the pediatric surgical patient. *Surg Clin North Am* 2012; 92:471–485.

11. S.C. Lawrie, D.W. Forbes, T.M. Akhtar, *et al.* Patient-controlled analgesia in children. *Anaesthesia* 1990; 45:1074–1076.

Chapter

50

PACU emergencies

Robert F. Olszewski Jr.

- Prompt intervention in postoperative complications reduces morbidity and mortality.
- Most serious adverse events occurring immediately after surgery involve hypoxia.
- Emergencies presenting after surgery are often influenced by the residual effects of anesthesia and/or surgery and require interventions unique to the perioperative period.

The Post-Anesthesia Care Unit (PACU) is a dynamic location serving a variety of patients of differing medical backgrounds that provides intensive care unit level of care for individuals recovering from anesthetic agents. The primary goal of the PACU is to provide close monitoring and support to these patients until they have returned to sufficiently normal physiological states to return to the hospital ward or to home. Because of the physiologic effects and stresses of anesthesia and surgery, the PACU is a unique location within the hospital in which emergencies of varying levels occur on a more regular basis than on the general hospital floor or in the general public.

The aim of this chapter is to provide an overview of some of the more common emergent situations encountered in the PACU and the initial steps that should be undertaken to mitigate these events and increase the chance of a favorable patient outcome. This chapter is by no means intended to be an exhaustive coverage of any of the topics herein. Most of the topics discussed here have been covered in greater detail elsewhere in this text, and I would encourage the reader to refer to the relevant chapters for more detail.

Respiratory arrest

Hypoventilation is a common concern in the PACU.[1] Many of the medications administered preoperatively (i.e. benzodiazepines, barbiturates, opioids, and other sedative hypnotics such as propofol and the potent inhaled anesthetics) depress respiratory drive. Increasing propensity towards obesity, lung disease, and obstructive sleep apnea only serves to compound this risk. A high index of suspicion should be raised for the effects of medications in contributing to post-anesthetic respiratory arrest.[2] Furthermore, hypercarbia will cause respiratory depression and possible arrest at $PaCO_2$ greater than 40 torr, as such hypoventilation itself can cause respiratory arrest.

Post-Anesthesia Care: Symptoms, Diagnosis, and Management, ed. James W. Heitz. Published by Cambridge University Press. © Cambridge University Press 2016.

Immediate initiation of the American Heart Association's Basic Life Support (BLS) protocol such as mask ventilation with 100% oxygen should occur. Any difficulty in mask ventilation by an experienced provider should prompt consideration for reintubation. Likely causes of respiratory depression should be ascertained and ruled out, starting with a review of recent medication administration with special attention paid to opioids. Consideration for measured administration of an intravenous opioid antagonist such as naloxone should be undertaken. Naloxone commonly is supplied in 0.4 mg/ml (400 mcg/ml) solution. The stock solution should be diluted 1 to 10 for a final concentration of 0.04 mg/ml (40 mcg/ml)and given in 0.5 to 1 ml aliquots every 2 to 3 minutes, titrated to the effect of return of spontaneous ventilation[3] with a rate of 12 to 14 breaths per minute. If, after a reasonably high dose has been administered, spontaneous respirations do not resume, other causes of respiratory depression such as benzodiazepine overdose or cerebral vascular accident should be considered. In this case reintubation and mechanical ventilation would be a reasonable course of action. Administration of the benzodiazepine antagonist flumazenil can be considered, but extreme care should be taken in patients on chronic benzodiazepine therapy as antagonism can precipitate withdrawal seizures. If opioid or benzodiazepine antagonism is initiated, continued close monitoring of the patient is warranted because of the difference in pharmacological half-lives of the initial agents and their respective antagonists.

Cardiac arrest/circulatory arrest

Cardiac arrest in the PACU is a rare (perioperative incidence of 19.7 per 10,000 anesthetics) but potentially devastating occurrence.[4] Upon recognition of this condition, BLS protocol with high-quality CPR should be instituted immediately as the Advanced Cardiac Life Support (ACLS) or "code" cart is retrieved. As soon as arrest events in the PACU are witnessed, immediate identification of "shockable" rhythms and early defibrillation will increase favorable patient outcomes. The American Heart Association's ACLS protocol should be initiated without delay, but the causes of sudden cardiac arrest differ in the perioperative population than in the pre-hospital setting, and therefore a more focused assessment of the possible causes of the event can be undertaken. The generic ACLS algorithm may not be the most appropriate for perioperative patients.[4] The most common electrocardiogram (ECG) rhythms noted during perioperative arrests are bradycardia (23%), asystole (22%), ventricular tachyarrhythmias (14%), and normal (i.e. pulseless electrical activity or PEA). Common causes of arrest in perioperative patients can be divided into the categories: anesthetic, respiratory, and cardiovascular.[4]

Refer to Table 50.1 for common causes of perioperative cardiac arrest and suggested treatments.

The importance of early initiation of BLS cannot be stressed highly enough. Return of coronary perfusion is of the utmost importance for the return of cardiac function and spontaneous circulation.

Cardiac ischemia

The incidence of cardiac ischemia may be exacerbated by general anesthesia, owing to decrease in perfusion from cardiac depression and vasodilation that predominates with the majority of anesthetic agents. Furthermore, the depressed mental state that often occurs during the post-anesthetic period has a high likelihood of masking the subjective

Table 50.1 Common causes of perioperative cardiac arrest[4]

Causes	Treatment
Anesthetic causes	
Anesthetic overdose	Stop the offending medication. Administration of chemical pacemakers such as epinephrine, transcutaneous/transesophageal pacing, intubation and mechanical ventilation until return of spontaneous circulation and ventilation
Sympathectomy from neuraxial anesthesia	Administration of chemical pacemakers such as epinephrine, transcutaneous or transesophageal pacing, intubation and mechanical ventilation until return of spontaneous circulation and ventilation
Local anesthetic toxicity	Immediate intubation. Administration of lipid emulsion such as intralipid (1.5 ml/kg load followed by 0.25 ml/kg/hr), avoid epinephrine bradycardia treated with atropine. Consideration of initiation of extra corporeal membrane oxygenation (ECMO) until return of spontaneous circulation occurs
Malignant hyperthermia (MH)	Initiation of MH protocol, administration of dantrolene, cool patient using ice or active cooling devices
Drug administration error	Varies, stop offending medication, administer antagonist if available otherwise supportive measures
Respiratory causes	
Hypoxemia	Initiate oxygen therapy with 100% oxygen via bag-valve mask, strongly consider reintubation and mechanical ventilation
Auto-PEEP*	If intubated, increase expiratory time. Consider brief disconnect of breathing circuit to allow release of trapped air. Administer bronchodilators
Bronchospasm	Administer bronchodilators such as beta-agonists and nebulized racemic epinephrine
Cardiovascular causes	
Vaso-vagal reflex	Administer atropine; if unsuccessful administer epinephrine, consider transcutaneous pacing
Hypovolemic shock	Fluid resuscitation, control bleeding source
Abdominal compartment syndrome	Emergent surgical intervention, decompressive laparotomy
Pneumothorax	Needle decompression, chest tube insertion
Transfusion reaction	Cease transfusion, supportive care
Anaphylaxis	Administer epinephrine
Acute coronary syndrome (ACS)	Begin ACS protocol, urgent interventional cardiology consultation

Table 50.1 (cont.)

Causes	Treatment
Pulmonary embolism	Surgical intervention, consider ECMO
Prolonged QT syndrome – Torsades de pointes	Intravenous magnesium therapy, defibrillation, antiarrhythmics
Pacemaker failure	Transcutaneous or transesophageal pacing.
Severe pulmonary hypertension	Intubation and initiation of pulmonary vasodilator such as nitric oxide
Acute electrolyte imbalance	Correct imbalance

* Positive end-expiratory pressure

symptoms of cardiac ischemia (i.e. chest pain, arm pain, feelings of dysphoria, etc.). This, coupled with the low incidence of postoperative ECG, necessitates a high index of suspicion for cardiac ischemia in perioperative patients.

Indications of cardiac ischemia include chest pain, arrhythmia, tachycardia, bradycardia, hypotension, abdominal discomfort, changes in continuous ECG monitor, and cardiac arrest. Early identification and intervention is essential in patients exhibiting signs and symptoms of cardiac ischemia as sequelae of this condition are severe.

The *sine qua non* of evaluation of chest discomfort and signs of cardiac ischemia is the 12-lead ECG. Although changes may be seen on the continuous telemetry monitor, these are often influenced by non-standard lead placement, patient movement, etc. and cannot be considered definitive. Twelve-lead ECG is an inexpensive, rapid, and sensitive method to rule out serious or massive cardiac ischemia that allows differentiation between ischemia requiring urgent invasive intervention such as percutaneous coronary intervention (PCI) from episodes that warrant medical management alone. It is important to note that early involvement of an expert in cardiology should be sought in cases of known or suspected cardiac ischemia.[5] In cases of cardiac ischemia, early intervention should include treatments that maximize oxygen delivery to affected myocardium, decrease myocardial oxygen demand, and minimize further impairment of coronary blood flow. The traditional mnemonic for the treatment of cardiac ischemia is the MONA-B, with the corresponding letters representing Morphine, Oxygen, Nitroglycerin, Aspirin, and Beta Blockade.[5]

Morphine is recommended to control the anxiety and pain associated with cardiac ischemia, decreasing catecholamine release, tachycardia, and increased contractility associated with this state. In postoperative patients, control of the pain associated with the recent procedure is also important. Therefore, administration of the opioid pain medication most appropriate for the individual patient should be undertaken to minimize the hemodynamic effect of the pain response.[5]

Supplemental oxygen should be provided to all patients in the PACU owing to the propensity for hypoventilation after receiving general anesthetics, and is often provided in the form of nasal cannula. However, in patients with suspected or confirmed cardiac ischemia, oxygen should be provided more aggressively to obtain an arterial hemoglobin saturation of at least 90% to maximize available oxygen at the ischemic site. Oxygen therapy should be continued for 6 hours after presentation of ischemic symptoms.[5]

Nitroglycerin causes coronary vasodilation and increases coronary perfusion. It has the secondary effect of decreasing blood pressure primarily by vasodilation of the venous system with a minor effect on arterial vasodilation. The result is a net increase of myocardial perfusion with a decrease in preload, and a minor decrease in afterload, thus simultaneously increasing coronary blood flow while decreasing myocardial oxygen demand. However, nitrates should be avoided in patients with systolic blood pressure less than 90 mmHg or who exhibit a decrease in systolic blood pressure greater than 30 mmHg below their baseline. Nitroglycerin therapy is also contraindicated in patients who have taken a phosphodiesterase inhibitor within 24 hours.[5]

Aspirin therapy is a staple of the treatment of acute coronary syndrome (ACS) in non-perioperative patients, owing to its platelet-inhibiting effects.[5] In patients in the immediate postoperative period, however, it is important to weigh the benefits of aspirin's antithrombotic effects against the possibility of increased postoperative bleeding. Perioperative Aspirin administration remains controversial. As mentioned earlier, it is important to involve the surgical team as early as possible in the care of postoperative or post-anesthetic complications so that the relative risks and benefits of antithrombotic treatment can be effectively assessed. However, in general, non-steroidal anti-inflammatory drug (NSAID) therapy should be avoided in patients who have undergone procedures in areas where a small amount of bleeding can cause excessive damage, such as neurosurgical patients.[6]

Because of the high risk of postoperative bleeding, thrombolytic therapy such as the administration of tissue plasminogen activator is most likely contraindicated in the majority of post-surgical patients. In centers where PCI is not immediately available considerations for stabilization, initiation of the above supportive measures, and transfer to a facility capable of interventional cardiac catheterization should be made. The mantra of the American Heart Association with regards to PCI is "door to needle in 30 minutes or less."[5]

Cerebrovascular accident/stroke

Perioperative stroke is an acknowledged risk of general anesthesia in susceptible populations. Early recognition, diagnosis, and supportive therapy should improve outcomes. Work-up of a patient with signs of stroke includes non-contrast head CT scan,[7] full blood labs including blood glucose, basic metabolic panel, complete blood count, cardiac biomarkers, prothrombin time / partial thromboplastin time (PT/PTT), a 12-lead ECG, and continuous oxygen saturation monitoring, as well as a complete set of vital signs.[8]

For reasons acknowledged in the previous section, thrombolytic therapy is most likely contraindicated in the postoperative population except with perhaps the most minor and superficial surgeries. Measures to increase blood flow and oxygen delivery to the affected neural tissue should be instituted. Maintenance of mean arterial blood pressures at or slightly above the patient's baseline is highly recommended; however, hypertension is common in the setting of ischemic stroke and systolic blood pressures greater than 160 mmHg are seen in greater than 60% of stroke patients. Systolic pressures greater than 180 mmHg and/or diastolic pressures greater than 110 mmHg have been linked to worsening outcomes and should be treated with intravenous labetalol, nitroglycerin, or nicardipine drip as deemed clinically appropriate.[8] Oxygen therapy to maintain hemoglobin saturation greater than 90% is also advisable. Early involvement of the surgical team and prompt neurology consultation is likewise advisable.

Seizure

Seizure can occur in susceptible patient populations in the perioperative period. Causes include but are not limited to: withholding of chronic anti-seizure medication, pro-seizure medication administration, intracranial hemorrhage, and hypoxia. Offending medications should be eliminated. Administration of a benzodiazepine such as lorazepam should be considered. Efforts to minimize the risk of injury to the patient should be instituted. In instances of extended seizure or status epilepticus, intubation and mechanical ventilation should be considered, as the greatest risk from extended grand mal seizure after injury is hypoxia due to lack of respiration. In patients without known seizure history, CT scan can be obtained after initial management to rule out intracranial hemorrhage or mass.[9]

In patients who are seizing, it is important to distinguish between seizures secondary to existing seizure disorder, stroke, and those caused by local anesthetic toxicity. Large amounts of local anesthetic are often instilled into the wound at the end of the surgical procedure, often after skin closure, and seizure in the recovery room could represent toxicity from these medications. If local anesthetic toxicity is suspected, seizure should be halted with benzodiazepine treatment; institution of lipid emulsion therapy is reasonable as side effects are minimal and the potential benefits are high. Intralipid emulsion should be administered as a bolus dose of 1.5 ml/kg followed by 0.5 mg/kg/min infusion. During and after initiation of this treatment, general anti-seizure medications such as lorazepam should be administered and supportive measures instituted. Careful monitoring for ECG changes and cardiac arrhythmias should be instituted as cardiovascular collapse is a potential consequence of local anesthetic toxicity.[10]

Hypoxia

Mild hypoxia is common in the postoperative period because of hypoventilation secondary to the effects of anesthetics, pain, and opioid pain medications.[11] Severe hypoxia is a less common but serious occurrence. Atelectasis is common in the post-surgical population and is often the cause of hypoxemia. Administration of increased oxygen therapy up to and including 100% oxygen via a non-rebreathing mask should be instituted. If the patient is conscious, encourage deep breaths to recruit alveoli and decrease intrapulmonary shunt.[10] If the patient is obtunded or otherwise unable to comply, initiate positive pressure ventilation via bag-valve mask ventilation, and consider endotracheal intubation.

Pulmonary embolism (PE) is a serious and common cause of hypoxia in hospitalized patients, and a high index of suspicion is prudent especially after long procedures, extended hospitalization, trauma, or after orthopedic procedures involving long bones (fat embolism). Supportive therapy such as intubation should be instituted immediately if PE is suspected, and diagnostic modalities such as spiral CT angiography obtained as soon as possible to determine whether surgical intervention is warranted.

Hypoxia can also be caused by residual weakness from non-depolarizing neuromuscular blocking agents. Although apparent normal ventilation may be observed in these patients, even mild airway obstruction can overcome the impaired respiratory reserve of these patients. Routine reversal of these agents with cholinesterase inhibitors such as neostigmine is common in the operating room, but if reversal has not occurred it can be administered in the PACU.[12] If weakness persists in spite of reversal, sedation and reintubation until full return of muscular function after clearance of the offending agent is advisable.

Pulmonary edema is a common cause of hypoxia in hospitalized patients. Cardiogenic pulmonary edema from either over-aggressive fluid resuscitation or acute decrease in cardiac function is most commonly the cause; however, non-cardiac pulmonary edema can occur as well from either adult respiratory distress syndrome (ARDS)[13] or negative pressure pulmonary edema secondary to forceful inhalation against a closed glottis in the setting of laryngospasm. Treatment of mild to moderate cardiogenic pulmonary edema includes use of diuretics and fluid restriction. More severe cases should be treated with intubation and mechanical ventilation. Suspected ARDS should be treated with intubation and ARDSnet (www.ARDSnet.org) or similar protocol mechanical ventilation. Negative pressure pulmonary edema is self-limiting, but severe cases may require temporary positive pressure ventilation.

The importance of pain control after major abdominal and/or thoracic procedures cannot be overstated. Often hypoventilation is secondary to pain limiting inspiratory effort. Increased doses of pain medication, although counterintuitive, may help increase respiratory effort. In the setting of decreased effort and low respiratory rate, regional or neuraxial analgesia and non-opioid pain medications for a multimodal approach should be considered to augment pain control while decreasing the need for opioid pain medication.[10]

Hypoglycemia

Hypoglycemia is common in diabetic patients who have fasted for surgery. Mild hypoglycemia can manifest as lethargy or malaise. Severe hypoglycemia can rapidly progress from coma, to irreversible global brain injury, to death. It should therefore be considered as dangerous as severe hypoxia. A high index of suspicion for hypoglycemia should be maintained in all diabetic patients displaying changes in mental status or slow emergence from anesthesia. Rapid determination of blood glucose level using point-of-care testing should occur. Hypoglycemia should be aggressively treated with intravenous dextrose therapy.

Malignant hyperthermia

Malignant hyperthermia (MH) is a dreaded complication of general anesthesia with the potent inhaled anesthetics and/or neuromuscular blockade with succinylcholine. MH is a genetic disorder of calcium channels (most often at the ryanodine receptor site) in skeletal muscle and is most commonly transferred in an autosomal dominant fashion. Exposure to a trigger agent in susceptible individuals causes an uncontrolled calcium flux from the sarcoplasmic reticulum to the cytoplasm of muscle cells, causing uncontrolled contraction. This results in a hypermetabolic state causing greatly increased oxygen consumption, carbon dioxide production, and heat production, quickly overwhelming the body's ability to compensate and if untreated leading to circulatory collapse.

Treatment of MH involves *getting help*, removal of the offending trigger agent, administration of dantrolene sodium, control of hyperpyrexia by packing the patient in ice, correction of the acidosis by intubation and hyperventilation along with administration of sodium bicarbonate, and managing dysrhythmias caused by electrolyte imbalance, especially hyperkalemia. Aggressive fluid resuscitation is advisable when not contraindicated to prevent renal damage from the inevitable rhabdomyolysis. Administration of an osmotic diuretic is also advisable for renal protection, although it should be noted that most formulations of dantrolene contain mannitol for this purpose. Supportive treatment for organ dysfunction should be instituted as well. Early and aggressive treatment is essential to maximize patient chance of survival as mortality in this condition can be as high as 80% if not treated effectively. Malignant hyperthermia kits must be available in any location that trigger agents are routinely used and should contain all of the supplies necessary to administer dantrolene in a timely fashion, including dantrolene itself as well as sterile water for reconstitution.[14] For more information, contact the Malignant Hyperthermia Association of the United States (www.mhaus.org, current emergency numbers: United States: 1+800-644-9737 or outside the USA 00+1+209-417-3722).

Laryngospasm

Laryngospasm is a common complication of general anesthesia. It occurs when stimulation is applied to the vocal cords in a patient in stage 2 or the hyperexcitable stage of anesthesia. Although it is of low prevalence in a PACU at adult institutions where patients are awakened fully in the operating room before transport to the recovery area, in some locations, especially pediatric facilities, it is common to bring patients to the PACU in a heavily sedated and/or fully anesthetized state. In these centers, mild to severe laryngospasm is an ever-present danger. The definitive treatment of laryngospasm is the administration of a neuromuscular blocking agent, most often succinylcholine owing to its rapid onset and short duration of action. Other methods have, however, been shown to be successful in the treatment of mild to moderate laryngospasm, such as continuous positive airway pressure via bag-valve mask or, ideally, anesthesia hyperinflation set, and deepening the anesthetic by administration of an intravenous sedative hypnotic such as propofol.[15] In transporting pediatric patients following minor procedures in which intravenous access is not available, pre-measured succinylcholine in a syringe supplied with an intramuscular delivery needle is imperative.

Hypotension

Hypotension is a side effect of the majority of anesthetics in use today, as the most commonly used agents are vasodilators as well as cardiac depressants. Neuraxial anesthetics likewise act to produce sympathectomy at the anesthetized levels, contributing to hypotension directly, as well as blunting the physiological response to normal stimuli. Serious causes of hypotension should also be considered, such as decreases in cardiac output due to cardiac ischemia, arrhythmia, or hypovolemic shock secondary to bleeding or underresuscitation.

In patients who have received neuraxial anesthetics, peripheral vasodilation is most likely the cause of hypotensive episodes. Judicious use of fluid bolus should be a mainstay of treatment in these patients with the ultimate goal of return of intravascular euvolemia. In patients who demonstrate signs of fluid overload, or who do not respond to fluid bolus, use of vasoactive agents such as α-adrenergic receptor agonists (phenylephrine or norepinephrine) or sympathomimetics such as ephedrine can be used as temporizing measures. In extreme cases, infusion of phenylephrine or norepinephrine can be instituted until the blockade level recedes and normal sympathetic function returns, although the necessity of doing so is relatively rare.

In all post-surgical patients with hypotension, a high index of suspicion for bleeding should exist. Careful physical exam for signs of bleeding such as swelling or increased drain output should be undertaken, and early involvement of the surgical team should be sought. Laboratory values such as hemoglobin and hematocrit are not good indicators of early acute bleeding as this represents a loss of whole blood. These values may not change appreciably until fluid resuscitation and equilibration have occurred. Patients who respond to fluid boluses only to require repeated bolus shortly thereafter should be observed carefully for signs of blood loss.

References

1. J.T. Moller. Hypoxemia in the PACU: an observer study. *Anesthesiology* 1990 73:890–895.

2. D.K. Rose, M.M. Cohen, D.F. Wigglesworth, D.P. DeBoer. Critical respiratory events in the postanesthesia care unit. *Anesthesiology* 1994 81:410–418.

3. Naloxone Hydrochloride Injection USP Narcotic Antagonist *Package Insert.*

4. V.K. Moitra. Anesthesia advanced circulatory life support. *Canadian Journal of Anaesthesia* 2012 59:586–603.

5. E.M. Antman, D.T. Anbe, P.W. Armstrong *et al.* ACC/AHA guidelines for the management of patients with ST-elevation myocardial infarction. *Circulation* 2004, 110:588–636.

6. N.S. Gerstein, P.M. Schulman, W.H. Gerstein *et al.* Should more patients continue aspirin therapy perioperatively?: clinical impact of aspirin withdrawal syndrome. *Annals of Surgery* 2012 255:811–819.

7. R.E. Latchaw, M.J. Alberts, M.H. Lev *et al.* Recommendations for imaging of acute ischemic stroke. *Stroke* 2009 40:3646–3678.

8. H. Adams, G. del Zoppo, M.J. Alberts *et al.* Guidelines for the early management of adults with ischemic stroke. *Stroke* 2007 38:1655–1711.

9. C.L. Harden, J.S. Huff, T.H. Schwartz *et al.* Reassessment: neuroimaging in the emergency patient presenting with seizure. *Neurology* 2007 69:1772–1780.

10. J.M. Neal, C.M. Bernards, J.F. Butterworth *et al.* ASRA Practice Advisory on local anesthetic systemic toxicity. *Regional Anesthesia and Pain Medicine* 2010 35:152–193.

11. B.E. Marshall, M.Q. Wyche. Hypoxemia during and after anesthesia. *Anesthesiology* 1972 37:178–209.

12. B. Plaud, B. Debaene, F. Donati, J. Marty. Residual paralysis after emergence from anesthesia. *Anesthesiology* 2010 112:1013–1022.

13. N.D. Ferguson, E. Fan, L. Camporota *et al.* The Berlin definition of ARDS. *Intensive Care Medicine* 2012 38:1573–1582.

14. J. Zhou, P.D. Allen, I.N. Pessah, M. Naguib. Neuromuscular disorders and malignant hyperthermia. Chapter 37 in *Miller's Anesthesia* 7th edition (ed. R.D. Miller) Philadelphia: Churchill Livingston Elsevier, 2010, 1181–1190.

15. G.A. Orliaguet. Case scenario: perianesthetic management of laryngospasm in children. *Anesthesiology* 2012 116:458–471.

Index

Page numbers in italics refer to illustrations; numbers in bold refer to tables.